Instructor's Manual and Test Questions for Jarvis

Physical Examination and Health Assessment

Third Edition

Keith O. Plowden, PhD, RN, CCRN
Assistant Professor
School of Nursing
University of Maryland, Baltimore
Baltimore, Maryland

Janice Donaldson Hausauer, RN, MS
Adjunct Assistant Professor
Montana State University College of Nursing
Bozeman, Montana

W.B. SAUNDERS COMPANY
A Division of Harcourt Brace & Company
Philadelphia London Toronto
Montreal Sydney Tokyo

W.B. SAUNDERS COMPANY
A Division of Harcourt Brace & Company
The Curtis Center
Independence Square West
Philadelphia, Pennsylvania 19106-3399

Instructor's Manual and Test Questions for
Jarvis
PHYSICAL EXAMINATION AND HEALTH ASSESSMENT
Third Edition

ISBN 0-7216-8430-0

Printed in United States of America

Last digit is the print number: 9 8 7 6 5 4 3 2 1

Introduction

The content in this Instructor's Manual is designed to aid instructors teaching health assessment using *Physical Examination and Health Assessment, 3e* by Carolyn Jarvis.

The following table is a general guide for programs using the text and employing a functional health patterns approach to assessment.

Functional Health Patterns	Potential Correlating Chapters
Health Perception - Health Management	Chapter 2, Developmental Tasks and Health Promotion Across the Life Cycle Chapter 4, The Interview Chapter 5, The Complete Health History
Nutritional - Metabolic	Chapter 7, Nutritional Assessment Chapter 9, General Assessment, Measurement, Vital Signs Chapter 10, Skin, Hair, and Nails Chapter 14, Nose, Mouth, and Throat Chapter 19, The Abdomen
Elimination	Chapter 19, The Abdomen Chapter 22, Male Genitalia Chapter 23, Anus, Rectum, and Prostate Chapter 24, Female Genitalia
Activity - Exercise	Chapter 16, Thorax and Lungs Chapter 17, Heart and Neck Vessels Chapter 18, Peripheral Vascular System and Lymphatics Chapter 20, Musculoskeletal System
Sleep - Rest	Chapter 5, Complete Health History
Cognitive - Perception	Chapter 6, Mental Status Assessment Chapter 11, Head and Neck, Including Regional Lymphatics Chapter 12, Eyes Chapter 13, Ears Chapter 14, Nose, Mouth, and Throat Chapter 21, Neurologic System
Self-Perception - Self-Concept	Chapter 2, Developmental Tasks and Health Promotion Across the Life Cycle Chapter 6, Mental Status Assessment
Role-Relationship	Chapter 2, Developmental Tasks and Health Promotion Across the Life Cycle Chapter 3, Transcultural Considerations in Assessment
Sexuality - Reproductive	Chapter 15, Breasts and Regional Lymphatics Chapter 22, Male Genitalia Chapter 24, Female Genitalia Chapter 25, The Pregnant Female
Coping - Stress Tolerance	Chapter 2, Developmental Tasks and Health Promotion Across the Life Cycle
Value - Belief	Chapter 2, Developmental Tasks and Health Promotion Across the Life Cycle Chapter 3, Transcultural Considerations in Assessment

Table of Contents

INSTRUCTOR'S MANUAL

UNIT 1 Assessment of the Whole Person

UNIT 2 Physical Examination

UNIT 3 Integration of the Health Assessment

ASSESSMENT VIDEO SERIES

Body Systems

Head-To-Toe

TEST MANUAL

UNIT 1 Assessment of the Whole Person

UNIT 2 Physical Examination

UNIT 3 Integration of the Health Assessment

Instructor's Manual

Chapter 1

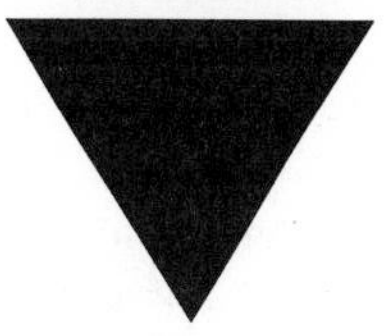

Assessment for Health and Illness

ANNOTATED LEARNING OBJECTIVES

At the completion of this chapter the student will:

Discuss the expanded concept of health and relate it to the process of data collection.

The concept of health has expanded over time and is based on the practice model used. Because of this expanded definition, the list of data to be collected varies based on the practice model used. The biomedical model of Western medicine views health as the absence of disease. With this view, the focus of data collection is on biophysical signs and symptoms and on curing disease. If health is viewed as wellness, assessment will encompass the whole person, that is mind, body, and spirit. Each interacts within the person and with the environment. With health viewed as wellness, data on all of these aspects of the individual and environment must be assessed. Consideration of the whole person is referred to as holistic health.

The concept of health has also been expanded to include the concept of health promotion and disease prevention. The behaviors that promote health or may cause illness must be identified. Counseling is provided to promote or enhance health-promoting behaviors.

Use the purpose of assessment as a guide for data collection and health evaluation.

The purpose of assessment is to make a judgment or diagnosis about the health of an individual. Factors assessed will influence the diagnosis. These factors must therefore be comprehensive and address all aspects of the individual and his/her life style, such as culture and role, in addition to performing an examination of the body. The list of factors to be assessed is identified by the American Nurses' Association and is cited in Chapter 1. Its discussion differentiates among the terms *subjective data*, *objective data*, and *data base*.

While the practitioner may collect subjective and objective data concurrently, it is important to distinguish between the two and to recognize that both are part of the data base. Subjective data is the information provided by the affected individual. Objective data is the information obtained by the health care provider through physical assessment, the client's record, and laboratory studies. The data base is the totality of information available about the client.

Contrast medical diagnosis with nursing diagnosis.

Medical diagnosis and nursing diagnosis are independent but interrelated. Medical diagnosis is concerned with the etiology of disease. Nursing diagnosis is concerned with the impact of the health problem on the whole person and with the individual's response to the problem. Both the nursing diagnosis and classification systems for intervention and outcome provide a common language with which to communicate.

Relate the client situation to the amount of data collected.

The practitioner must modify the approach to data collection based upon the presenting clinical situation. A health care provider in an emergency department will need to assess airway, breathing, and circulation and complete a problem-focused exam. An individual gathering data for a complete history and physical examination will usually examine each system in depth. There are four different types of clinical situations and related data bases identified: complete, or total data base; episodic or problem-centered; follow-up; and emergency. After identifying the type of data base indicated, the practitioner must proceed to gather the correct data. The data base will form the bases of one or more nursing diagnoses.

Relate the client age and health status to the frequency of health assessment.

At one time, periodic health examinations, frequently yearly, were recommended for all adults. Frequency of health visits is now based upon preventive services for each age group and individualized for each client. This change in frequency is more reflective of considering the whole person when providing health care. The age-specific charts for periodic health examination can be used as a schedule for health care. The focus is on major risk factors specific for each age group.

KEY TERMS

Subjective data
Objective data
Data base
- Total health data base
- Episodic/problem-centered
- Follow-up
- Emergency

Diagnosis
- Medical
- Nursing

Environment
Health promotion
Holistic health
Wellness
Prevention

TEACHING STRATEGIES

- ▼ Using the list of assessment factors listed in Chapter 1, have students discuss how each factor affects his/her own health status.
- ▼ Have students obtain examples from professional journals, newspapers or magazines of occupations that have actual or potential health risks.
- ▼ Using the occupations identified above, have students discuss health teaching or environmental changes that might be implemented for each of the health risks identified. For example, Universal Precautions have been instituted to provide a safer environment for health care providers.
- ▼ Have students obtain examples from newspapers or magazines of environmental factors that have actual or potential health risks (i.e., second-hand smoke, lead in house paint).
- ▼ Using the environmental factors identified above, have students discuss health teaching or environmental changes that might be implemented to decrease the identified risk(s).
- ▼ Using the NANDA diagnoses listed, have students identify a nursing diagnosis for each of the health risks discussed.
- ▼ Using the identified health risks, discuss the difference in approach between a nurse and physician for each risk/problem.
- ▼ Again using professional journals, newspaper or magazine articles as a basis for identifying health problems, have students describe the type of data collection indicated: complete, episodic, follow-up, or emergency.
- ▼ Using the age-specific chart for periodic health examination, have students identify a client and design a recommended frequency of health visits and preventive services for that individual client.

CRITICAL THINKING EXERCISES

Application to Clinical Practice

For each of the following case studies have students identify the subjective and objective data, at least one nursing diagnosis, additional factors that might need to be described and, if the situation indicates, a complete, problem-centered, follow-up, or emergency data base. Design a periodic health examination schedule for each client based on the age-specific chart. If other than a complete examination is required, have students identify the body system(s) that must be focused upon. Have students also discuss age, socioeconomic, and transcultural considerations for each situation.

- ❑ P.D. is brought to the emergency department complaining of a sore shoulder. He states that he was forced off the road while riding his motorcycle and sideswiped a telephone pole. P.D. did not lose consciousness. A urine specimen reveals gross hematuria. P. D. also states that a tape player in the right pocket of a leather jacket is shattered.

❑ A family of two adults, mother age 33 and father age 29, and two children, ages 6 months and 3 years, come to the local health clinic. The adults state that they have recently relocated to this area and are interested in finding a health care provider. When asked, the mother says there are no known health problems. During the interview with the parents, you note the 3-year-old playing with a puzzle.

❑ M. G., known to the health care provider, comes to the local diabetes center. The last visit was 6 months prior to this visit. M. G. brings a record of blood glucose levels and insulin dosages for the past 6 months. When asked how she has been feeling, she states she had a sore elbow from playing tennis 2 weeks ago but otherwise feels well.

❑ G. M., known to the health center, calls for an emergency appointment. G. M. is complaining of a sore throat and an ear ache. Upon examination both the pharynx and eardrum are seen to be reddened.

❑ J. P. is a 65-year-old African American man who comes into the clinic for a periodic health visit. He has a history of hypertension. During the visit, he has no other complaints other than having to wake up frequently to urinate.

WEB SITES OF INTEREST

Academy of Medical-Surgical Nurses- ***www.amsn.com***

American Nurses Association- ***www.ana.org***

National League for Nursing- ***www.nln.org***

National Student Nurse Association- ***www.nsna.org***

American Hospital Association- ***www.aha.org***

Case Management Society of America- ***www.cmsa.org***

Chapter 2

Developmental Tasks and Health Promotion Across the Life Cycle

ANNOTATED LEARNING OBJECTIVES

At the completion of this chapter the student will:

Describe expected physical, psychosocial, cognitive, and behavioral milestones of client based on developmental stage.

Growth is continuous and change is perpetual throughout the life cycle. Physical, cognitive, personality, and behavior changes occur as an individual progresses through these stages. Qualitative changes in thinking and behavior occur during particular times of development. Because the focus of holistic care is the individual within the environment, the knowledge of developmental stages is needed to place the data base into a meaningful frame.

Differentiate developmental stages for each group.

While various theorists may approach the physical, psychosocial, cognitive, and behavioral development of an individual from different perspectives or foci, the general framework for human developmental stages are those described in the beginning of Chapter 2.

Each developmental stage has tasks that are usually accomplished within the identified time frame. It must be remembered that both the stages and tasks are guidelines. Each person grows at his/her own best rate.

Compose a periodic health examination schedule for an individual in each of the nine developmental stages, given the individual enjoys good general health. Develop a periodic health screening schedule for a client based on the age of the client and expected developmental stages, given that the individual enjoys good general health.

Visits to the health care practitioner should be planned, based upon the needs of the individual. For children, this may be based on an immunization schedule; for older adults, it may be based on recommended periodic health screening measures.

Consider growth and developmental stage when evaluating health data.

While each child grows at his/her own best rate, developmental tables provide a guide for the health practitioner for the identification of potential or actual health problems.

Incorporate the use of major developmental frameworks in conducting a holistic health assessment.

The various theories serve as a general guide for the assessment of clients at each stage of the life cycle. Each portrayal considers the holistic development of individuals. These portrayals offer a general framework for assessment.

Relate the behavioral development observed in each child to the expected behaviors identified by the tables in Chapter 2. Also, relate observed behavioral development in clients to the expected behaviors identified in the chapter.

Knowledge of behavioral milestones will assist the practitioner to differentiate between behavior that is expected for a given age and identify the presence or absence of behavior that may signal an actual or potential health problem. This knowledge will also serve as a guide for counseling of the clients.

KEY TERMS

Developmental stages
Physical development
Cognitive development
Behavioral development
Psychosocial development

TEACHING STRATEGIES

- ▼ Based on availability of clients/family members in various developmental stages, assign students to complete a developmental assessment of an individual. Try to have each of the nine stages represented within the student group. Have each student present a brief description of the individual.
- ▼ Based on the above descriptions, have the students describe the relevant developmental tasks and determine whether the individual is engaged in those tasks. If not, why not?
- ▼ Again using the identified individuals, have students plan a periodic examination schedule for each.
- ▼ Have students relate developmental tasks as identified by various theorists to the games played by/with children of various ages. Have students consider how these games are culture related.
- ▼ Using the clients identified in the Chapter 1 exercises, have students identify health counseling needs based on the age of the individual.

CRITICAL THINKING EXERCISES

Application to Clinical Practice

For each of the individuals described in the situations below, have students discuss the expected developmental stage (physical, cognitive, psychosocial, and behavioral). Also, have the students describe socioeconomic and transcultural considerations that should be considered during the gathering of data and the provision of health care. Does the choice of theorist affect the structure of the interview or the health care provided? For each situation, have the students design a periodic examination schedule.

- ❑ J. J. is a 16-year-old female quadriplegic from an auto accident. She has been through an intensive rehabilitation program and attends the local high school. Her reason for the visit to the clinic is frequent headaches.
- ❑ M. G., a 35-year-old graphic artist, is known to your facility for 5 years with type I diabetes. He is married with 2 young children. His reason for scheduling this visit is blurred vision.
- ❑ M. C. is a 10-year-old brought to your facility by her mother because of excessive thirst and frequent urination. Her blood glucose level is 250.
- ❑ B. K., age 55, brings her 5-year-old granddaughter to your clinic for a preschool examination. Since she is known to your facility, you are surprised by her bringing the child, who you thought lived several states away. Upon discussion, B. K. states that because of the illness of her daughter, she now has custody of the child.
- ❑ B. D., age 8 months, is brought to the family clinic for routine immunizations. Have students describe the developmental tasks that should be assessed and the parent teaching indicated.
- ❑ You are visiting your sister and her 18-month-old child. During the visit, a neighbor, who frequently watches the child for your sister stops in to visit. Suddenly, the child runs across the room while saying, "I get it—shoes." Have students discuss the developmental stage of this child.
- ❑ L. M. comes to your facility for a periodic health examination. She is 60 years old and is known to your facility. She has a 34-year-old son who has post-traumatic brain disorder. Although he has completed college, he holds an entry-level, low-paying position and has limited social skills. L. M. is complaining of insomnia, headaches, and depression. Describe the developmental tasks associated with the son of L. M. Does he appear to be accomplishing the tasks successfully? Support answer with theorists from the chapter.
- ❑ M. D. is observed at a local day care center playing "dress-up." What is the probable developmental stage for this child and what other tasks are included in this stage?

Chapter 3

Transcultural Considerations in Assessment

ANNOTATED LEARNING OBJECTIVES

At the completion of this chapter, the student will:

Describe the basic characteristics of culture.

Culture, which is dynamic and ever changing, has four characteristics: namely, it is (1) learned from birth through language acquisition and socialization, (2) shared by all members of the same cultural group, (3) adapted to specific conditions related to environmental and technical factors and (4) adapted to the availability of natural resources. Value is a perception of the worth of an act, belief, or object.

Culture is a belief system that guides the day-to-day behavior of individuals. Before a student can integrate an acceptance of the impact of culture on health and health practices of clients, the elements of their clients' culture must be identified. The manner in which these beliefs affect acceptance or rejection of biomedical/scientific health practices can then be addressed.

Discuss areas of potential cultural conflicts between nurses and clients of different ethnic groups.

According to demographics, minority groups will soon make up more than one-half of the population of the United States. Attention to the cultural aspects of health and illness must therefore be considered by health care providers. Before a student can begin to integrate the role that beliefs and values play in the clients' lives, awareness of both culturally dominant values and personal values must be identified. The major areas in which cultural conflicts between nurses and clients from culturally diverse backgrounds occur is in differences in time and relationship perceptions. For some cultures, the attention to past or present may influence health practices. When making decisions about health, clients may rely on relationships with others, and behavior may depend on the opinion of others.

Discuss the influence of religion and spirituality on health and illness perception.

In times of illness, religion and spirituality may be a source of comfort for clients and their significant others. Religion and spiritual leaders may exert considerable influence on perception of health, illness, and practices. Spirituality may be used to find meaning and purpose for illnesses. Data regarding the client's religious affiliation and spiritual beliefs should be gathered.

Discuss components of the health belief system and their influence on health practices and illness expressions.

While it is impossible for a health care professional in a multicultural country such as the United States, with such a large and diverse representation of various cultural and ethnic groups, to be knowledgeable about the beliefs and practices of each patient assigned for care, the health care professional can accept that differences exist and be open to the importance of these practices to the client.

The meaning of health and illness to the patient is, in part, determined by the way in which members of his or her cultural group define them. The perceived causes of illness and symptoms can be culturally based and may be viewed as biomedical, naturalistic, and/or magico-religious. All cultures have their own preferred lay or popular healers, recognized symptoms of disease, acceptable sick role behavior, and treatments. Patients may seek help from biomedical/scientific health professions and traditional healers. It is important to be aware of the existence of traditonal folk practices and include this as part of your assessment.

Examine the sources that influence the culture and beliefs the student embraces.

Each individual probably belongs to more than one primary group or subgroup. Identification of the various influences within his or her life will assist the student in acknowledging influences within the patient population served. For example, one student may be a member of a recognized religion, have parents or grandparents who are migrants from the south, and live in the inner city, while a classmate may have a family that has been in this country for many generations, have grown up in the suburbs, and not attend church. While each of these students will be influenced by the same school culture and professional socialization, each comes with a different perspective and expectation of that shared experience.

Provide care that reflects an acceptance of the client as a unique individual.

Each individual will respond differently to the same stimuli, regardless of primary culture and value system. The health professional must continually strive to resist prejudgment of anyone. However, to state that each client is a unique individual is valueless unless the care provided reflects respect for this uniqueness, and culture is but one aspect of this uniqueness. It is imperative to guard against categorizing or stereotyping individuals.

KEY TERMS

Culture assessment
Subculture
Cultural competence
Ethnocentrism
Ethnicity
Culture shock
Culture competence
Family
Values
Religion
Spirituality

TEACHING STRATEGIES

- Discuss the health beliefs held by each student and the influence on beliefs and behavior.
- Have students interview an individual from a culture different from their own to identify health practices/beliefs.
- Have each student draw a Ven diagram as a graphic representation of the various cultural influences and beliefs that are part of his/her value system.
- Have students search the Web to identity various cultures in their geographic region. Have them identify the health patterns and beliefs of these groups.
- Break students into small groups. Have each group develop questions that may be used during a cultural assessment. Major topics that may be considered include the following:

  Self-reported race and ethnicity
  Religious beliefs and practices
  Roles within the family/significant others
  Verbal and nonverbal communication patterns including primary language
  Environmental influences
  Beliefs and practices regarding food
  Beliefs and practices regarding health and illness
  Attitudes toward pain
  Use of traditional healers
  Methods of treating illnesses

- Have students compare their questions to those listed in the Cultural Assessment Guide at the end of Chapter 5. Have students discuss and critique these questions.
- Using the minority groups identified above, have students describe the implications for health care.
- In the clinical area, have students complete a cultural assessment for an assigned client.
- In the clinical area, have students complete a pain assessment on an assigned client. Include in the data collected the client's cultural group influence on health behavior and perception of pain.
- Have students describe how care for the client identified above was individualized based on data gathered through the cultural assessment.

CRITICAL THINKING EXERCISES

Application to Clinical Practice

For each of the following case studies, have students (1) describe how they would assess the client for health practices and beliefs that are outside of the biomedical/scientific model, (2) describe the possible impact of these practices on the care that might be indicated, (3) identify any age or socioeconomic considerations and (4) debate whether nursing should support the practices and beliefs of the client.

- ❑ You are a public health nurse on a Reservation for Native Americans. Your client has type I diabetes. When you arrive for a visit, the Shaman is also present.
- ❑ G. D., age 64, has come to the health clinic for follow-up care for hypertension. You are the primary health care provider for G. D. While G. D. appears to be following the prescribed regimen for the hypertension, you note a lack of eye contact and a noted decrease in verbal responses to questions. Further exploration reveals that G. D. recently admitted his mother to a nursing home following 5 years of providing her care at home. G. D. reveals that although he could no longer provide the care needed, he feels guilty because he had promised at the onset of his mothers' illness that he would not admit her to a nursing home.
- ❑ You are an Emergency Department nurse. A Middle Eastern client is brought in with vaginal bleeding. The woman appears to be battered. She has bruised eyes, bruising around the neck, and lacerations on her arms. The husband refuses to leave the room for you to interview the client.
- ❑ As an obstetrical clinical specialist, you must inform your Irish American client that the results of prenatal testing indicate that the fetus has hydrocephalus and myelomeningocele. Because of the location of the myelomeningocele, the child will probably be paralyzed from the hips down. You offer to discuss terminating the pregnancy. The client and her husband refuse because of their religious beliefs.
- ❑ T. J. P., a second semester sophomore in college, has come to the student health center with complaints of fatigue, headache, and insomnia. From your initial contact with this student you remember that the student is a member of a local church that is not in the majority in the region or school.
- ❑ N. C. is 13 years old and has just started menses. She has come to the family clinic complaining of fatigue. The conjunctiva and mucous membranes are pale. Hematocrit and hemoglobin are dangerously low. A nutrition assessment reveals that N. C. is a member of the Seventh Day Adventist Church and does not eat meat.

WEB SITES OF INTEREST

Center for Disease Control and Prevention- ***www.cdc.gov***

Department of Health and Human Services Disparity in Health Statistics- ***www.hhs.gov***

U.S. Census Bureau- ***www.census.gov***

Transcultural Nursing Society- ***www.tcn.org***

Chapter 4

The Interview

ANNOTATED LEARNING OBJECTIVES

At the completion of this chapter the student will:

Demonstrate the ability to establish the parameters for a health interview.

A health interview is a structured interaction between the health care provider and the patient. It is important that the rules governing this interaction be clearly outlined and agreed upon by the interviwer and interviewee at the beginning of the interview. While outlining the parameters for a structured interview may seem second nature to the seasoned practitioner, a beginning practitioner may have difficulty in clearly communicating the limits and expectations for the interview, especially if the client is senior in age to the student.

The parameters that must be addressed are outlined in the beginning of the chapter.

State facilitators and blockers of effective communication.

In a two-person interaction, there are usually two roles, that of sender and that of receiver. During the exchange of information, both individuals engage in both verbal and nonverbal communication. In addition to awareness of the roles of each individual, also consider the context of the exchange and any internal and external factors that may have an impact on the interview. Adding yet another dimension is the fact that for each interaction between two people, there is an intellectual response and a feeling response. The interviewer must monitor both of these responses within him/her self, and when possible, within the interviewee. Finally, the interviewer must be aware of facilitators and blockers of effective communication. Other internal and external factors to be considered by the interviewer are outlined in the chapter.

Use the outlined communication techniques appropriately to gather data.

Facilitation, silence, reflection, empathy, clarification, confrontation, interpretation, explanation, and summary each elicit a different response from the client. The perspective shifts from the client to the health care provider with the last four. Each has a role in the interview process; however, practice is required to use each effectively and move from one response to another smoothly.

State the 10 traps of interviewing.

In addition to practicing the use of appropriate verbal responses, the practitioner must develop an awareness of various traps and guard against inadvertently using any of them.

Discuss the meaning of common nonverbal modes of communication.

Physical appearance, posture, gestures, facial expression, eye contact, voice, and touch each convey a variety of messages from sender to receiver. The health care practitioner must develop the skill to "read" the nonverbal behavior of clients and to monitor his/her own nonverbal communication.

Modify communication techniques as indicated by the clients' developmental stage, special needs, or cultural practices.

The practitioner needs to develop the skill to establish rapport not only with adults but also with parents, young children, adolescents, older individuals, and clients with special needs. Each may require some modification in approach. Behaviors that are viewed in a positive manner in one culture may have different, possibly negative connotations, in another. Individuals experiencing a health crisis will also need to be interviewed in a manner that will expedite their receiving appropriate health care.

KEY TERMS

Communication
Verbal communication
Nonverbal communication
Active listening
Facilitation
Reflection
Confrontation
Interpretation
Subjective
Empathy

TEACHING STRATEGIES

Divide students into pairs. Have the student acting as client identify a concern/problem he/she would like to discuss. This does not need to be something intimate: it could be a test coming up, transportation to school, what movie to see over the weekend; anything that may involve choices on the part of the individual. Have the student as practitioner interview the student/client regarding the identified concern. At the completion of the interview, have the student with the concern give feedback to the interviewer. Did the student/client feel the interviewer clearly understood the concern? Did the interviewer try to "solve" or "fix" the problem rather than assist the client to find a solution? Have students identify facilitators and barriers. Did the interviewer provide structure for the interview? (see Performance Checklist)

- ▼ After the critique suggested above, have students change roles and repeat the process.
- ▼ If a videorecorder is available, have students video record the interview described above. Critique of the tape may be done by the individuals involved or the instructor. Use the Performance Checklist as a basis for the critique. Note: Permission should be obtained prior to audio or video recording any interaction with another individual.
- ▼ If a video recorder is not available, have students practice interviewing with an audio recorder. One or both may critique the tape using the Performance Checklist.
- ▼ Divide students into pairs. Give the student in the role of client one of the case studies found in this manual. Have the second student conduct an interview to elicit further information about the problem supplied to the first student.
- ▼ Assign students to watch a TV news magazine and identify the verbal and nonverbal interview responses used by the news correspondent and the interviewee.
- ▼ Assign a student to a client with special needs, and have the student identify facilitators used to overcome barriers to communication. Using the Web, have the students identify community resources available to assist the client. What facilities are available within the facility?

CRITICAL THINKING EXERCISES

Application to Clinical Practice

For each individual described in the situations below, have students discuss the developmental, age, socioeconomic, and transcultural considerations that should be considered during an interview.

In addition, have students name the appropriate and inappropriate behavior employed by the interviewer, and discuss alternatives for any inappropriate behavior identified. Finally, ask students to describe how they would "feel" if they were the interviewee.

- ❑ C. M. has come to the health center for a follow-up visit for hypertension. While the practitioner is writing in the chart, C. M. states, "My brother had a stroke yesterday." The practitioner responds, "I'm sorry to hear that. Your blood pressure is being controlled by the medication. I'll need to see you again in six months."
- ❑ M. D. stops by a faculty office during posted office hours with the intent of asking for help with a diffi-

cult concept. While M.D is at the office door, without looking up, the instructor asks, "Did you need something?"

- ❑ The health practitioner is visiting a client who had abdominal surgery yesterday. The practitioner closes the chart, looks at the client, and asks, "I see that you have been having frequent injections for pain. Is the medication relieving your pain? If so, how long does the relief last?"
- ❑ S. M. walks into a client's room on the oncology unit prepared to take vital signs and notes that the client is crying. S. M. sets down the equipment, walks over to the client, takes the client's hand and observes, "you look upset." S. M. then remains silent while holding the client's hand.
- ❑ As G. L. is walking up to a client's room, the physicians are leaving. The client has diabetes, and G.L. is aware that amputation of the right lower leg is being considered. When G. L. enters the room, the client states, "They want to cut it off." G. L. responds, "That is too bad, but don't be too concerned; with physical therapy you will recover quickly."
- ❑ S. S. receives a phone call from a friend who states, "Kevin has been in an automobile accident and is in intensive care." S. S. responds "I know you are very upset. What can I do to help?"
- ❑ M. A. has come into the Emergency Department with difficulty breathing. X-ray films reveal fractured ribs. The radiologist also reports evidence of previous fractures. The practitioner asks the husband of M. A. to leave the examining room before beginning the intake interview.
- ❑ B. H. calls the assigned faculty advisor for an appointment to discuss a personal problem. The instructor states, "It is now 12:30. I have a meeting at 1:30. If you can come over right away, I will be glad to see you."
- ❑ W.S. has been seeing a counselor for depression. During an interview, W.S. begins describing specific suicidal ideation. The counselor states, "I am concerned that you may harm yourself. Do you have a plan to kill yourself? I must inform the psychiatrist with our practice of your plans."

WEB SITES OF INTEREST

Federation for the Blind- ***www.afb.org***

American Speech-Language-Hearing Association- ***www.asha.org***

Deafness Research Foundation- ***www.drf.org***

Self-Help for Hard of Hearing People- ***www.shhh.org***

PERFORMANCE CHECKLIST

INTERVIEW—Essential Behaviors

	Yes	No	Comments
Create an appropriate physical environment.			
Provide privacy.			
Greet client by proper name.			
Introduce self.			
Refuse interruptions.			
Wear appropriate attire.			
Provide a clear introduction to the interview.			
State the time available for the interview.			
State the purpose of the interview.			
Indicate the role of each participant.			
If an adolescent or adult, ask permission from client for other health care providers or family members to be present.			
Indicate confidentiality of the interview and any limitations.			
State any costs that may be incurred.			
Use the nine types of verbal response appropriately.			
Use appropriate nonverbal behavior.			
Respond appropriately to client's nonverbal behavior.			
Provide client time to respond.			
Use appropriate terminology/language.			
Close the interview with a summary or other polite signal that the interview is complete.			
Consider special needs of the client.			

Chapter 5

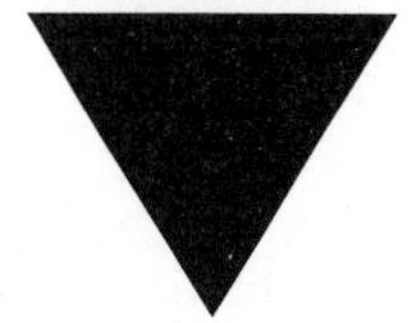

The Complete Health History

ANNOTATED LEARNING OBJECTIVES

At the completion of this chapter the student will:

State the purpose of the complete health history.

The collection of subjective data or learning what a person says about him- or herself is the purpose of the health history. Through combining the subjective information with objective information obtained through the physical examination and relevant diagnostic studies, the health care provider strives to view the client as a whole individual functioning within the environment. The data is used to make a judgment about the health status of the person.

The health care provider conducting the interview must also keep in mind that others will refer to his/her documentation. Completeness, accuracy, and clarity of the recording will assist all who refer to the client's record.

List the categories of information contained in a health history.

Although the form itself may vary among health care settings, the following information is usually obtained: biographical data, reason for seeking care, present health or history of present illness, past history, family history, review of systems and functional assessment or activities of daily living (ADL). It should be noted that in the past the reason for seeking care was referred to as the "Chief Complaint" (CC). Because change in behavior occurs slowly over time, this term may still be noted when reading health histories written by other health care providers.

Describe the data/information that must be gathered for each category of a health history.

Because the health history, combined with objective data obtained through physical examination and diagnostic studies, provides the base on which a judgment or diagnosis regarding the health status of the individual is made, obtaining accurate and complete information is critical. While the depth of information obtained for each category may vary from one setting to another, all must be addressed before a diagnosis is made. The categories addressed in a health history are listed in the Performance Checklist.

Describe the eight characteristics included in the summary of each client symptom.

As can be seen, the health history provides the basis for decisions regarding the health and wellness care needs of each client. To ensure the completeness of data collected, eight characteristics that should be addressed for each symptom have been identified. These characteristics are as follows: location, character or quality, quantity or severity, timing, setting, aggravating or relieving factors, associated factors, and client's perception of the symptom. Note that for each body system assessed for symptomatology, health-promoting behaviors are also assessed. The student might find it helpful to organize the symptom analysis into the pneumonic PQRSTU (Provocative or palliative, quality or quantity, region or radiation, severity scale, timing, and understanding patient's perception of the problem).

Relate the developmental considerations to be addressed during a health history for a child or older adult.

The same structure is followed for a child as for an adult with pertinent modifications/additions. The additions include prenatal and perinatal history, parents' description of the present problem, any childhood illnesses or accidents, immunization data, developmental overview, and nutritional history. When assessing functional abilities, the child's environment and his/her function/role within the environment must be considered.

Additional questions may also need to be added to the health history of an older adult. Note questions that explore changes in ADL that may be caused by the aging process or chronic illness. The impact of disease or disease burden may be more important to the older adult than the actual disease diagnosis or pathology. The health care provider must therefore be alert to record the person's reason for seeking care, not the care provider's assumption of the problem.

KEY TERMS

Cultural assessment

Disease burden

ADL

IADL

Symptom

Sign

TEACHING STRATEGIES

- ▼ Have the students search the Internet for health assessment documents and have the students critique them.
- ▼ Using the form obtained from the Internet or a health history form from the agencies used by your school, assign students working in pairs to obtain a health history from each other.
- ▼ Discuss the interviewing techniques implied by the health history form.
- ▼ Have students identify whether the interviewing techniques implied by the form were helpful or obstructive when gathering data.
- ▼ Have students identify the interviewing techniques that were most helpful in obtaining the data; least helpful.
- ▼ After the interview is complete, have the interviewee indicate whether anything of significance was not addressed with the form used. If so, how would the data best be obtained?
- ▼ Using the Checklists from Chapters 4 and 5, have students create a "matching" test. Which steps of an interview best relate to each of the categories in a health history?
- ▼ Using an audio or video recorder, record a health history interview. Critique it for completeness using the Checklists provided at the end of Chapters 4 and 5. Note: Remind students about obtaining permission for the recording.
- ▼ Assign each student to construct a genogram for the individual interviewed.

CRITICAL THINKING EXERCISES

Application to Clinical Practice

For each individual described in the situations below, have students discuss the developmental, age, socioeconomic, and transcultural considerations that should be considered during the gathering of subjective and objective data. Since discharge planning begins upon admission, ask students to identify discharge planning concerns that need to be considered.

Ask students to identify the categories of the health history that have been addressed and those for which additional data must be obtained. Using the Checklists provided for Chapters 4 and 5, assign students to work in pairs to supply the missing data and write at least one relevant nursing diagnosis for any actual or potential problem identified. Have students discuss whether the missing data affected the identification of the problem(s).

- ❑ A. H., age 55, is being admitted for a cholecystectomy. History reveals a 1-pack-a-day cigarette habit and family members inform the care provider that A. H. has been addicted to alcohol for 15 years. A. H. is 5'4" and weighs 102 pounds. Rales and rhonchi are noted upon auscultation of the lungs. No other significant findings are noted during the physical examination.
- ❑ T. C. has come for her first prenatal visit. This is the first pregnancy for this 24-year-old European American. While history and a review of systems does not reveal any personal health problems, family history includes a sister with von Willebrand's

disease, and a grandmother who is a twin. She states that the paternal grandparents are both first generation Irish and that she has not been taking folic acid.

- ❑ B. H., a 50-year-old female, is being admitted to the short procedure unit for removal of a ganglia on the left wrist. Interview reveals she has no health problems that would affect anesthesia. B. H. is 5'6", weighs 190 pounds and lives alone.
- ❑ H. N. is being admitted for an abdominal hysterectomy and salpingo-oophorectomy. She is 40 years old, lives with her daughter, and states that she has had asthma for 10 years. Interview reveals no other health problems. She performs monthly self breast examinations.
- ❑ C. C., age 55, is admitted for an ankle fusion to improve her gait. She has a benign tumor in the spinal cord at T 10, which has gradually impaired her gait over a period of 15 years. She has never married and lives alone. Currently she uses two Canadian crutches for ambulation. Review of systems reveals asthma for 20 years and one-pack-a-day use of cigarettes.
- ❑ T. S. is being seen by the home health nurse at 8 a.m. This is the first visit after the discharge of T. S. from the local community hospital, where an insulin regimen and blood glucose testing for type II diabetes mellitus was begun. The disease was first diagnosed 10 years ago. T. S. is 45 years old and employed as a broker for a real estate firm. T. S. states that her father is alive and in good health, and that her mother also has type II diabetes and has had a below-the-knee amputation for complications of the disease. She is 5'7" and weighs 200 pounds.
- ❑ G. S. is brought to the Emergency Department by ambulance. His son states that he had a "fit." Since the client is unable to answer questions, the son is interviewed for relevant health problems. The son states that there is no prior history of neurologic problems and other than a compound fracture of the elbow at age 30, past history is unremarkable. Both parents of G. S. are alive. Father is well and mother has hypertension and congestive heart disease controlled by medication. No history of neurologic problems for either of G. S.'s parents are known to the son.
- ❑ C. H., age 17, is admitted to the pediatric unit of a rehabilitation hospital. For 2 months she has been hospitalized in her local community hospital following a head injury from a motor vehicle accident. Initial examination reveals a tracheotomy, contractures of leg and arm on the left side, and withdrawal from painful stimuli; her eyes open to verbal stimuli, and her pupils react to light. Her mother states that there are three siblings alive and well, ages 22, 24, and 26. The mother's breath smells of alcohol, but the mother denies any health problems for her or the child's father.

WEB SITES OF INTEREST

American Hospital Association- ***www.aha.org***

American College of Nurse Practitioners- ***www.nurse.org/acnp***

American Academy of Nurse Practitioners- ***www.aanp.org***

Physicians for Prevention- ***www.pfprevention.com***

PERFORMANCE CHECKLIST

HEALTH HISTORY

	Yes	No	Comments
Initial assessment: history			
Date			
Source of history			
Reliability of historian			
Biographical data			
Reason for seeking care			
Present health or history of present illness (including critical characteristics)			
Past history			
Family history			
Review of systems			
Functional assessment			
ADL			
IADL			
Developmental considerations (if indicated)			
Discharge needs			

Chapter 6

Mental Status Assessment

ANNOTATED LEARNING OBJECTIVES

At the completion of this chapter the student will:

Define the behaviors that are considered in an assessment of an individual's mental status.

Consciousness, language, mood and affect, orientation, attention, memory, abstract reasoning, thought process, thought content and perceptions all need to be considered when assessing mental status. For some aspects of the assessment, direct questions may need to be asked such as "Where are you?", while for others, the examiner can gather the data indirectly through the way in which the client responds to questions asked during the health assessment.

Describe relevant developmental considerations of the mental status examination.

Consciousness, the use of language, attention span, and the ability to use abstract thinking all develop over time and must be considered from a developmental perspective when examining infants and children. While the process of aging leaves the parameters of mental status mostly intact, a slower response time may affect new learning. The examiner must also be cognizant of the impact of age-related physical changes such as alterations in vision or hearing that may affect the mental status of the older adult.

State the purpose of a mental status examination.

The full mental status examination is a systematic check of emotional and cognitive function. The purpose is to determine mental health strengths and coping skills and to screen for any dysfunction. Usually, mental status can be assessed through the context of the health history interview. A full mental status examination would be conducted if family members express concern about a person's behavior, if the presence of cerebral pathology or aphasia is observed, or if the symptoms of psychiatric mental illness are noted. The examiner must be aware of factors that might affect findings such as pre-existing illnesses and medications. These factors are included in the health history.

List the four components of mental status assessment.

Appearance, behavior, cognition, and thought processes are the four main components addressed during the mental status assessment. The letters A, B, C, & T may help the practitioner to remember these categories.

Complete a Mini-Mental State examination.

The Mini-Mental State is a quick and easy means of assessing cognitive function, not mood or thought processes. It may be used for both initial and serial measurement to follow a client over time. The exam is used to detect dementia and delirium. In addition, the exam is used to differentiate organic disorders from psychiatric illnesses. As with other skills, practice increases both competence and self confidence. Using the form under the guidance of an instructor will assist in this development.

Discuss developmental considerations for infants, children, and the aging adult.

The focus of the mental status assessment of infants and children addresses the behavioral, cognitive, and psychosocial development of the child in coping with his or her environment. The Denver II screening test can be used to assess the mental status of young children. In addition to this, use the A, B, C, & T guidelines outlined for the adult and review expected developmental milestones for children. The omission or lack of achievement of a milestone may be an indication for further exploration. The Behavioral Checklist provided in the text can be used as an assessment tool for school-age children. For the aging adult, the set (FACT) test is useful for assessing mental status. In this test, the person is asked to name 10 items in each of four categories or sets: fruits, animals, colors, and towns. Before assessing mental status in older adults, sensory status must be checked and deficits corrected, if possible.

KEY TERMS

Mental status
Mental disorder
Consciousness
Mood
Affect
Orientation
Organic disorder
Psychiatric disorder
Language

TEACHING STRATEGIES

- Have the students search the Web for available mental status assessment instruments. For each instrument, have the students assess the instrument for completeness.
- Working in trios, have students role play various types of clients that may be encountered. (Shy, angry, fearful, disoriented, etc.). One student is the interviewer, one is interviewee, and the third uses the checklist to follow the interview. Both the Interview Checklist and the Checklist for this chapter may be helpful. At the conclusion of the interview, have each student describe the strengths and weaknesses of the interview.
- Using the form provided in the text, assign students to work in pairs and each complete a Mini-Mental State Examination on the assigned partner. At the completion of the exercise, discuss interviewing techniques that facilitated the completion of the exam.
- Use segments of movies or other visual materials and ask students to describe the mental status of the personality portrayed using A, B, C, & T in the segment viewed. Some suggestions for movies might include "The Over the Hill Gang" with George Burns for viewing older adults, "Forest Gump" for the educationally challenged, "Rainman" for a psychiatric disorder and "Terms of Endearment" for anger.
- Write brief descriptions of various alterations in mental status that students might encounter in the clients of various clinical agencies. Ask one or two students to provide a role play based on the supplied description and have the rest of the group complete a mental status assessment on the "client."
- At the end of the assigned class or lab period, have each student briefly (providing a 1/2 piece of paper will limit length of response) answer the question, "The area in which I would like additional clarification is . . ."
- Assign students to complete a mental status assessment of an assigned client in a clinical setting, using responses to health history questions as the basis for the exam.
- Have students document the results of the above assessment and associated nursing diagnosis.

CRITICAL THINKING EXERCISES

Application to Clinical Practice

For each individual described in the situations below, have students discuss the developmental, age, socioeconomic, and transcultural considerations that should be addressed during the gathering of subjective and objective data and the implications for the provision of health care. Ask students to determine whether information is provided regarding appearance, behavior, cognition, and thought processes (A, B, C, & T). Because clients with alterations in mental status may be unable to meet his/her own physical needs, have students also discuss the implications for the family member providing care or community social services that may be required. Have students describe any additional data that might be needed before a judgment/diagnosis can be made, and cite at least one relevant nursing diagnosis for any actual or potential problem identified.

❑ H. M. visits the social center where congregate meals are provided at lunch time. He is known to the health care provider and has been alert and oriented X's 3 in the past. Today, the provider notes that although it is 30° outside, he has come without a coat or jacket, is unshaven, and has difficulty obtaining food in the cafeteria line.

❑ D. J. suffers form Parkinson disease and is therefore seen every 6 months for follow-up evaluation. In the past, her husband has accompanied and been present during the examination. Because he was unable to accompany her today, a neighbor has brought D. J. for the visit, and D. J. is therefore in the examining room alone. When the health care practitioner comes into the room, D. J. is still in her street clothes and when asked to put on the examining gown seems confused about how to proceed with the task. She is unable to recall what she had for breakfast and cannot state her phone number.

❑ T. R. comes 5 days a week to an outpatient clinic for physical therapy and occupational therapy for strengthening and gait training following an auto accident that resulted in a head injury. She has been prescribed thorazine by a psychiatrist. Today she is angry, unwilling to follow the directions of the therapist, and her tremors seem to be more pronounced. She evades orientation questions by responding, "Why do you need to know that?"

❑ C. C., a college student, is in her advisor's office because she has been issued a clinical jeopardy form. The advisor is aware that C. C. has a history of manic depression and is under the care of a psychiatrist. C. C. is crying uncontrollably, looks unkempt in appearance and her speech is not completely coherent. The advisor asks C. C. whether she is considering suicide and C. C. answers "yes" and reveals that she has been saving her medications.

❑ T. C. is recovering from abdominal surgery and is receiving narcotics for pain. When the nurse comes to complete an assessment at the beginning of the day, T. C. tells the nurse about the moving pictures he is seeing on the wall. Interview reveals that T. C. is oriented to place and person, and review of admission data does not indicate a history of mental illness.

❑ D. S. is admitted to the unit via the Emergency Department where a diagnosis of CVA was made. The nurse performing the health history notes the inability of the client to answer questions, but D. S. responds correctly when given simple commands. Because of right-sided paralysis, D. S. is unable to write.

❑ A. H. has come for a follow-up visit for pneumonia. The practitioner is aware that her daughter was recently killed in a motor vehicle accident that involved alcohol. During the examination, the practitioner notes the smell of mints on A. H.'s breath, slurred speech, and a disheveled appearance.

WEB SITES OF INTEREST

American Federation for Aging Research- ***www.afar.org***

American Psychological Association- ***www.apa.org***

Association of Child and Adolescent Psychiatric Nurses- ***www.acapn.org***

PERFORMANCE CHECKLIST

MENTAL STATUS

	Yes	No	Comments
Appearance			
Posture			
Body movements			
Dress			
Grooming & hygiene			
Behavior			
Level of consciousness			
Facial expression			
Speech			
Mood and affect			
Cognitive functions			
Orientation			
Time			
Person			
Place			
Attention span			
Recent memory			
Remote memory			
New learning—four unrelated words test			
Aphasia assessment			
Word comprehension			
Reading			
Writing			
Judgment			
Thought processes and perceptions			
Thought processes			
Thought content			

(Continued)

PERFORMANCE CHECKLIST

MENTAL STATUS (cont'd)

	Yes	No	Comments
Perceptions			
Suicidal thoughts			
Supplemental Mental Status Examination—Mini-Mental			
State Examination			
Developmental consideration			
Document findings			

Chapter 7

Nutritional Assessment

ANNOTATED LEARNING OBJECTIVES

At the completion of this chapter the student will:

Define nutritional status.

The degree of balance between nutrient intake and nutrient requirement is referred to as nutritional status. As with all aspects of assessment, several factors may affect the health status of an individual. For nutrition assessment, the physiologic, psychosocial, developmental, and cultural aspects of the individual's life must be considered. The health practitioner needs to determine whether the client has optimal nutrition, undernutrition, or overnutrition.

Describe the unique nutritional needs for various developmental periods throughout the life cycle.

While nutritional assessment should be included consistently in the provision of health care, recognition of nutritional needs for each stage of development will enable the health care provider to better meet those needs. Each of the following have special nutritional needs: infancy and childhood, adolescence, pregnancy and lactation, adulthood, and older adulthood.

Describe the role cultural heritage and values may play in an individual's nutritional intake.

While each client must be viewed as an individual within his/her environment, a knowledge of the role of food in the cultural groups within the health care service area will increase the ability of the health care provider to meet individual needs. Some areas to be considered when completing an individual nutritional assessment include the role of cultural values and heritage in addition to occupation, socioeconomic group, religion, health awareness, patterns of eating, and dietary practices.

State the purposes of a nutritional assessment.

Three purposes for completing a nutritional assessment are (1) to identify individuals who are malnourished, including over- and undernutrition or to identify individuals who are at risk for developing malnutrition; (2) to obtain data for developing a nutrition plan that will prevent or decrease the development of malnutrition; and (3) to establish a baseline of data for the evaluation of nutritional care.

Describe the components of a nutritional assessment.

A comprehensive nutritional assessment is used for individuals identified at nutritional risk. Nutrition screening is the first step in the nutritional assessment. Based on the data obtained, patients at risk for altered nutrition can be identified. Weight and weight history, conditions associated with increased nutritional risk, dietary history, direct observation, anthropometric measures, and routine laboratory data are used as parameters for screening.

Discuss the strengths and limitations of the methods used for collecting current dietary intake.

The 24-hour diet recall can be obtained during the nutritional assessment and is therefore easy to use. Sources of error with this method include the following:

the historian may be unable to recall the type or amount of food eaten; the last 24 hours may be atypical of usual intake; the historian may alter the truth or underestimate serving size; and snack items and gravies, sauces and other additives may be underreported. A food frequency questionnaire can also be completed during the nutritional assessment interview and is therefore easy to use. Limitations of this method include the absence of quantity or serving size of food eaten and the dependence upon the historian's memory. Food diaries have the potential to be a more accurate representation of dietary intake. However, potential problems also exist for this method. These include noncompliance, inaccurate recording, atypical intake on the recording days, and conscious alteration of diet during the recording period.

Use anthropometric measures and laboratory data to assess the nutritional status of clients.

Various methods of determining nutritional status through body measure and laboratory data have been described in the text. Accurate identification of nutritional problems allows for earlier intervention.

Use nutritional assessment in the provision of health care.

As with all aspects of health assessment, the goal of nutritional assessment is to identify actual or potential health problems and provide individualized care toward resolution of the problem.

KEY TERMS

Anthropometry
Nutritional status
Mid-upper arm circumference (MAC)
Mid-upper arm muscle circumference (MAMC)
Mid-arm muscle area (MAMA)
Arm span
Waist-to-hip ratio
Body Mass Index
Cultural stereotyping

TEACHING STRATEGIES

- ▼ Have the students search the Internet for dietary assessment instruments.
- ▼ Discuss the impact of economic factors/living situation on food choices.
- ▼ Have students relate the results of a personal 24-hour record of food intake to the food pyramid.
- ▼ Using the suggested questions provided at the end of this section and the nutritional assessment forms provided in the text, have students complete a screening and comprehensive nutritional assessment on a peer.
- ▼ Using the suggested questions provided at the end of this section and the nutritional assessment forms provided in the text, have students complete a nutritional screening and/or assessment on a client.
- ▼ Using the charting formats of the clinical agencies used by the school, have students document the results of the above screening/assessment and other relevant data. See Performance Checklist.
- ▼ Assign students to provide nutrition counseling to a client based on the above assessment. When possible, use a variety of clinical settings: acute care, long-term care, rehabilitation, community, home. Have students discuss the similarities/differences of their findings.
- ▼ Assign students to examine frozen and prepackaged food for nutritional value.
- ▼ Assign students to examine the nutritional value of the foods available in local fast food establishments.
- ▼ Discuss the implications of the above examination for clients on various special diets such as low sodium, calorie restriction, low fat, etc.
- ▼ Discuss drug/diet interactions that must be included in client teaching.
- ▼ Assign students to conduct a nutritional assessment on an individual from a different culture. Have them describe the nutritional implications of the cultural values of the individual.
- ▼ Have nursing students visit a grammar school or high school and assess the school lunch program in relation to the food pyramid. Is good nutrition provided? Do they have suggestions for change? Are food machines in the school? If so, evaluate choices.

CRITICAL THINKING EXERCISES

Application to Clinical Practice

For each individual described in the situations below, have students discuss the developmental, age, socioeconomic, and transcultural considerations that should be considered during the gathering of subjective and objective data and the provision of health care.

In addition, have students relate findings to the food pyramid for adequacy of diet or the identification of nutritional deficiencies. Calculate anthropometric measures using data provided. Use the screening nutritional assessment form found in the text to determine whether additional information is needed in order to make a judgment and individualize the plan of care. When indicated, identify at least one relevant nursing diagnosis for any actual or potential problem identified, and in particular, address any health teaching needs of the client.

❑ K. B., age 30, is 5'5" and weighs 350 pounds. She has two children, ages 3 and 5. K. B. is employed as a secretary, earning $20,000 a year. A 24-hour food record reveals the use of prepackaged food, snacks with high-fat, high-salt content.

❑ L. R., age 16, was in an auto accident 2 months ago in another state. He was hospitalized a total of 5 weeks, 4 of which were in an intensive care unit. He was on a ventilator for 3 weeks and did not receive tube feedings. Weight prior to accident was 195 pounds and height is 6'1". Current weight is 155 pounds. Appetite is good, and he is able to eat now at pre-accident ability. He has been referred to the home health agency for care of a heel decubitus that developed during hospitalization.

❑ P. S. has been transferred to a cardiac step-down unit. She is complaining of nausea and vomiting since her physician changed her medications. After reporting her symptoms to the physician who adjusted her medications, the nurse begins a health interview. P. S. indicates that she and her husband have two to three martinis each evening. Albumin is noted to be 3.3 g/dl.

❑ H. M. has come to the health clinic for a follow-up visit. Her primary health problem is asthma. Medications include aminophylline begun at the last visit. Interview reveals anorexia, and the health practitioner notes a weight loss of 20 pounds since the last visit.

❑ K.K. has been admitted to a long-term care facility. He suffered a CVA 1 month ago resulting in right-sided paralysis. Review of the record indicates that fluids were initially provided IV. Following swallowing studies, the client was placed on a pureed diet. The client is right handed. Comparison of weight prior to illness as reported by the client's wife and admitting weight reveals a weight loss of 30 pounds. The client is 5'8" and weighed 180 pounds prior to onset of illness. Albumin is 3.1 g/dl, hemoglobin is 12 and hematocrit is 35.

❑ R. M. has brought her 5-month-old infant to the health clinic for a routine visit. Weight at birth was 9 pounds 1 ounce and height was 21 inches. Current weight is 30 pounds and height is 24 inches. When asked, R. M. states that the child takes between 9 and 10 bottles of formula a day in addition to solid foods three times a day.

❑ T. G., age 75, has come to his health care provider complaining of insomnia and abdominal pain. Examination reveals a weight loss of 20 pounds since his last visit 6 months ago. The health care provider is aware that T. G.'s wife, who did the shopping and cooking for both of them, died 5 months ago. Income is social security and a small pension.

WEB SITES OF INTEREST

American Heart Association- ***www.americanheart.org***

American Diabetes Association- ***www.diabetes.org***

American Dietetic Association- ***www.eatright.org***

CDC- Diabetes Home Page- ***www.cdc.gov***

National Institute of Diabetes and Digestive and Kidney Disease- ***www.niddk.nih.gov***

PERFORMANCE CHECKLIST

NUTRITION

	Yes	No	Comments
Assess for general factors that may influence nutrition:			
Socioeconomic factors			
Psychological factors			
Culture/values			
Religion/religious practices			
Food preferences			
Drug and alcohol intake			
What is the general appearance of the client?			
Request a description of typical eating patterns.			
Does the client have dentures? If yes, do they fit? Are they used?			
Is the client on a special diet? If yes, are adequate nutrients provided by the diet?			
Does the client use prepackaged and prepared foods?			
Does the client eat fast foods often?			
Assess diet for adequacy of vitamin and mineral intake.			
Has there been a recent change in diet? If yes, was this intentional?			
Has there been a recent increase or decrease in caloric intake? If yes, was this intentional?			
Has there been a recent change in bowel habits, mobility, physical exercise?			
Have the client describe his/her life style as active, sedentary etc.			
Does the client have a regular exercise regimen?			
Has the client experienced recent physical or emotional stress such as surgery, trauma, burns, infection, loss of spouse or job, retirement or other changes that may affect nutrition?			

(Continued)

PERFORMANCE CHECKLIST

NUTRITION (cont'd)

	Yes	No	Comments
Does the client take any over-the-counter medications, especially vitamin or mineral supplements or appetite suppressants? If yes, obtain reason, dose and beginning date.			
Does the client use any health foods? Describe.			
Review the client's current medication regimen, including over-the-counter preparations.			
Have the client describe his/her alcohol, tobacco, snuff or caffeine intake.			
Does the client have any eating disorder?			
Is there any family history of food allergy, intolerance?			
Does the client have a history of cardiovascular disease, Crohn's disease, diabetes mellitus, GI tract disorders, sickle-cell anemia, allergies, food intolerance, obesity?			

Chapter 8

Assessment Techniques and Approach to the Clinical Setting

ANNOTATED LEARNING OBJECTIVES

At the completion of this chapter the student will:

Describe the use of inspection as a physical examination technique.

Inspection is critical observation of the client in a systematic, deliberate manner that begins as a "general survey" the moment the practitioner first meets the client. It is the first technique used in the performance of a physical assessment. While conducting an inspection, the practitioner uses the client's body as his or her own control to determine symmetry between the right and left sides of the body. Good lighting, adequate exposure and, at times, the use of special instruments aid in the completion of a good inspection.

Describe the use of palpation as a physical examination technique.

Palpation is the use of touch to determine the texture, size, consistency, and location of body parts. Temperature, moisture, change in size, vibrations, pulsations, rigidity or spasticity, crepitation, presence of lumps or masses, and the presence of tenderness or pain may also be noted.

Describe the use of auscultation as a physical examination technique.

Auscultation (listening to sounds produced by the body) is done with both the unassisted sense of hearing and with special instruments, usually a stethoscope. Sounds heard with the ear alone include speech, percussion tones, difficult breathing, coughing, and loud abdominal sounds. Areas most commonly assessed with a stethoscope are the heart, blood vessels, lungs, and abdomen. Because the stethoscope does not amplify sound but blocks out extraneous room sounds, a quiet environment is required. The examiner listens for the presence or absence of sound and the quality of sound heard.

Describe the use of percussion as a physical examination technique.

Percussion is the technique of striking a part of the body with short, sharp taps of the fingers. Location, size, position, and density of the underlying organs can be assessed through noting the change in percussion notes elicited. Percussion is used most frequently to assess the thorax and abdomen.

Describe direct and indirect percussion.

Direct percussion, most commonly used to assess the adult sinuses and thorax of an infant, is the technique of striking the finger or hand directly against the body. With indirect percussion the examiner's interphalangeal joint is placed firmly against the client's skin with the remainder of the hand lifted off the skin. The middle finger of the dominant hand is used as the striking force (plexor). The striking finger, using the action of the wrist, hits directly at right angles to the stationary finger on the portion in contact with the skin surface. NOTE: To elicit the best tones and to avoid pain, short fingernails are a must.

Identify the components of a percussion note.

Amplitude is the intensity of the sound produced. The louder the sound, the greater the amplitude. Both the force of the blow and the structure's ability to vibrate affect the amplitude. Pitch or frequency describes the number of vibrations per second. More rapid vibrations produce a high-pitched tone, slower vibrations yield a low-pitched tone. Quality or timbre is a subjective difference due to a sound's distinctive overtones. Duration is the length of time the note lingers.

Relate the parts of the hands to palpation techniques used in assessment.

Fine tactile discrimination is best achieved with the fingertips. Position, shape, and consistency of an organ or mass is determined through the use of the opposition of the fingers and thumb. Temperature is best determined with the dorsa (back) of the hands and fingers. Vibration is assessed with the base of the fingers (metacarpophalangeal joints).

Differentiate between light, deep, and bimanual palpation.

Light palpation, a downward pressure of approximately 1 to 2 cm, is used to evaluate surface characteristics and identify any areas of tenderness. Deep palpation, a downward pressure of 2 to 4 cm, is used to palpate an organ or mass deeper within a body cavity Bimanual palpation is the use of both hands to envelope or capture certain body parts or organs such as the kidneys.

Discuss appropriate infection control measures used to prevent spread of infection.

Stethoscope and other equipment can become a common vehicle for transmission of infection. Designate a "clean" versus a "used" area for handled equipment. All equipment carried by the examiner should be cleaned with alcohol between patients. The single most important step to decrease the risk of microorganism transmission is a thorough hand wash after physical contact with patients or body fluids. Standard precautions are used for all patients, and standard-based precautions are used with patients with documented or suspected transmissible infections. As the examiner enters the room, hands should be washed in the patient's presence.

Discuss developmental consideration needed for patients.

Special consideration is given to position and preparation of patients. The order of developmental stage must be considered in determining the sequence of the examination. For children, a less threatening approach is needed, and parents are encouraged to be present for infants, toddlers, and preschoolers. Privacy is essential for other age groups and must be maintained. The examination must be paced to meet the possible slowed pace of the aging person. A mini data base may be needed for patients in distress.

KEY TERMS

Inspection
Palpation
Percussion
Auscultation
Otoscope
Ophthalmoscope
Resonance
Tympany
Nosocomial infection

TEACHING STRATEGIES

- ▼ Assign students to create a crossword puzzle for the new terms found in this chapter.
- ▼ Obtain two styrofoam cups with lids. Fill one with water or sand. Leave the other empty. Have students percuss the tops of the two cups. Although the sounds are exaggerated, it will allow students to begin to differentiate between the sound heard over an air-filled organ and a solid organ. It also allows the instructor to observe the percussion technique of the student.
- ▼ Instruct students to come to lab in shorts and t-shirts. Working in pairs, have students practice the techniques used in a physical examination. Be sure to observe each student, especially for hand position with indirect percussion and the proper use of the stethoscope.
- ▼ Arrange for each student to observe a physical examination performed by an experienced practitioner.

- Bring an otoscope/ophthalmoscope to class or lab and allow students to practice handling the equipment.
- Discuss techniques that enhance the comfort of the client and improve the quality of findings during a physical examination: for example—wetting the hair on the chest of a male to decrease the interference with sound transmission, having a warm room to increase the physical comfort of the patient, providing sufficient lighting and privacy. Advise students to avoid bumping tubing together and to focus on one sound at a time when auscultating the chest.
- Discuss universal precautions and infection control issues for the protection of both the client and the examiner.
- Have students purchase a stethoscope for personal use. Review the use of the diaphragm and bell, discuss fit of the ear pieces and look at the length of the tubing. Having scissors handy might also be helpful since some less expensive scopes come with very long tubing. A length of 12 inches is usually recommended. Discuss modifications needed for pediatric and elderly patients.

CRITICAL THINKING EXERCISES

Application to Clinical Practice

For each situation described below, have students discuss the developmental, age, socioeconomic, transcultural, and infection control considerations that should be addressed when applicable. Ask students to discuss the technique(s) used to obtain the data or identify factors that may alter the data obtained.

- ❑ After visiting all assigned patients, the nurse records the following for one patient: "B.P. 120/70, P. 68, R. 16, T. 99°, skin warm and dry, dressing dry and intact."
- ❑ P. G.. is a client recovering from an abdominal resection performed yesterday. On the chart the nurse has written, "Abdomen soft, non-tender, B. S. (Bowel Sounds) present in all 4 quadrants."
- ❑ L. J. has come to the dermatology clinic complaining of itching. The health care provider charts "erythematous areas 1 cm x 2 cm on dorsal surface of left hand."
- ❑ P. C. is recovering from an appendectomy. History includes use of 1 package of cigarettes a day. The nurse has come to complete a postoperative assessment at the beginning of the afternoon shift. When the nurse asks to turn down the TV, P. C. responds, "No, I have to see my soap operas."
- ❑ O. W. has been admitted for general malaise. Interview reveals a history of excessive intake of alcohol for 20 years. The nurse documents "dullness to percussion in rt. quadrant from 5th intercostal space to 4 cm. below the costal margin, + fluid wave."
- ❑ F. N. has come to the clinic with complaints of pain in her right great toe. The practitioner documents "V. S. (vital signs) B. P. 180/98, P. 78, R. 20, T. 99.6°, small ulcer on the plantar surface of right great toe 3 cm in diameter, necrotic edges with yellow center, thick purulent, foul-smelling drainage; complains of pain to touch."
- ❑ The night nurse is making initial rounds on assigned postoperative patients. J. K. had an open reduction of a hip fracture that morning. The client has a cast, a Foley catheter, and an IV running. Have students write a note that would reflect pertinent findings for this patient.

EQUIPMENT NEEDED FOR PHYSICAL EXAM

Platform scale with height attachment
Skinfold calipers
Sphygmomanometer
Stethoscope with bell and diaphragm (adult or pediatric)
Thermometer
Penlight
Tangential lighting
Otoscope/ophthalmoscope
Tuning fork
Nasal speculum
Tongue depressor
Disposable sharp object or split tongue blade
Pocket vision screener
Skin-marking pen
Flexible tape measure
Ruler marked in centimeters
Reflex hammer

Cotton balls
Bivalve vaginal speculum
Examination gloves
Materials for cytologic study
Water-soluble lubricant
Hemoccult test equipment

WEB SITES OF INTEREST

Centers for Disease Control and Prevention- ***www.cdc.gov***

Latex Allergy Homepage- ***www.allergy.mcg.edu/physician***

Association of Professionals in Infection Control and Epidemiology, Inc.- ***www.apic.org***

American Association of Occupational Health Nurses- ***www.aaohn.org***

PERFORMANCE CHECKLIST

ASSESSMENT TECHNIQUES—Essential Behaviors

	Yes	No	Comments
Gather equipment			
Provide privacy			
Wash hands			
Explain procedure to patient			
Obtain basic measurement			
Height			
Weight			
Blood pressure			
Temperature			
Pulse			
Respiration			
Additional nutritional measurements if indicated			
Provide proper lighting			
Describe each step			
Proceed in a head-to-toe fashion			
Summarize findings with patient			
Document findings			

Chapter 9

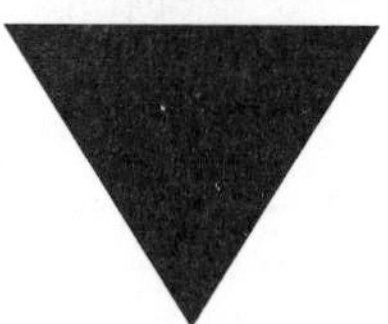

General Survey, Measurement, Vital Signs

ANNOTATED LEARNING OBJECTIVES

At the completion of this chapter the student will:

List the information considered in each of the four areas of a general survey—physical appearance, body structure, mobility, and behavior.

The general survey is an overall impression of each client and begins when the practitioner first encounters the individual. Four areas are considered in this overview. *Physical appearance* includes an assessment of age, sex, level of consciousness, skin color, facial features, and signs of distress. *Body structure* addresses stature, nutritional status, symmetry, posture, position and body build, and notation of any obvious physical deformities. *Mobility* is concerned with gait and range of motion. *Behavioral* assessment considers facial expression, mood and affect, speech, dress, and personal hygiene. Changes in any of these areas may be indicative of an illness.

Discuss relevant developmental considerations in relation to a general survey.

For a child, interaction with the accompanying adult should be observed. Unexpected behavior on the part of either the adult or child may be clues to possible child abuse, mental illness, or a developmental disability or disorder on the part of either the child or the adult. In the aging adult, posture, appearance, and mobility may change. A flexion of the spine may be noted by the eighth decade, an angulation of features and a redistribution of body proportions may be noted. Gait may be wider-based to compensate for change in balance.

Describe various routes of temperature measurement and special consideration for each route

The routes of temperature measurement reflect the body's core temperature. The oral temperature is accurate and convenient. Oral route may not be appropriate for comatose or confused persons, wired mandible, facial dysfunction, or for those who cannot close the mouth. Axillary temperature is safe and accurate for infants and young children when the environment is reasonably controlled. Rectal route is used when other routes are not practical. Disadvantages are patient discomfort, time-consuming and disruptive activity, and risk of cross-contamination. Tympanic membrane thermometer is a noninvasive, nontraumatic device that is quick and efficient. This method is most reflective of core temperature. Special consideration is needed for patients with ear disorders.

Describe the four qualities considered when assessing the pulse.

The four qualities included in a pulse assessment are rate, rhythm, force, and elasticity. Normal rates range between 60 and 100 beats per minute but vary with age and sex. Rhythm, in relation to the heart, refers to the pattern of beats and the pauses between; normal pulse rhythm is regular. Force or amplitude of the pulse refers to the quality of the pulse in relation to the strength of the heart's stroke volume. Pulse force is recorded using a three- or four-point scale, depending on agency policy. Elasticity refers to the flexible quality of the artery, which usually feels springy, straight and resilient.

Describe appropriate procedure for assessing normal respirations.

Because breathing is normally relaxed, regular, automatic, and silent, respirations are counted while the hand is still in position for taking the pulse and the client is unaware that respirations are being counted. Respirations are counted for 30 seconds unless an abnormality is suspected; the rate is then counted for a full minute. A ratio of 4:1 for pulse rate to respiratory rate is common. Assessment findings may be altered based on the patient's condition.

Describe the relationships among the terms blood pressure, systolic pressure, diastolic pressure, pulse pressure, and mean arterial pressure (MAP).

Blood pressure is the pressure of the blood against the wall of the blood vessels. The term usually refers to the pressure of the blood within the arteries. Systolic pressure is the maximum pressure felt on the artery during left ventricular contraction. The diastolic pressure is the elastic recoil, or resting pressure the blood exerts constantly between each contraction. The pulse pressure is the difference between the systolic and diastolic pressures and reflects the stroke volume. The mean arterial pressure is the pressure forcing blood into the tissue, averaged over the cardiac output.

List factors that affect blood pressure.

Several interrelated factors affect blood pressure: the pumping action of the heart or cardiac output, the resistance to the flow of blood in the arterioles, the elasticity of the walls of the main arteries, the blood volume, extracellular fluid volume, and the blood's viscosity.

Relate the use of an improper size blood pressure cuff to the possible findings that may be obtained.

The width of the rubber bladder of the cuff should equal 40 percent of the circumference of the person's arm. The length of the bladder should equal 80 percent of this circumference. A cuff that is too narrow yields a falsely high pressure; a cuff that is too wide yields a falsely low pressure.

KEY TERMS

Bradycardia
Tachycardia
Sphygmomanometer
Eupnea
Tachypnea
Bradypnea
Cheyne-Stokes
Apnea

TEACHING STRATEGIES

- Have each student observe a peer and document findings as a "general assessment."
- Discuss Infection Control Practices in relation to measuring vital signs.
- Refer the students to the web sites of interest in order to identify new recommendations for blood pressure.
- Relate institutional isolation policies to vital sign measurement.
- Have each student take vital signs on a peer. The use of a teaching stethoscope is helpful with new students learning to take blood pressures. Practice with height and weight on a platform scale must be at the instructor's discretion. If obese students are in the class, the activity may be embarrassing to them.
- Have various size sphygmomanometers available. Have students take pressure on the same individual using inappropriate size cuffs and note the difference in readings obtained.
- Be sure to have students take blood pressure on both arms and also practice taking blood pressure on a leg.
- Having "client" raise the arm being assessed for a few seconds helps empty the veins and may aid in hearing a difficult pressure.
- Discuss contraindications for taking a blood pressure in a particular extremity.
- Obtain graphic sheets from various clinical agencies. Have students record findings using the various forms.
- After students have obtained a baseline assessment on each other, have the students in the role of client perform an activity that will alter vital signs, such as rapidly climbing stairs or jumping in place, and have the students in the role of nurse repeat the assessment. Note how long it takes for the signs to return to baseline.

- ▼ Discuss the advantages of charting BPs on a graph versus writing the findings as a number on the chart.
- ▼ Using a baby mannequin, have students practice measuring length, weight, and head circumference.
- ▼ In the clinical setting, assign students to write a general survey description of a client.

CRITICAL THINKING EXERCISES

Application to Clinical Practice

For each individual described in the situation below, have students discuss the developmental, age, socioeconomic, and transcultural considerations that should be considered during the gathering of subjective and objective data and the provision of health care.

In addition, have students relate expected findings to those described, discuss any additional information that might be needed before a judgment/diagnosis can be made, and identify at least one relevant nursing diagnosis for any actual or potential problem identified.

- ❑ It is December in a northern state. S. A. has brought her two children, ages 3 and 5, to the health clinic for the first time. She states that she recently immigrated from India. She is wearing a Sari with a light coat and each of the children is wearing a light jacket. Interaction between parent and children is appropriate. The children both fall at the 4th percentile for both height and weight. Overall nutrition status appears to be satisfactory.
- ❑ P. H., age 18, has been admitted to the intensive care unit with diabetic ketoacidosis. Vital signs are: BP 110/60, P. 56, R 30, T. 99°. Discussion with his mother reveals that he is a member of the high school track team.
- ❑ H. N. has come into the Emergency Department with epistaxis of two hours duration. Vital signs are: B. P 160/90, P. 76, R. 16, T. 97°. Client states normal pressure is 110/70.
- ❑ Nursing Assistant Dana has come into M. K.'s room to take morning vital signs. The client had a right-sided mastectomy yesterday. When Dana begins to apply the cuff to M. K.'s right arm, M. K. objects. As the professional nurse responsible for M.K.'s care, what would you say to Dana regarding M.K.'s objection?
- ❑ R. M. has come for follow-up care for hypertension. She is taking medications. Describe how vital signs should be taken and the results expected.
- ❑ E. H., age 80, stops in to see the health care provider in the senior center she attends every day. She is complaining of general malaise, and a productive cough. Vital signs are: B.P. 150/90, P. 76, R. 20 and T. 99.2°F. Should any of these findings be a cause for concern?
- ❑ B. D., age 9 1/2 months, has come for her first well baby checkup at this facility. The family has recently been transferred. An assistant obtained the following screening information: H. 27 inches, W. 20 lbs, 9 oz, and head circumference 46 cm. Plot these findings and discuss any additional information that may be needed.

WEB SITES OF INTEREST

American Heart Association- ***www.americanheart.org***

NIH- National Heart, Lung, and Blood Institute (NHLBI)- ***www.nhlbi.nih.gov***

PERFORMANCE CHECKLIST

GENERAL SURVEY

	Yes	No	Comments
Physical appearance			
Age			
Sex			
Level of consciousness			
Skin color			
Facial features			
Signs of distress			
Body structure			
Stature			
Nutritional status			
Symmetry			
Posture			
Position			
Body build			
Physical deformation			
Mobility			
Gait			
Range of motion			
Behavior			
Facial expression			
Mood and affect			
Speech			
Dress			
Personal hygiene			
Temperature			
Appropriate instrument			
Sufficient time			

(Continued)

PERFORMANCE CHECKLIST

GENERAL SURVEY (cont'd)

	Yes	No	Comments
Pulse assessment—taken for a minimum of 30 seconds; describe:			
Rate			
Rhythm			
Force			
Elasticity			
Respiration—taken for 30 seconds			
Blood pressure			
Appropriate cuff size			
Appropriate stethoscope			
Systolic determined prior to taking pulse			
Weight			
Standardized balance scale			
Shoes and heavy outer clothes removed			
Appropriate method for age and condition			
Height			
Headpiece aligned with top of head			
Patient's shoes removed			
Appropriate method for age and condition			
Documentation of findings			
All findings explained to client			

Chapter 10

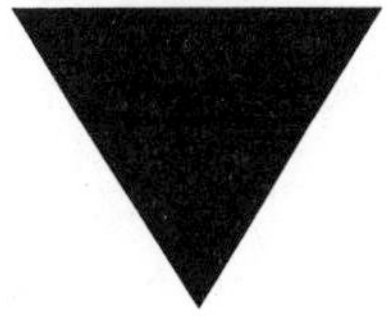

Skin, Hair, and Nails

ANNOTATED LEARNING OBJECTIVES

At the completion of this chapter the student will:
Relate the anatomical structures of the skin to its functions.

Skin is part of the body's neurosensory system. As the body's largest organ system, the skin functions as the sentry of the body, protecting it from environmental stress and serving as a warning of danger. Intact skin protects the body from invasion by pathogens and loss of fluid and electrolytes. Sebum secreted through the hair follicles lubricates the skin and retards water loss. Through the evaporation of sweat or shivering, the skin acts as part of the body temperature regulatory system. Review the structure and function of the skin presented in the text as needed to efficiently perform this assessment.

Describe the significant differences between the skin of the very young, the older adult, and healthy adult skin.

Because of its immaturity, the skin of the very young is unable to effectively prevent fluid loss or function in temperature regulation. The stratum corneum of older skin thins and flattens, allowing chemicals easier access to the body. Wrinkling occurs because of the loss of elastin, collagen and subcutaneous fat as well as reduced muscle tone.

Cite examples of health care implications presented by skin alterations.

Clients of any age with burns, incisions, or lacerations must be protected from infection. Any procedure that alters the integrity of the skin makes the client vulnerable to infection. The young must be protected from loss of body heat and the older patient from shearing and tearing injuries. All clients must be examined for skin changes that may be indicative of cancer.

Describe the differentiation between normal and abnormal skin color for various ethnic groups.

Skin color varies from one part of the body to another, from one individual to another, and from one ethnic group to another. The ability to effectively assess the skin of each individual who may present for health care and to differentiate between normal and abnormal findings must be developed through experience with many individuals. Each client serves as his/her own normal measure for skin color.

State the significance of skin tone changes.

The examiner must be alert to subtle skin tone changes and their relationship to the general health of the client. Skin tone changes may be indicative of underlying disease. In addition to examining for symmetry in general, mucous membranes, lips, nail beds, and sclera must be examined for changes that may not be visible to the casual observer. For example, the sclera may be the first area in which jaundice is noted. Decreased perfusion or anemia is exhibited as cyanosis. Bruising that does not match the history provided by the client may be indicative of abuse. Careful, tactful questioning of the client or family member may assist the the practitioner with this step in skin assessment.

Complete an assessment of hair, skin, and nails using appropriate technique for all developmental stages.

Inspection and palpation are the primary methods used to examine the hair, skin, and nails. Each practitioner must develop a systematic manner for this examination to ensure completeness. Documentation following the example provided in the text is the final phase of the examination necessary to convey the results of the examination to other health professionals.

KEY TERMS

Alopecia
Cyanosis
Erythema
Jaundice
Lesion
Pallor
Pruritus

TEACHING STRATEGIES

- ▼ Have the students search the Internet for a skin assessment instrument. Have them critique the instrument for completeness.
- ▼ Using a copy of the picture of the skin provided in the text, have students label the structures of the skin.
- ▼ Divide students into pairs or trios to complete a history, examination and documentation of an examination of the hair, skin, and nails. One student may be the patient, one may conduct the examination, and one may read the text to guide the examiner. Rotate roles as time permits.
- ▼ If possible, have members of various ethnic groups work together so students may begin to recognize normal skin color and tone for groups other than their own.
- ▼ Have paper rulers available so students can measure any lesions/marks found during the assessment.
- ▼ Provide a diagram/silhouette of a person for students to indicate the location of the lesions/marks assessed.
- ▼ Provide a list of terms used in the inspection of hair, skin and nails. The terms may be written on the blackboard, on an overhead or in a handout. Have students describe each term (i.e., freckle, nevus, birthmark etc.).
- ▼ Create a game of "password." Working in pairs, have one student hold a set of cards containing the terms and definitions. The partner must guess each term from the clues provided. In addition to the Key Terms listed here, additional terms may be found in the text.
- ▼ In the clinical area, assign students to clients from various ethnic groups and have them complete an assessment including the submission of a completed history and description of findings. Students might complete this assignment singly or in pairs.
- ▼ Simulate erythema. Working in pairs or trios, have each student slap his or her left hand and compare its tone to that of the right hand. Students may need especially good lighting to note the difference between the two hands, but there will be a noticeable difference. This exercise underscores the need for good lighting. A change will occur regardless of each student's basic skin color. This is one way to teach students how to assess for the phlebitis that may be associated with IVs.

CRITICAL THINKING EXERCISES

Application to Clinical Practice

For each individual described in the situations below, have students discuss the developmental, age, socioeconomic, and transcultural considerations that should be considered during the gathering of subjective and objective data and the provision of health care. In addition, have students relate expected (normal) findings to those described, discuss any additional information that may be needed before a judgment/diagnosis can be made, and identify at least one relevant nursing diagnosis for any actual or potential problem identified.

- ❑ R. H. presents to the local health clinic stating that two red, scaly patches on her left hand started about 8 weeks ago. She states that the first lesions appeared to be poison ivy. After the vesicles cleared, the itching and scaling remained. Additional lesions now appear over her left eyebrow, right eye, and a small patch appears over her right upper lip. She states that the lesions have not cleared with OTC preparations. Steroids, antibacterials, and antifungals have been tried. In order to relieve the itching, she has placed a transparent dressing over the lesions on the hand.

❑ B. K. is brought to the Emergency Department accompanied by his son. A towel is wrapped around his right hand and an ice pack is applied to his left eye. The eye has a deep laceration. Ecchymotic areas are developing under the left eye and on the chin. In addition, B. K. has abrasions to the right shoulder and left knee. He states that the wounds were acquired from tripping and falling while he was walking his large dog down a steep hill.

❑ A father brings a 4-year-old child to the family clinic in January. The child has a "mosquito" bite on the abdomen. The child has been in good health prior to this time and immunizations are up to date.

❑ T. M. is in the family clinic for a routine physical. During the initial interview, you ask whether there have been any health changes since her last visit. After pausing a moment, she states that there is a pimple on her forehead that seems to be taking a long time to heal. You know T. M. likes to garden.

WEB SITES OF INTEREST

Dermatology Nurses Association- ***www.dna.nurse.com***

Wound, Ostomy, and Continence Nursing Society- ***www.wocn.org***

National Psoriasis Foundation- ***www.psoriasis.org***

American Academy of Dermatology- ***www.aad.org***

PERFORMANCE CHECKLIST

SKIN, HAIR, AND NAILS

	Yes	No	Comments
Wash hands			
Provide for privacy			
Explain procedure to client			
Obtain proper lighting			
Obtain history			
Don gloves if indicated			
Inspect and palpate the hair for:			
Texture			
Condition (any infestation)			
Distribution			
Inspect and palpate the skin for:			
Tone			
Symmetry			
Hydration/turgor			
Temperature			
Lesions			
Inspect and palpate the nails for:			
Condition			
Nail base angle			
Irregularities			
Symmetry			
Document findings			

Chapter 11

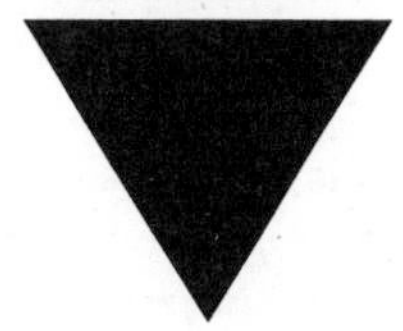

Head and Neck, Including Regional Lymphatics

ANNOTATED LEARNING OBJECTIVES

At the completion of this chapter the student will:

Describe the significant features of the head.

The skull, a rigid, bony box, protects the brain and special sense organs. Seven cranial bones (frontal, parietal, occipital, and temporal) unite at immovable joints called *sutures*. The cranium is supported by the cervical vertebrae. Fourteen facial bones also articulate at sutures, except the mandible—which has a movable joint, the temporomandibular—anterior to each ear. The temporal artery lies superior to the temporalis muscle and has a palpable pulsation, anterior to the ear. The sublingual and submandibular salivary glands are accessible to examination while the parotid glands are not normally palpable.

Identify the structures and landmarks of the neck.

The neck is delimited by the skull, inferior border of the mandible above, and by the manubrium sterni, the clavicle, the first rib, and the first thoracic vertebrae below. The carotid artery and internal jugular vein lie beneath the sternomastoid muscle, while the external jugular vein runs diagonally across this muscle. Parts of the respiratory and digestive systems, in addition to nerves and lymphatics, pass through the neck. The major neck muscles are the sternomastoid and the trapezius, innervated by cranial nerve XI. The sternomastoid muscle divides each side of the neck into two triangles. The anterior triangle extends to the mandible above and the midline of the body medially. The posterior triangle lies behind the sternomastoid muscle and in front of the trapezius. The thyroid gland straddles the trachea in the middle of the neck. The thyroid cartilage with a small palpable notch, lies above the thyroid isthmus.

List the names of the lymph nodes of the neck and their locations.

Preauricular: in front of the ear
Posterior auricular mastoid: superficial to the mastoid process
Occipital: base of the skull
Submental: midline, behind the tip of the mandible
Submaxillary: submandibular halfway between the angle and the tip of the mandible
Jugulodigastric: under the angle of the mandible
Superficial cervical: overlying the sternomastoid muscle
Deep cervical: deep under the sternomastoid muscle
Posterior cervical: in the posterior triangle along the edge of the trapezius muscle
Supraclavicular: just above and behind the clavicle, at the sternomastoid muscle

Describe the assessment that would follow the palpation of an abnormal lymph node.

The examiner should be familiar with the direction of the drainage patterns of the system. The area proximal (upstream) to the location of the abnormal node is explored.

Identify relevant developmental consideration for the head and neck.

At birth, the head is larger than the chest circumference. During infancy, trunk growth predominates, and head size changes in proportion to body height. Lymphoid tissue is well developed at birth and reaches adult size by age 6. At age 10 or 11, the lymph tissue exceeds adult size and then slowly atrophies. During pregnancy, the thyroid enlarges due to hyperplasia and increased vascularity. In the older adult, the facial bones and orbits appear more prominent due to decreased elasticity and subcutaneous fat.

KEY TERMS

Bruit
Crainotabes
Crepitation
Lymphadenopathy
Palpebral fissure
Normocephalic

TEACHING STRATEGIES

- ▼ Have students search the Internet for community resources available to clients with head and neck disorders. Have them design a resource book for clients.
- ▼ Using a baby mannequin, have students identify the location of the cranial bones, the sutures, and fontanels.
- ▼ Assign students to work in groups of three: one to follow the checklist and textbook, one to perform the exam, and one to act as client. Allow sufficient time for students to rotate roles so each has an opportunity to be the examiner.
- ▼ Have students palpate the salivary glands, the thyroid, location of lymph nodes and anterior and posterior triangles of the neck on a partner.
- ▼ If possible, bring a young child into the lab for students to practice palpating lymph nodes that are palpable.
- ▼ Have students locate C7 on each other.
- ▼ Encourage students to verbalize the names of the structures being examined to assist in the memorization of the structures' names and locations.
- ▼ Using the rationale for the examination questions presented in the text, create "headache case studies." Provide a copy to the student in the role of client. Instruct the student in role of examiner to interview the client based on the "clues" provided by the client.
- ▼ Using forms from clinical agencies used by the school, have students document the data obtained from the history and examination of the head and neck.

CRITICAL THINKING EXERCISES

Application to Clinical Practice

For each individual described in the situations below, have students discuss the developmental, age, socioeconomic, and transcultural considerations that should be considered during the gathering of subjective and objective data and the provision of health care.

In addition, have students relate expected (normal) findings to those described, discuss any additional information that might be needed before a judgment/diagnosis can be made, identify at least one relevant nursing diagnosis for any actual or potential problem identified, and identify community resources available.

- ❑ A.M. has come for a routine visit for hypertension. During the course of the exam, she complains of a recent, sudden decrease in hearing.
- ❑ T. J. , age 45, has come for a follow-up visit for minor surgery. The health practitioner observes T. J. with insurance forms and notes that he is holding the papers at arm's length.
- ❑ D. C., a farmer, has come to the clinic with complaints of a buzzing sound in the left ear; sudden onset 2 days ago.
- ❑ M. N., age 57, is at the health clinic for monitoring of Chronic Obstructive Pulmonary Disease (COPD). During the exam, M. N. complains of frequent headaches since the last visit, at which time the medication regimen was changed to include a bronchodilator.
- ❑ P. D., age 18 months, has been brought to the health practitioner by his mother. He has a temperature of 102.4 degrees F per tympanic membrane. The child is listless; the skin is warm and dry.

- ❑ T. D., age 31, has just moved to the area served by the health center. History includes an auto accident at age 15. Inspection of the face reveals ptosis of the left eye.
- ❑ S. M., age 6, has been brought to the health center by her parent because of a temperature elevation and loss of appetite. History and exam reveal the following information: headache, T. 103°F; enlarged, right parotid gland that is painful on palpation. S. M refused the orange juice served with breakfast.
- ❑ B. D., age 9 1/2 months, has come for her first well-baby check-up at this facility. The family has recently been transferred. An assistant obtained the following screening information. Height, 27 inches; weight, 20 lbs, 9 oz; and head circumference 46 cm. Bossing of the forehead is noted, and the sclera are visible above the pupils. Palpation of the anterior fontanel reveals bulging.

WEB SITES OF INTEREST

American Council for Headache Education-
www.achenet.org

PERFORMANCE CHECKLIST

HEAD AND NECK, INCLUDING REGIONAL LYMPHATICS

	Yes	No	Comments
Obtain relevant history			
The Head			
Inspect skull			
Palpate:			
Skull			
Temporal artery			
Temporomandibular joint			
Inspect the face for:			
Expression			
Symmetry			
Involuntary movements			
Edema			
Lesions			
The Neck			
Inspect			
Palpate for:			
Symmetry			
Range of motion			
Lymph nodes			
Salivary glands			
Trachea			
Thyroid gland			
Auscultate the thyroid			
Document findings			

Chapter 12

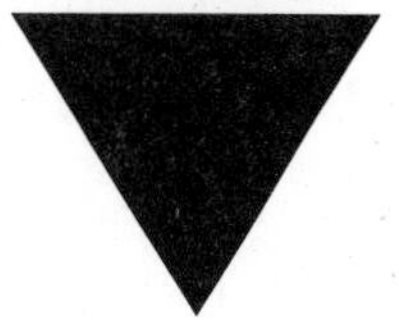

Eyes

ANNOTATED LEARNING OBJECTIVES

At the completion of this chapter the student will:

Identify the external anatomic features of the eye.

Each eye is protected by the bony orbital cavity and is surrounded with a cushion of fat. The eyelids, like two movable shades, further protect the eye from injury, strong light, and dust. The upper eyelid is larger and more mobile. Eyelashes curve outward from the lid margin to filter out dust and dirt. When closed, the lid margins approximate completely. The limbus is the border between the cornea and sclera. The canthus is the corner of the eye, the angle where the lids meet. The caruncle is a small fleshy mass containing sebaceous glands and is located at the inner canthus. A stripe of connective tissue, the tarsal plate, gives shape to the upper lid. Within the tarsal plates are the meibomian glands, modified sebaceous glands that secrete an oily lubrication material onto the lids. The conjunctiva, a thin mucous membrane, is a transparent protective covering of the exposed part of the eye. Constant irrigation is provided by the lacrimal apparatus. Tears drain into the puncta, located on the upper and lower lids at the inner canthus. Six muscles attach the eyeball to its orbit: the superior, inferior, lateral, and medial rectus muscles and the superior and inferior oblique muscles. These muscles serve to direct movement of the eye and are stimulated by cranial nerves III, IV, and VI.

Describe the internal anatomy of the eye.

The eye has three concentric coats or layers. The sclera is a tough, protective, white covering, continuous anteriorly with the smooth, transparent cornea. The cornea, part of the refracting media of the eye, covers the iris and pupil. Touching the cornea with a wisp of cotton stimulates a blink referred to as the *corneal reflex.* Cranial nerves V and VII innervate this reflex. The middle layer contains the choroid, which has dark pigmentation to prevent light from reflecting internally and is highly vascular to deliver blood to the retina. The choroid is continuous with the ciliary body and the iris. The lens, which divides the eye into the anterior and posterior segments, is a transparent structure located behind the pupil. The lens keeps viewed objects in continual focus on the retina. The inner layer contains the retina, which is the visual receptive layer of the eye. In the retina, light waves are changed into nerve impulses.

Name the functions of the ciliary body, the pupil, and the iris.

The ciliary body controls the thickness of the lens, the iris serves as a diaphragm, varying the opening at its center, the pupil, to control the amount of light admitted onto the retina. The muscle fibers of the iris contract and dilate the pupil.

Describe the compartments of the eye.

The anterior compartment, behind the cornea and in front of the iris and lens, has two chambers—anterior and posterior. It contains a clear liquid called *aqueous humor*, produced by the ciliary body. The continuous flow of fluid serves to deliver nutrients to the surrounding tissues and to drain metabolic waste. Intraocular pressure is determined by the balance between the amount of aqueous produced and resistance to its outflow at the angle of the anterior chamber. The posterior compartment is filled with a clear gel-like substance called *vitreous humor*.

Identify the structures viewed through the ophthalmoscope.

The retinal structures viewed with an ophthalmoscope are the optic disc, the retinal vessels, the general background, and the macula. Fibers from the retina converge at the optic disc to form the optic nerve. The color of the disc (optic papilla) varies from creamy yellow-orange to pink. It is round or oval in shape, has margins that are distinct and sharply demarcated, especially on the temporal side, and has a physiologic cup where blood vessels exit and enter.

Define pupillary light reflex, fixation and accommodation.

Pupillary light reflex is the normal constriction of the pupils when bright light shines on the retina. Fixation is a reflex direction of the eye toward an object attracting a person's attention. Accommodation is the adjustment of the eye for seeing objects at various distances; accomplished by the ciliary muscle.

Identify age-related changes in the eye.

At birth, eye function is limited. Peripheral vision is intact in newborns. The macula is absent at birth but is mature by age 8 months. Eye movement is poorly coordinated but matures by age 3-4 months. The structure of the eyeball reaches adult size by age 8 years. With aging, the skin loses its elasticity, causing wrinkling and drooping; fat and muscles atrophy; and involution of the lacrimal glands causes decreased tear production and a feeling of dryness and burning. Pupil size decreases, the lens loses elasticity causing presbyopia. The normally transparent fibers of the lens begin to thicken and yellow, resulting in senile cataract. Visual acuity may diminish gradually after age 50.

Discuss the three most common causes of decreased visual functioning in the older adult.

Cataract formation, or lens opacity, can be expected by age 70. Glaucoma or increased ocular pressure increases with age. Chronic, open-angle glaucoma is the most common type and involves a gradual loss of peripheral vision. Macular degeneration is a breakdown of the cells in the macula lutea, resulting in a loss of central vision in the affected eye; peripheral vision is not affected.

KEY TERMS

Cataract
Glaucoma
Macular degeneration
Presbyopia
Fixation
Accommodation
Limbus
Canthus
Caruncle

TEACHING STRATEGIES

- ▼ Have students search the Internet for community resources available for clients with visual impairment and for visual assessment instruments.
- ▼ Demonstrate the proper use of the ophthalmoscope.
- ▼ Observe students using the ophthalmoscope to visualize objects in the room.
- ▼ Discuss ways of grossly checking visual acuity in the bedridden client.
- ▼ Obtain a model of the eye. Assign one student to read the names of the anatomic structures from the text while another identifies these structures on the model.
- ▼ Encourage students to verbalize the names of the structures being examined to assist in the memorization of the structures' names and location.
- ▼ Using a color copier, copy the pictures of eye disorders in the text. Make flash cards of the disorders by pasting one picture per card on 3" by 5" cards and writing the name and description of the disorder on the back. This may be used to practice learning to diagnose the disorders, to document what is observed, and as a test to describe what is observed.
- ▼ Assign students to work in groups of three: one to follow the checklist and textbook, one to perform the examination, and one to act as client. Allow sufficient time for students to rotate roles so that each has an opportunity to be the examiner.

- ▼ Instruct students to document the results of the above exam.
- ▼ Encourage students to practice using the ophthalmoscope on friends and family members.
- ▼ If students from various ethnic groups are in the class, encourage students to examine one another's eyes to learn the variations that occur among individuals.
- ▼ Assign students to create visual materials that could be used for teaching good health practices for the eye, especially at a health fair.

CRITICAL THINKING EXERCISES

Application to Clinical Practice

For each individual described in the situations below, have students discuss the developmental, age, socioeconomic, and transcultural considerations that should be considered during the gathering of subjective and objective data and the provision of health care.

In addition, have students relate expected (normal) findings to those described, discuss any additional information that might be needed before a judgment/diagnosis can be made and identify at least one relevant nursing diagnosis for any actual or potential problem identified.

- ❑ M. D. has come to the health office at school for an emergency appointment. He states that when he awoke this morning his eye was red, swollen, and itchy with yellow drainage.
- ❑ J. M. has been brought to the family practice clinic by her mother. She has a patch on her left eye. She states something flew into her eye during school wood shop.
- ❑ C. N., age 55, provides the following information during the interview as part of an annual physical: Lights appear to have halos, a blind spot has been noticed, and she relates that she seems to have increased difficulty with night driving. She has no complaints of pain.
- ❑ M. N., a 68-year-old Floridian, has come to the health center with complaints of decreasing vision , especially in the right eye. Interview further reveals that she no longer drives at night because of the lights from other cars, and she now obtains large print books from the library in order to have something to read.
- ❑ A. W. has come to the Emergency Department with complaints of a sudden onset of loss of vision in the left eye. He was playing racquetball at the time the loss of vision occurred.
- ❑ The health practitioner is examining the eyes of M. H., a type II diabetic. Visualization of the retina reveals thickened capillary walls, microaneurysms, and tortuous veins.

WEB SITES OF INTEREST

American Foundation for the Blind- ***www.afb.org***

Eye Bank Association of America- ***www.restoresight.org***

PERFORMANCE CHECKLIST

EYES

	Yes	No	Comments
Wash hands			
Obtain relevant history			
Provide privacy			
Position the client			
Test visual acuity			
Test visual fields			
Inspect extraocular muscle function			
Corneal light reflex (Hirschberg test)			
Cover test			
Diagnostic positions test (six cardinal positions of gaze)			
Inspect external eye structures			
Eyebrows			
Eyelids and lashes			
Eyeballs			
Conjunctiva and sclera			
Eversion of the upper lid			
Lacrimal apparatus			
Inspect anterior structure of the eye			
Cornea and lens			
Iris and pupil			
Pupillary light reflex			
Accommodation			
Inspect the ocular fundus			
Optic disc			
Retinal vessels			
General background			
Macula			

(Continued)

PERFORMANCE CHECKLIST

EYES (cont'd)

	Yes	No	Comments
Special considerations			
Transcultural			
Developmental			
Document findings			

Chapter 13

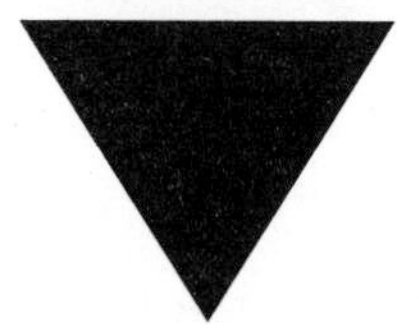

Ears

ANNOTATED LEARNING OBJECTIVES

At the completion of this chapter the student will:

List the anatomic landmarks of the external ear.

The external ear, called the auricle or pinna, has six anatomic landmarks: the helix, antihelix, external auditory meatus, tragus, antitragus, and lobule. The landmarks are used as reference points when documenting findings. (See text for photograph).

Describe the tympanic membrane and its anatomic landmarks.

The tympanic membrane, or eardrum, separates the external and middle ear. It is translucent with a pearly gray color. On inspection with an otoscope, a prominent cone of light is visible—a reflection of the otoscope light. The malleus pulls at the center of the ear, causing it to appear oval and slightly concave. The umbo, almost in the center, the most depressed point, is the location of the attachment of the first ossicle; the pars flaccid is the small, slack, superior section of the membrane, and the remainder of the drum, which is thicker and more taut, is the pars tensa. The thickened border is referred to as the annulus.

List the functions of the middle ear.

The middle ear conducts sound vibrations from the outer ear to the central hearing apparatus in the inner ear and protects the inner ear by reducing the amplitude of loud sounds. The eustachian tube allows equalization of air pressure on each side of the tympanic membrane.

State the functions of the inner ear that can be assessed.

The ear transmits sound and converts its vibrations into electrical impulses, which can be analyzed by the brain. The inner ear contains the bony labyrinths, which hold the sensory organs for equilibrium and hearing. Although the inner ear is not accessible to direct examination, its function can be assessed.

Differentiate among the types of hearing loss.

Anything that obstructs the transmission of sound impairs hearing. Hearing loss may be conductive, sensorineural, or mixed. Conductive hearing loss involves a mechanical dysfunction of the external or middle ear. If the sound amplitude is increased enough, the person is able to hear. Cerumen and otosclerosis are two possible causes of this type of hearing loss. Sensorineural or perceptive hearing loss indicates pathology of cranial nerve VIII. Presbycusis, a gradual degeneration of the nerve, may be the cause. When hearing loss is the result of both conductive and sensorineural causes, the loss is referred to as mixed.

Relate the anatomic developmental differences that alter hearing.

In the infant, the eustachian tube is relatively shorter and wider and is in a more horizontal position than it is in an adult. This allows pathogens to migrate to the middle ear from the nasopharynx. In addition, the lumen, surrounded by lymphoid tissue, is easily occluded. Otosclerosis is a common conductive hearing loss in young adults between ages 20 and 40 years. Hearing acuity may be decreased in the elderly because of coarse and stiff cilia lining the ear, impacted cerumen, and nerve degeneration in the inner ear.

KEY TERMS

Otosclerosis
Cerumen
Presbycusis
Otalgia
Tinnitus

TEACHING STRATEGIES

- Demonstrate the use of the otoscope.
- Discuss relevant infection control practices.
- Assign students to work in groups of three: one to follow the checklist and textbook, one to perform the examination, and one to act as client. Allow sufficient time for students to rotate roles so that each has an opportunity to be the examiner.
- Assist students with the positioning of the otoscope in the client's ear.
- Discuss examination modifications needed for clients at various developmental stages.
- Instruct students to document the results of the above examination.
- Encourage students to practice using the otoscope on friends and family members.
- If students from various ethnic groups are in the class, encourage students to examine one another's ears to learn the variations in cerumen that may occur among individuals.
- Assign students to list intrauterine exposures that may affect hearing.
- Discuss clues to hearing loss in individuals of varying ages.
- Assign students to prepare teaching materials that identify environmental factors that may cause hearing loss and devices used to decrease the risk, if available.

CRITICAL THINKING EXERCISES

Application to Clinical Practice

For each individual described in the situations below, have students discuss the developmental, age, socioeconomic, and transcultural considerations that should be considered during the gathering of subjective and objective data and the provision of health care.

In addition, have students identify additional information required and examinations that should be carried out before a judgment/diagnosis can be made and identify at least one relevant nursing diagnosis for any actual or potential problem identified.

- ❑ C. D., age 14, has come to the school health office complaining of pain in his left ear. Vital signs are T 99°F, P 64, R 16, BP 110/74. Review of his records indicates that he is on the swim team.
- ❑ B. B. is in for a routine health examination. History elicits complaints of tinnitus and an increase in the use of aspirin because of joint pain.
- ❑ A. G., age 79, complains of a rather recent decrease in the ability to hear.
- ❑ B. F. has been brought to the Emergency Department following a bicycle accident. B. F. was not wearing a helmet. Examination of the ear reveals clear watery drainage that tests positive for glucose.
- ❑ During a routine health visit, the provider notes that the pinna of the ears of M. J., age 2, are not in alignment with an imaginary line extending from the corner of the eye, and that the vertical angle is greater than 10°.
- ❑ M. A.'s mother has brought him to the clinic because he has been fussy all night. Examination reveals the pinna and tragus are painful to the touch, and redness and swelling of the canal with purulent discharge is noted.

WEB SITES OF INTEREST

American Speech-Language-Hearing Association- ***www.asha.org***

Deafness Research Foundation- ***www.drf.org***

Meniere's Network of the Ear Foundation- ***www.hearfound.org***

Self-Help for Hard of Hearing People- ***www.shhh.org***

PERFORMANCE CHECKLIST

EARS

	Yes	No	Comments
Obtain relevant history			
Gather equipment			
Provide privacy			
Wash hands			
External ear			
Inspect:			
Size and shape			
Skin condition			
External auditory meatus			
Palpate:			
Pinna			
Tragus			
Mastoid process			
Otoscopic examination			
External canal			
Tympanic membrane			
Color			
Characteristics			
Position			
Integrity of membrane			
Hearing acuity			
Voice test			
Rinne			
Weber			
Special considerations			
Developmental			
Transcultural			
Document findings			

Chapter 14

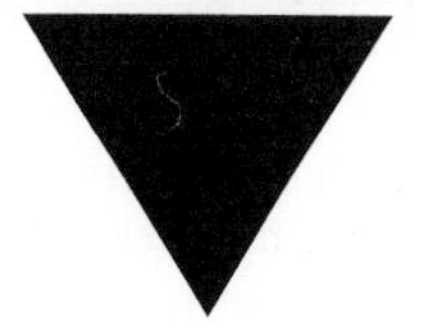

Nose, Mouth, and Throat

ANNOTATED LEARNING OBJECTIVES

At the completion of this chapter the student will:

Name the functions of the nose.

The nose, the first segment of the respiratory system, warms, moistens, and filters inhaled air. It is also the sensory organ of smell, innervated by cranial nerve I.

List the anatomic landmarks of the external nose.

The external nose, shaped like a triangle, consists of: the bridge or superior part; the free corner or the tip; the openings at the base of the triangle, the nares; and (inside the nares) a vestibule, the columella that divides the two nares and is continuous inside with the nasal septum; and the ala, the lateral outside wing of the nose on each side.

Describe the nasal cavity.

The nasal cavity extends back over the roof of the mouth. The anterior edge is lined with coarse nasal hairs that filter the coarsest matter from inhaled air. The remainder of the cavity is lined with ciliated mucous membrane that filters out dust and bacteria. Because of its rich blood supply, the nasal mucosa appears redder than the oral mucosa. The increased blood supply warms inhaled air. Kiesselbach's plexus is located in the anterior part of the septum, which divides the nasal cavity into two air passages. Kiesselbach plexus is the most common site of nosebleeds. The superior, middle, and inferior turbinates increase the surface area of the nose so that more blood vessels and mucous membrane are available to warm, humidify, and filter the inhaled air. Under each turbinate is a cleft, the meatus, named for the turbinate above. The sinuses drain into the middle meatus and tears from the nasolacrimal duct drain into the inferior meatus.

Name the paranasal sinuses and their functions.

There are four pairs of sinuses, two of which are accessible to examination—the frontal and maxillary sinuses. The ethmoid and sphenoid sinuses are not accessible to examination. The sinuses lighten the weight of the skull bones, serve as resonators for sound production, and provide mucus.

Identify the structures of the oral cavity.

The lips, insides of both cheeks, the roof of the mouth or palate, the mandible, and maxilla form the oral cavity. The teeth, both sets, begin development in utero. Children have 20 deciduous, or temporary teeth. All 20 should appear by 2 _ years of age. An adult mouth has 32 teeth, the tongue, gums, and openings for three pairs of salivary glands, (parotid, submandibular, and sublingual) and the uvula. The palatine tonsils are in the posterior end of the oral cavity, the lingual tonsils are at the base of the tongue bilaterally and the pharyngeal tonsils (adenoids) are in the posterior nasopharynx.

List the functions of the mouth.

The mouth is the first segment of the digestive system and an airway for the respiratory system. In addition, the mouth contains taste buds and aids in speech production.

Identify the effects of some of the age-related changes that take place in the mouth.

Nasal stuffiness and epistaxis may occur during pregnancy. Also, the gums may be hyperemic and softened. Loss of subcutaneous fats makes the nose appear more prominent in some people. A decrease in smell may diminish after age 60 because of a decrease in the number of olfactory nerve fibers. Tooth loss causes a series of difficulties including temporomandibular joint pain and osteoarthritis. A decrease in the sensation of smell and taste may affect appetite and contribute to malnutrition. The problems created by tooth loss may also cause the older person to eat soft foods, high in carbohydrates, and to decrease meat and fresh vegetable intake, adding to the risk of malnutrition.

KEY TERMS

Fetid
Caries
Malocclusion
Dysphagia
Xerostomia
Halitosis
Rhinitis
Leukoplakia

TEACHING STRATEGIES

- ▼ Demonstrate the use of the otoscope and the nasal speculum to examine the nose.
- ▼ Discuss relevant infection control practices.
- ▼ Assign students to work in groups of three: one to follow the checklist and textbook, one to perform the examination, and one to act as client. Allow sufficient time for students to rotate roles so each has an opportunity to be the examiner.
- ▼ Instruct students to document the results of the above examination.
- ▼ Ask students to share unusual observations with peers.
- ▼ Discuss effective approaches to the examination of an infant, toddler, and child.
- ▼ Encourage students to practice doing examinations on friends and family members.
- ▼ Discuss with students potential barriers to completing a thorough examination of the nose, mouth, and throat and ways of overcoming those barriers.
- ▼ Assign students to prepare teaching materials that address care of the teeth and mouth.

CRITICAL THINKING EXERCISES

Application to Clinical Practice

For each individual described in the situations below, have students discuss the developmental, age, socioeconomic, and transcultural considerations that should be considered during the gathering of subjective and objective data and the provision of health care.

In addition, have students relate expected (normal) findings to those described, discuss any additional information that might be needed before a judgment/diagnosis can be made and identify at least one relevant nursing diagnosis for any actual or potential problem identified.

- ❑ P. M. has come to the local health center complaining of a lesion in the left cheek that has not healed. He states that he has been aware of the lesion for 6 weeks. Interview reveals the use of chewing tobacco.
- ❑ C. M., age 3, has been brought to the clinic by her mother. She has been refusing to eat. Examination of the mouth reveals inflammation of the gums with bleeding and multiple caries in the teeth. The child's breath is fetid.
- ❑ C. N. has come into the Emergency Department complaining of a nose bleed that has persisted for 1 hour. History includes the use of high doses of ibuprofen for arthritis.
- ❑ M. D. has come to the family health practitioner complaining of the inability to breathe through her nose for 2 weeks. History includes seasonal allergies. Upon questioning, she reveals that she has been frequently using nose drops because of her allergies.
- ❑ F. N. , age 55, is at the clinic for an annual physical. Examination of the mouth reveals white plaque in the mouth that cannot be wiped off. F. N. is known to be a pipe smoker.
- ❑ C. R. has been brought to the Emergency Department by ambulance. His friends state he was mugged. His face is bruised, bloody, and appears asymmetrical.

WEB SITES OF INTEREST

American Thyroid Association-Montefore Medical Center-
www.thyroid.org

American Cancer Society- ***www.cancer.org***

Cancer Information Hotline-
www.cdc.gov/nccdphp/osh/tobacco.htm

Voice Center- ***www.voice-center.com/laryngectomy.html***

Speaking after a laryngectomy-
www.ama-assn.org/sci-pubs/journals/archive/otol/vol_123/no_5/oa6363.htm

PERFORMANCE CHECKLIST

NOSE, MOUTH, AND THROAT

	Yes	No	Comments
Obtain relevant history			
Gather equipment			
Provide privacy			
Wash hands			
Inspect the nose for symmetry, deformity, lesions and patency			
External nose			
Nasal cavity; use speculum for:			
Color			
Integrity			
Septum			
Deviation			
Perforation			
Bleeding			
Turbinates			
Color			
Exudate			
Swelling			
Polyps			
Palpate the external nose			
The sinus area			
Palpate			
Perform transillumination			
The mouth			
Inspect:			
Lips			
Teeth			
Gums			

(Continued)

PERFORMANCE CHECKLIST

NOSE, MOUTH, AND THROAT (cont'd)

	Yes	No	Comments
Tongue			
Buccal mucosa			
Palpate the palate			
Observe the uvula			
The throat			
Inspect and grade tonsils			
Special Consideration			
Transcultural			
Developmental			
Document findings			

Chapter 15

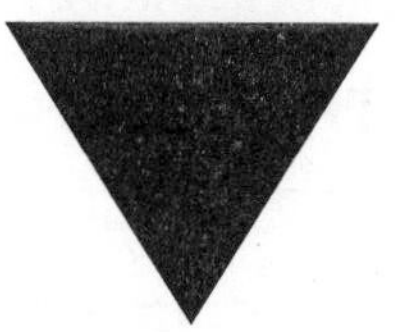

Breasts and Regional Lymphatics

ANNOTATED LEARNING OBJECTIVES

At the completion of this chapter the student will:

Identify significant breast anatomy.

The breasts (paired mammary glands) are located between the second and sixth ribs and lie anterior to the pectoralis major and serratus anterior muscles. They extend from the sternal margin to the midaxillary line. The nipple is just below the center of the breast and is surrounded by the areola for a 1- to 2-cm radius. Montgomery's glands in the areola secrete a protective lipid material during lactation. The tail of Spence projects up and laterally into the axilla. The breast is composed of glandular, fibrous, and adipose tissue.

Describe the composition of breast glandular tissue.

The glandular tissue of the breast contains 15 to 20 lobes radiating from the nipple. Each lobe is composed of 20 to 40 lobules that contain the alveoli (acini cells) that produce milk. Each lobe empties into a lactiferous duct that carries milk to the lactiferous sinuses or ampullae. These serve as reservoirs for storing milk behind the nipple.

Relate the changes that occur in Cooper's ligaments with cancer.

Cooper's ligaments become contracted in cancer, producing pits or dimples in the overlying skin.

Describe the ways of documenting clinical findings from a breast examination.

For purposes of documenting findings, the breast may be divided into four quadrants with imaginary horizontal and vertical lines that intersect at the nipple. The quadrants are referred to as upper inner quadrant, upper outer quadrant, lower outer quadrant, and lower inner quadrant. Findings may also be described according to a clock and centimeters from the nipple. Note that the tail of Spence, which projects into the axilla, is the most frequent site of breast tumors.

Relate the anatomy of the breast lymphatic system.

Four groups of axillary nodes drain 75 percent of the lymph from the breast. The groups are: the central axillary nodes, high in the middle of the axilla; the pectoral nodes, along the lateral edge of the pectoralis major muscle; the subscapular, along the lateral edge of the scapula and the lateral nodes; along the humerus, inside the upper arm. A small amount of lymph flows up to the infraclavicular group, into the chest or abdomen or across to the opposite breast.

Review breast development in the adolescent female.

Estrogen hormones stimulate breast changes that occur between the ages of 8 and 9 years for African-Americans and 10 years for Caucasians. At this time the breasts enlarge, mostly due to extensive fat deposition. The duct system also grows and branches, and masses of small, solid cells develop at the duct endings, the potential alveoli. Tenderness is common. The reader is referred to the five stages of breast development presented in the text.

Review breast changes that occur during pregnancy.

An early sign of pregnancy for most women are breast changes that begin during the second month. Pregnancy stimulates the expansion of the ductal system and supporting fatty tissue as well as development of the true secretory alveoli. The breasts enlarge and feel more nodular; the nipples are larger, darker, and more erectile. The areolae enlarge and become a darker brown, the tubercles become more prominent. A venous pattern is prominent over the skin surface. Colostrum may be expressed after the fourth month.

KEY TERMS

Colostrum

Cooper's ligaments

Lactiferous

Tail of Spence

Montgomery's glands

TEACHING STRATEGIES

- Discuss relevant infection control practices.
- Give students a picture of a breast and have each sketch the position of the lymphatics and the direction of lymph flow.
- Arrange students in a U shape so that each student is within the instructor's line of vision. Supply a breast mannequin for each one or two students. While students perform an examination on the mannequins, observe for technique.
- Discuss the importance of examining the male breast and ways of creating an environment that will provide psychological comfort for both client and practitioner.
- Assign students to work in groups of three: one to follow the checklist and textbook, one to perform the examination, and one to act as client. Allow sufficient time for students to rotate roles so that each has an opportunity to be the examiner.
- Instruct students to document the results of the above examination using appropriate descriptions for the location of any unusual findings.
- Assign students to complete a breast examination on a client in the clinical area.
- Assign students to prepare or obtain teaching materials for breast self examination.
- Have the students search the Internet for community resources related to the breast. Using these resources, assign students to design and instruct a client or group of clients on breast self examination.
- Have students document the results of the breast examination on the client and, if applicable, the teaching provided.
- Assign students to clients of different ethnic groups. Have the students interview the clients for barriers to breast self examination.

CRITICAL THINKING EXERCISES

Application to Clinical Practice

For each individual described in the situations below, have students discuss the developmental, age, socioeconomic, and transcultural considerations that should be considered during the gathering of subjective and objective data and the provision of health care.

In addition, have students relate expected (normal) findings to those described, discuss any additional information that might be needed before a judgment/diagnosis can be made, and identify at least one relevant nursing diagnosis for any actual or potential problem identified.

- ❑ M. H. has come to the family practice clinic where she informs the care provider that she realized she was changing her position during sleep because of pain in her left breast. Self examination revealed a nodule at 2 o'clock at the edge of the areola. Her last mammogram was 1 year ago, which was reported as negative.
- ❑ C. K. has come in because she felt a large lump in the lower, outer quadrant of her right breast yesterday when doing her monthly breast examination. The area in question is surrounded by ecchymosis, and C. K states that she takes one aspirin a day per physician direction. She does not recall any trauma to her breast.
- ❑ During a routine examination, the health care provider notes what initially appears to be a mole on the chest wall below the right breast. Further examination reveals that it is a tiny nipple and areola.

- ❑ C. W., a 15-year-old male, high school student, has come to the family doctor for a school health physical. During the examination, breast enlargement is noted, and a smooth, firm, movable disc is felt in the area of the breast.
- ❑ K. D. has just raised both arms above her head during a breast examination. The practitioner notes retraction of the left breast in the area of the tail of Spence.
- ❑ T. W. has come for a yearly gynecologic examination. Breast examination reveals engorgement, tenderness to palpation, and a feeling of nodularity. The lobes feel prominent and their margins are distinct. A firm ridge is felt in the lower quadrants.
- ❑ B. H., 3 months postpartum, calls the family care provider complaining of an elevated temperature, and a red, swollen, tender right breast. She also complains of headache and malaise.

WEB SITES OF INTEREST

American Cancer Society- ***www.cancer.org***

Oncology Nursing Society- ***www.ons.org***

Breast Cancer Information Clearing House- ***http://hysemet.org/bcic***

National Cancer Institute- ***www.nih.gov/nci***

NCI's Cancer Net- ***www.nci.nih.gov***

Breastfeeding Task Force of Greater Los Angeles- ***www.breastfeedingtaskforla.org/***

PERFORMANCE CHECKLIST

BREASTS AND REGIONAL LYMPHATICS

	Yes	No	Comments
Provide privacy			
Obtain history relevant for life stage			
Complete breast cancer risk assessment, if indicated			
Wash hands			
Position client			
Inspect:			
General appearance of breasts			
Symmetry			
Skin			
Lymphatic drainage areas			
Nipples			
Areola			
Axilla			
Complete maneuvers to screen for retraction			
Palpate:			
Axillae			
Breast—all 4 quadrants			
Document findings			
Provide lifestage-appropriate health teaching, including demonstration/review of breast self exam			
Discuss approaches for examining the male breast			

Chapter 16

Thorax and Lungs

ANNOTATED LEARNING OBJECTIVES

At the completion of this chapter the student will:

Name the components of the thoracic cage.

The thoracic cage consists of the sternum, 12 pairs of ribs, 12 thoracic vertebrae, and the diaphragm, which forms the "floor." Further detail is found in the text.

Describe the surface landmarks on the thorax.

The surface landmarks on the thorax are the suprasternal notch, a U-shaped depression just above the sternum; the sternum or breastbone with three parts: the manubrium, the body, and the xiphoid process; the manubriosternal angle or angle of Louis, the bony ridge felt a few centimeters down the manubrium and continuous with the second rib; the costal angle, formed where the right and left costal margins form an angle at the xiphoid process; vertebral prominences; inferior border of the scapula, usually at the seventh or eighth rib; the twelfth rib, palpated midway between the spine and the side; and reference lines—midsternal, midclavicular, midspinal, vertebral, scapular, anterior axillary, posterior axillary, and midaxillary.

List the contents of the mediastinum.

The mediastinum is the middle section of the thoracic cavity. The esophagus, trachea, heart, and great vessels occupy the mediastinum.

Describe the borders of the lung.

The apex of the lung lies 3 or 4 cm above the inner third of the clavicles, the base rests on the diaphragm at about the fifth intercostal space in the right midclavicular line and at the sixth rib, midclavicular line on the left. Laterally, the lung extends from the apex of the axilla to the seventh or eighth rib and posteriorly, C7 marks the apex, and T10 usually corresponds to the base. On deep inspiration, the lungs expand their lower border to the level of T12.

Describe the anatomic demarcation of the five lobes of the lungs.

The lung is divided into the upper and lower lobes by the right and left oblique fissures. A line drawn from T3 to the fifth rib at the mid axillary line and continued to the sixth rib identifies the oblique fissure. On the right, a second line, the horizontal fissure, from the 5th rib midaxillary line to the right sternal border at the level of the 4th rib outlines the fissure of the third lobe on the right side.

Describe the pleura and its function.

The pleura is a serous membrane investing the lung and lining the walls of the thoracic cavity. The pleura has a vacuum, negative pressure that holds the lungs tightly against the chest, and its lubricating fluid allows the lungs to move without friction during respiration.

List the structures that comprise the respiratory dead space.

The respiratory dead space consists of the airways of the mouth, nose, pharynx, larynx, trachea, bronchi, and bronchioles. This space holds about 150 ml in an adult.

Discuss the location and functions of the trachea and bronchial tree.

The trachea, 10 to 11 cm long and 2.5 cm in diameter, lies anterior to the esophagus. Anteriorly it begins at the level of the cricoid cartilage in the neck and bifurcates just below the sternal angle. Posteriorly, the tracheal bifurcation is at the level of T4 or T5. The right bronchus is shorter, wider, and more vertical than the left. The bronchial tree protects the alveoli from small particulate matter with mucous, secreted by the goblet cells and the cilia, which sweep particles upward to where they can be swallowed or expelled. The functional unit of the respiratory tract is the acinus.

Summarize the mechanics of respiration.

The lungs supply oxygen to the blood and eliminate excess carbon dioxide through inspiration, an increase in the size of the thoracic cavity that creates a negative pressure, and expiration, a primarily passive act.

Discuss developmental considerations associated with the thoracic cavity.

The primitive lung buds emerge during the first 5 weeks of fetal life. By 16 weeks, the conducting airways reach the same number as in the adult. Surfactant is present in adequate amount by 32 weeks. Although developed in utero, the respiratory system does not function until birth. Respiratory development continues throughout childhood and reaches adult size by adolescence.

The enlarging uterus elevates the diaphragm 4 cm during pregnancy. The vertical diameter decreases, but this decrease is compensated for by an increase in horizontal diameter. The growing fetus creates increased oxygen demands on the mother's body. This is met by increasing the tidal volume.

In the elderly, the costal cartilages become calcified. The respiratory muscle strength declines after age 50 and continues to decrease into the 70s. The elastic properties within the lungs decrease, making them less distensible and lessening their tendency to collapse and recoil. These changes lead to a decrease in vital capacity and an increase in residual volume. With aging, there is a gradual loss of intraalveolar septa and a decreased number of alveoli.

KEY TERMS

Fissure
Angle of Louis
Dead space
Hypercapnia
Hypoxemia
Dyspnea
Eupnea
Tachypnea
Bradypnea
Vital capacity

TEACHING STRATEGIES

- Have students play "password" with the names of the thoracic landmarks. These terms need to be committed to memory in order to clearly communicate findings either verbally or in writing.
- Obtain a diagram of the thorax and have students label the structures and anatomic landmarks, or have students draw a sketch of the thorax and label appropriately.
- Have each student locate and name each of the surface landmarks on the thorax.
- Assign students to listen to audio tapes of normal and abnormal respiratory sounds.
- Discuss the clinical significance of the posterior chest consisting of almost all lower lobe.
- Discuss the clinical significance of hypercapnia as the normal respiratory drive.
- Discuss the significance of the difference in structure between the right and left main bronchus.
- Obtain styrofoam cups with lids. Fill one with water or dirt and leave the other empty. Have students practice hearing the difference in percussion notes with these. The sounds will be exaggerated, but it is a useful beginning.
- Assign students to work in groups of three: one to follow the checklist and textbook, one to perform the examination, and one to act as client. Allow sufficient time for students to rotate roles so that each has an opportunity to be the examiner.

- Observe students and assist them with correct percussion and palpation technique and the proper use of the stethoscope.
- Instruct students to document the results of the above exam using appropriate descriptions for the location of any unusual findings.
- Assign students to complete a respiratory assessment on a client in the clinical area.
- Have students document the results of the respiratory assessment completed on a client.

CRITICAL THINKING EXERCISES

Application to Clinical Practice

For each individual described in the situations below, have students discuss the developmental, age, socioeconomic, and transcultural considerations that should be considered during the gathering of subjective and objective data and the provision of health care.

In addition, have students relate expected (normal) findings to those described, discuss any additional information that might be needed before a judgment/diagnosis can be made, and identify at least one relevant nursing diagnosis for any actual or potential problem identified.

- ❑ N. C. has been suffering from a cold. This morning she is complaining of dyspnea, and wheezes are heard bilaterally. Cough is productive; sputum is thick and green in color.
- ❑ T. W. has just returned from a visit to her sister. She has come to the health center complaining of having red, itchy eyes. She is wheezing and having difficulty breathing. Interview reveals that her sister had acquired a kitten prior to the visit. T. W has no pets in her home.
- ❑ M. D. has come to the health center with an acute upper respiratory infection. Wheezes are heard in both lower lobes but decrease after cough. His health record indicates that he is a one-pack-a-day cigarette smoker.
- ❑ M. O., a Mexican migrant farm worker, has come to the health center complaining of flu-like symptoms, including cough and some shortness of breath that have persisted for 3 weeks.
- ❑ S. C. is recovering from a cholecystectomy. The nurse giving report indicates that he was not receiving good pain relief with the medications prescribed. During the A.M. assessment, the nurse notes rales in both lower lobes.
- ❑ P. W. has come to the health care center complaining of night sweats, a recent weight loss, and a decrease in energy level. Sputum is blood tinged.
- ❑ During a routine examination on M. C., a school age child, the right shoulder is noted to be higher than the left, the hips are at unequal levels, the rib interspaces are flared on the right side and vertebrae are not straight when the individual bends from the waist.
- ❑ E. R. has come to the health center complaining of a productive cough with bloody sputum and shortness of breath. A unilateral wheeze is heard on auscultation.
- ❑ S. B. has come for his first physical in several years. History includes the use of 1–2 packs of cigarettes a day for 20 years. Examination reveals increased AP diameter, decreased tactile fremitus, hyperresonance on percussion, and decreased breath sounds.
- ❑ D. D., a newborn, is being examined in the newborn nursery. The nurse notes that he breathes through the nose, his chest is barrel shaped and respiratory rate is 46. Bronchovesicular breath sounds are heard in the peripheral lung fields.

WEB SITES OF INTEREST

American Thoracic Society Nursing Assembly- ***www.thoracic.org/nur***

American Lung Association- ***www.lungusa.org***

Cystic Fibrosis Foundation- ***www.cff.org***

PERFORMANCE CHECKLIST

THORAX AND LUNGS

	Yes	No	Comments
Obtain history			
Gather equipment			
Provide privacy			
Position appropriately for area to be examined			
Ensure a quiet environment			
Wash hands			
Explain procedure to client			
Use stethoscope appropriately			
Identify landmarks			
Suprasternal notch			
Angle of Louis			
2nd rib			
C7			
T1			
Location of lung fields			
Follow a logical sequence			
Inspect posterior and anterior chest for:			
Shape and configuration			
Symmetry			
Anteroposterior ratio			
Placement of scapulae			
Angle of ribs			
Neck & trapezius muscles			
Quality of respirations			
Observe:			
Position for breathing			
Skin color and condition			

(Continued)

PERFORMANCE CHECKLIST

THORAX AND LUNGS (cont'd)

	Yes	No	Comments
Facial expression			
Level of consciousness			
Palpate:			
Entire chest wall			
Posterior and anterior chest for:			
Symmetric chest expansion			
Tactile fremitus			
Percuss posterior and anterior chest			
Determine predominant note over lung fields			
Determine diaphragmatic excursion			
Auscultate posterior and anterior chest			
Systematically evaluate presence and quality of:			
Breath sounds			
Normal			
Adventitious			
Voice sounds			
Measure forced expiratory time			
Document findings			
Hair distribution			
Venous pattern			

Chapter 17

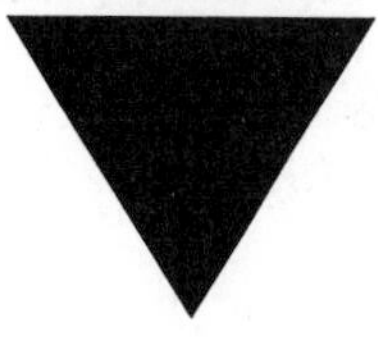

Heart and Neck Vessels

ANNOTATED LEARNING OBJECTIVES

At the completion of this chapter the student will:

Relate anatomic structures to the correct landmark/ anatomic location.

Structure	Location
Apex	5th I C space, MCL
Right atrium	to the right and above the right ventricle
	anterior cardiac surface
	right cardiac border
Left ventricle	behind the right ventricle
	left cardiac border
Left atrium	behind the right atrium
Great vessels	base of the heart
Superior and inferior	
Vena cava	
Pulmonary artery	
Aorta	

List the significant anatomic features of the heart.

The significant anatomic features of the heart are as follows: the pericardium, pericardial fluid, myocardium, endocardium, right and left atria, right and left ventricles, valves, and chordae tendineae.

Relate the name of the heart sound to the physiologic cause.

Sound	Cause
S1	closure of the tricuspid and mitral valves
S2	closure of the aortic and pulmonic valves
M1	closure of the mitral valve
T1	closure of the tricuspid valve
A2	closure of the aortic valve
P2	closure of the pulmonic valve
S3	vibration of the ventricles that resist early, rapid filling
S4	vibration of the ventricles that resist forceful filling

State why two distinct components to each heart sound exist.

Two distinct components to each heart sound exist because cardiac depolarization occurs slightly later on the right side of the heart than on the left side.

List three conditions that result in cardiac murmurs.

The three conditions that cause cardiac murmurs are an increase in the velocity of blood flow, a decrease in the viscosity of blood, and structural defects in the valves or unusual openings in the chambers.

Describe the characteristics of heart sounds.

Heart sounds are described by frequency, intensity, duration, and timing. See text for definitions.

Summarize the spread of the cardiac impulse through the heart.

The cardiac impulse originates in the S-A node and spreads through the atria and to the A-V node where it is delayed. The impulse travels to the bundle of His, the right and left bundle branches and then to the ventricles.

Relate the components of the jugular pulse to the cardiac events that are reflected.

The **a** wave reflects atrial contraction, the **c** wave reflects ventricular contraction, the **x** descent reflects atrial relaxation, the **v** wave reflects passive atrial filling, and the **y** descent reflects passive ventricular filling.

Describe the function of the foramen ovale and the ductus arteriosus.

The foramen ovale, an opening in the atrial septum, allows oxygenated blood from the placenta to be shunted to the left side of the heart and out to the general circulation. The ductus arteriosus, a shunt between the pulmonary artery and the aorta, allows any remaining blood being directed to the lungs to be shunted into the aorta.

Cite the risk factors associated with heart disease and stroke.

The major risk factors for heart disease and stroke are high blood pressure, smoking, high cholesterol levels, obesity, and diabetes.

KEY TERMS

Arrhythmia
Precordium
Mediastinum
Diastole
Systole
Murmur
Automaticity
Preload
Afterload
Bruit

TEACHING STRATEGIES

- Obtain a diagram of the heart and have students label the structures or have students draw a sketch of the heart and great vessels with labels.
- Using the above diagram, have students trace the flow of blood through the heart.
- This is another system with which the game of Challenge and Response can be played. Using the names of the anatomic structures as challenges, the responder must provide a brief description within 30 seconds.
- Challenge and Response may also be used to learn the various heart sounds and their physiologic causes.
- A game of jeopardy may be created. Divide students into two teams. Create a Jeopardy grid on transparencies. Give each team a bell. The instructor makes answers and questions for each number on the grid. The instructor reads the answer for the number requested by the students. The team wishing to provide the question rings the bell. For example: "For 100 points the answer is—carries unoxygenated blood to the lungs." Question. What is the pulmonary artery?
- A pneumonic that may help students remember which valve they are hearing is Ape To Man.

Aortic	2nd Intercostal Space, right sternal border
Pulmonic	2nd Intercostal Space, left sternal border
Erbs point	3rd Intercostal Space, left sternal border (aortic and pulmonic sounds)
Tricuspid	5th Intercostal Space, left sternal border
Midclavicle	5th Intercostal Space, left midclavicular line

- Another pneumonic to help remember which valves are on the left side of the heart is LAM—left aortic mitral.
- Assign students to listen to audio tapes of normal and abnormal heart sounds.
- Assign students to work in groups of three: one to follow the checklist and textbook, one to perform the examination, and one to act as client. Allow sufficient time for students to rotate roles so that each has an opportunity to be the examiner.

- ▼ Observe students and assist them with the proper use of the stethoscope, if necessary.
- ▼ Instruct students to document the results of the above examination using appropriate descriptions for the locations of any unusual findings.
- ▼ Assign students to complete a cardiac assessment on a client in the clinical area.
- ▼ Have students document the results of the cardiac assessment.

CRITICAL THINKING EXERCISES

Application to Clinical Practice

For each individual described in the situations below, have students discuss the developmental, age, socioeconomic, and transcultural considerations that should be considered during the gathering of subjective and objective data and the provision of health care.

In addition, have students relate expected (normal) findings to those described, discuss any additional information that might be needed before a judgment/diagnosis can be made, and identify at least one relevant nursing diagnosis for any actual or potential problem identified.

- ❑ J. J., aged 54, has come for a periodic health evaluation. He had an MI 1 year ago and is being treated with medication for hypertension. Interview reveals a change in his condition with the following symptoms: increase in number of pillows from two to four, decrease in activity tolerance, a dry, hacking cough, and a decrease in appetite.
- ❑ B. S has come to the family health care provider, at the insistence of his wife, because of recent episodes of epigastric discomfort that he believed to be indigestion. Interview elicits a relationship between exercise and a diffuse pain that sometimes radiates down the inner aspect of the left arm. The discomfort is relieved by rest.
- ❑ L. D., age 22 weeks, has been brought to the well-baby clinic for a periodic examination. Chart review indicates a normal growth and development pattern. Cardiac examination during this visit reveals a continuous grade ii murmur. A review of the prenatal health of the mother reveals an exacerbation of asthma with the use of prednisone to manage symptoms.
- ❑ S. D. was discharged yesterday after treatment for heart failure. She appears SOB when she answers the door for the home health nurse. The nurse also notes the following: rales unrelieved by coughing, +2 edema in both lower extremities, and a third heart sound.
- ❑ B. L., age 65, has come to the Emergency Department with complaints of increasing chest discomfort over the last few weeks, the worst episode happening this morning. History includes type I diabetes mellitus since age 7.
- ❑ L. R., age 70, returned to his home Friday following an extensive hospitalization for fractured ribs and adult respiratory distress syndrome. The injuries were incurred in a motor vehicle accident 6 weeks ago in another state. Although the air bag inflated on impact, the injuries were caused by the seat belt. On Monday, he visits his primary care provider complaining of SOB and dyspnea on exertion, which has gradually increased since his return home. Auscultation reveals diminished heart sounds over the entire precordium.
- ❑ M. J. has come for an evaluation following an episode of lightheadedness during a recent swimming session. Auscultation of the heart reveals a midsystolic click heard with the diaphragm at the apex of the heart. The click is high pitched and of short duration.
- ❑ A. C. has come for a monthly prenatal visit. While listening to her heart, the examiner notes an exaggerated splitting of S1, a loud, easily heard S3, and a grade ii systolic murmur. Other findings remain unchanged since the last visit.

WEB SITES OF INTEREST

NIH- National Heart, Lung, and Blood Institute (NHLBI)- ***www.nhlbi.nih.gov***

American Heart Association- ***www.americanheart.org***

American Heart Association Women's website- ***www.women.americanheart.org***

Heart Information Network- ***www.heartinfo.org***

Mended Hearts, Inc. ***www.mendedhearts.org***

PERFORMANCE CHECKLIST

HEART, LUNGS, AND BLOOD

	Yes	No	Comments
Obtain age-relevant history			
Determine presence of cardiac risk factors			
Gather equipment including light source			
Provide privacy			
Position appropriately for area to be examined			
Ensure a quiet environment			
Wash hands			
Explain procedure to client			
Use stethoscope appropriately			
Palpate:			
Carotid arteries			
Precordium			
Apical impulse			
Perform hepatojugular reflux			
Auscultate:			
Traditional listening areas and precordium using a Z pattern for:			
Rate			
Rhythm			
Identification of S1 and S2			
Assessment of S1			
Assessment of S2			
Extra heart sounds			
Murmurs			
Carotid arteries			
Determine apical rate			

(Continued)

PERFORMANCE CHECKLIST

HEART, LUNGS, AND BLOOD (cont'd)

	Yes	No	Comments
Inspect:			
Jugular venous pulse			
Estimate jugular venous pressure			
Precordium			
Percussion			
Determine borders of the heart			
Special considerations			
Transcultural			
Developmental			
Document findings			
The legs			
Inspect:			
Color			
Hair distribution			
Venous pattern			

Chapter 18

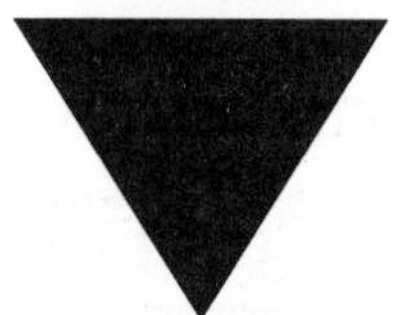

Peripheral Vascular System and Lymphatic System

ANNOTATED LEARNING OBJECTIVES

At the completion of this chapter the student will:

Relate the structure and functions of arteries and veins.

Arteries, which carry blood from the heart, are strong, tough, and tense, designed to withstand the pressure created with each heartbeat. Arteries contain elastic fibers that allow their walls to stretch with systole and recoil with diastole. Veins, which drain the deoxygenated blood and waste products from the tissues and return it to the heart, are thinner and more passive than the arteries. Veins contain intraluminal valves.

List the pulses accessible to examination.

The following arteries are accessible to examination: temporal, carotid, aorta, brachial, ulnar, radial, femoral, popliteal, dorsalis pedis, and posterior tibial.

Describe the mechanisms that keep blood moving toward the heart in the venous system.

Blood moves from the low-pressure system of the veins through the action of contracting skeletal muscles that milk the blood proximally back toward the heart, the pressure gradient caused by breathing, and the intraluminal valves that keep blood flowing in one direction.

Explain the term capacitance vessels.

Veins are called capacitance vessels because they are distensible and can therefore expand and hold more blood when blood volume increases. This compensatory mechanism reduces stress on the heart.

List the risk factors for venous stasis.

Standing, sitting, or bed rest contribute to the risk for venous stasis because of the absence of the milking action of walking. In addition individuals with hypercoagulable states and vein wall trauma are at risk. Varicose veins create incompetent valves that increase venous pressure. Obesity, pregnancy, and genetic predisposition are additional risk factors.

Relate the structure and functions of the lymph vessels.

The lymphatic system provides an axillary system for fluid to flow from interstitial spaces to the blood stream The lymphatic capillaries are permeable to substances of high molecular weight such as proteins. In addition, the lymphatic system forms a major part of the immune system and absorbs lipids from the intestinal tract. To achieve this special purpose, the lymphatic capillaries have a special structure; the endothelial cells are not connected to each other. The cells are attached by anchoring filaments to the connective tissue of the vessels, which start as microscopic open-ended tubes. The vessels have valves that cause them to appear as beads.

Describe the function of the lymph nodes.

Lymph nodes filter fluid before it is returned to the blood stream and filter out microorganisms that could be harmful to the body. The pathogens are exposed to lymphocytes in the lymph nodes, which mount an antigen-specific response to eliminate the pathogens. With local inflammation, the nodes in the affected area become swollen and tender.

Cite the location of superficial groups of lymph nodes that are accessible to examination.

The following four major groups of lymph nodes are accessible to inspection and palpation: the cervical nodes that drain the head and neck, the axillary nodes that drain the breast and upper arm, the epitrochlear node in the antecubital fossa, and the inguinal nodes in the groin.

Name the related organs and functions of the lymphatic system.

The spleen, located in the left upper quadrant of the abdomen, destroys old red blood cells, produces antibodies, stores red blood cells, and filters microorganisms from the blood. The tonsils (palatine, adenoid, and lingual), located at the entrance to the respiratory and gastrointestinal tracts, respond to local inflammation. The thymus, located behind the sternum in the mediastinum develops T-lymphocytes in the immune system in children but serves no function in adults.

KEY TERMS

Arteriosclerosis

Atherosclerosis

Homan's sign

Pulse

Ischemia

Varicose veins

TEACHING STRATEGIES

- ▼ Discuss relevant infection control practices.
- ▼ Have students come to lab in Tee shirts and running shorts or a bathing suit so all areas may be examined. Assign students to work in groups of three: one to follow the checklist and textbook, one to perform the examination, and one to act as client. Allow sufficient time for students to rotate roles so that each has an opportunity to be the examiner. Students frequently have difficulty palpating the pedal pulses, so be sure to verify the findings reported.
- ▼ At the end of the lab, give each student 1/2 of a piece of paper. Have each complete the following statement: At the next lab session, I would like additional help with the _________ part of this exam.
- ▼ Instruct students to document the results of the above examination, using appropriate descriptions for the location of any unusual findings.
- ▼ Assign students to complete a peripheral vascular examination on a client in the clinical area.
- ▼ Assign students to prepare or obtain teaching materials for individuals at risk for developing venous stasis.
- ▼ Assign students to instruct a client or group of clients on ways to decrease venous stasis.
- ▼ Encourage students to practice this assessment on their own bodies.

CRITICAL THINKING EXERCISES

Application to Clinical Practice

For each individual described in the situations below, have students discuss the developmental, age, socioeconomic, and transcultural considerations that should be considered during the gathering of subjective and objective data and the provision of health care.

In addition, have students relate expected (normal) findings to those described, discuss any additional information that might be needed before a judgment/diagnosis can be made, and identify at least one relevant nursing diagnosis for any actual or potential problem identified.

- ❑ A. M. has come to the health practitioner with complaints of leg wounds that have persisted for 4 weeks. A. M. works on a production line and is on his feet all day. On examination, the wounds are irregular with a bright red wound base and are not especially painful. There is moderate to heavy exudate and peripheral edema.
- ❑ H. G., age 45, has come to the health practitioner complaining of pain in both lower extremities. Visual examination reveals prominent, dilated veins in both lower extremities. She is a waitress.

- ❑ P. S. has come for a follow-up examination. She had a right mastectomy 6 weeks ago. Examination of the right arm reveals soft, pitting edema.
- ❑ E. A. has come to the health care provider with complaints of a sudden onset of pain in the left leg. Left distal pulses are absent, and the extremity is cold and pale.
- ❑ M. H. is recovering from a cholecystectomy. During the morning assessment, he complains of pain when the left knee is flexed and the left foot is plantar flexed. The calf circumference is 37 cm on the right and 40 cm on the left. The left calf is tender to palpation.
- ❑ B. D. has been referred to the home health agency for a painful wound on the dorsal aspect of the right foot. The wound is round, measuring 3 x 3 cm. The wound base is pale with well-defined edges; exudate is minimal.

WEB SITES OF INTEREST

AIDS Treatment Data Network- ***www.aidsnyc.org***

Allergy, Asthma, and Immunology Clinic- ***http://allergy.mcg.edu***

Center for Disease Control and Prevention- ***www.cdc.gov***

NIH- National Heart, Lung, and Blood Institute (NHLBI)- ***www.nhlbi.nih.gov***

PERFORMANCE CHECKLIST

PERIPHERAL VASCULAR SYSTEM AND LYMPHATIC SYSTEM

NOTE: While all of the examination may not be indicated for each client, have students practice all parts under supervision to increase confidence when the special maneuvers are needed.

	Yes	No	Comments
Obtain relevant history			
Provide privacy			
Wash hands			
Observe for symmetry			
Auscultate for bruit, when indicated			
The arms			
Inspect for:			
Color			
Temperature			
Texture			
Skin turgor			
Lesions			
Edema			
Clubbing			
Palpate:			
Capillary refill			
Upper extremity pulses			
Grade pulses			
Perform Allen's test			
The legs			
Inspect for:			
Color			
Hair distribution			
Venous pattern			

(Continued)

PERFORMANCE CHECKLIST

PERIPHERAL VASCULAR SYSTEM AND LYMPHATIC SYSTEM (cont'd)

	Yes	No	Comments
Size			
Swelling			
Atrophy			
Measure calf circumference			
Lesions			
Palpate:			
Temperature			
Inguinal lymph nodes			
Peripheral arteries			
Grade pulses			
Edema (grade if present)			
Perform:			
Manual compression test			
Test for Homan's sign			
Trendelenburg test			
Color change test			
Test for leg strength			
Doppler examination			
Ankle-Arm Index			
Special considerations			
Transcultural			
Developmental			
Document findings			

Chapter 19

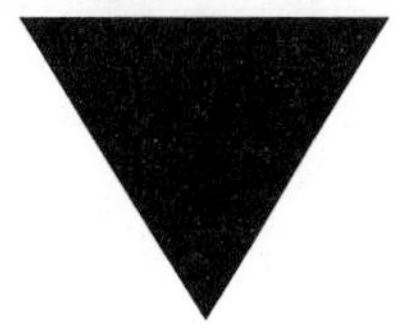

Abdomen

ANNOTATED LEARNING OBJECTIVES

At the completion of this chapter the student will:

Identify the organs located within each of the four abdominal quadrants.

The right upper quadrant contains the liver and gallbladder, the pyloric sphincter, the duodenum, the head of the pancreas, the right adrenal gland, a portion of the right kidney, the hepatic flexure of the colon, and portions of the ascending and transverse colon. The left upper quadrant contains the left lobe of the liver, the spleen, the stomach, the body of the pancreas, the left adrenal gland, a portion of the left kidney, the splenic flexure of the the colon, and portions of the transverse and descending colon. The right lower quadrant contains the lower pole of the right kidney, the cecum and appendix, a portion of the ascending colon, the right ureter, and the right ovary and fallopian tube, or right spermatic cord. The left lower quadrant contains the lower pole of the left kidney, the sigmoid colon, a portion of the descending colon, the left ureter, and the left ovary and fallopian tube or left spermatic cord. In addition, several structures lie in the midline: the abdominal aorta, the urinary bladder, and the uterus.

Identify pertinent topics that must be reviewed during the abdominal portion of the interview.

Subjective data obtained from the patient serves as a guide for the examiner in identifying actual or potential problems related to the gastrointestinal system. As the examiner gains experience, the depth of questioning will be based upon the prior responses of the patient. Topics that are of special relevance to the abdomen include nutrition and appetite, ability to chew and swallow foods, food intolerances or nausea and vomiting, and any pain associated with the abdomen. Questions to identify bowel habits and any laxatives used must be included. The interview must also obtain information regarding any present or past rectal problems and gastrointestinal problems. Because many medications are metabolized by the liver and/or have gastrointestinal side effects, a review of current medications is also indicated.

Employ measures that will enhance abdominal wall relaxation.

In order to accurately assess the abdomen, client relaxation is essential. The bladder must be empty, the room a comfortable temperature, the client comfortable with knees supported, arms at the sides, and good lighting and visualization of the entire abdomen available.

Employ the correct sequence of examining techniques.

The sequence for examining the abdomen is inspection, auscultation, percussion, and palpation. This is done because percussion and palpation can increase peristalsis and might give a false interpretation of bowel sounds.

Interpret findings obtained during inspection of the abdomen.

Contour, symmetry, shape of the umbilicus, condition of the skin on the abdomen, and presence of pulsations or movement all must be observed during inspection of the abdomen. The examiner must discriminate between normal and abnormal findings and use the information obtained through inspection as a basis for further exploration if indicated. The pattern of pubic hair growth and demeanor of the patient should be assessed with inspection.

Interpret findings obtained during auscultation of the abdomen.

Auscultation of the abdomen is an important nursing assessment, especially for postoperative clients. While the clicks of a normal bowel can occur anywhere from 5 to 30 times per minute, the nurse must listen for up to 5 minutes before deciding that bowel sounds are completely absent. In addition to bowel sounds, the examiner must note whether any vascular sounds or bruits are present.

Interpret findings obtained during percussion of the abdomen.

Knowledge of the location of various organs within the abdomen is especially important during percussion. This knowledge will assist the examiner in relating sounds heard to those expected from the organs in the region being percussed. Percussion reveals the relative density of the abdominal contents. Because of air in the intestines, tympany is the predominate sound. Dullness may be heard over a distended bladder, adipose tissue, fluid or a mass. A change in tone may be noted over the descending colon if there is a need for evacuation. A change from lung resonance to dullness will identify the borders of the liver, which ranges from 6 to 12 cm in width and, on some individuals, splenic dullness, which is 7 cm in width or less, may be noted between the 9th to 11th intercostal space behind the left midaxillary line.

Interpret findings obtained during palpation of the abdomen.

Light and deep palpation provide the examiner with the ability to distinguish between normal organs, enlarged organs, abnormal masses, and unusual sensations elicited.

KEY TERMS

Tympany
Bruit
Hernia
Viscera
Costovertebral angle
Epigastric region
Umbilical region
Hypogastric/suprapubic region
Pyrosis
Anorexia
Dysphagia
Anorexia nervosa
Purging

TEACHING STRATEGIES

- Obtain two styrofoam cups with lids. Fill one with water or sand. Leave the other empty. Have students percuss the tops of the two cups. Although the sounds are exaggerated, it will allow students to begin to differentiate between the sound heard over an air-filled organ and a solid organ.
- Using the photographs in the text as a guide, have students name the abdominal organs on a peer. This exercise may be done in groups of three, with students taking turns with each role. Student 1 is the client, student 2 follows the text, and student 3 acts as examiner.
- After all students feel knowledgeable with the text in view, have each locate and name each of the organs from memory.
- When students are knowledgeable regarding the anatomy and physiology of the abdomen, have students each complete an abdominal assessment using each other as patients.
- Have students practice using one hand, two hands (bimanual), and the hand of a client under their own for palpation.
- Have students document the results of the examination completed on a peer.
- At the completion of at least one complete abdominal examination, give students one half of a piece of paper and ask each to briefly describe the part(s) of the examination for which they most want to have additional practice. Discuss ways this can be achieved, such as on family members, classmates, additional patients in the clinical setting.
- Discuss normal and abnormal findings for an infant, a child, and an older adult.
- Assign students to complete an abdominal history and examination in the clinical setting.

- ▼ In the clinical setting, have students analyze the dietary history and abdominal assessment findings for an assigned client.
- ▼ Encourage students to practice on family members of various ages.

CRITICAL THINKING EXERCISES

Application to Clinical Practice

For each individual described in the situations below, have students discuss the age, socioeconomic, and transcultural considerations that should be considered during the gathering of subjective and objective data and the provision of health care. In addition, have students relate expected /normal findings to those described, discuss any additional information that might be needed before a judgment can be made, and identify at least one relevant nursing diagnosis for any actual or potential problem identified.

- ❑ M. S. has been coming to your health center for prenatal care. She is in the 24th week of gestation. During this visit, a weight loss of 5 pounds from the last visit of 1 month ago is noted. She states that she is having more difficulty with constipation, and "morning sickness" has not been totally resolved. Bowel sounds are diminished.
- ❑ A. Z., age 70, has come to the health center for follow-up care of type II diabetes, which seems to be well controlled. During the exam, A. Z. states that his wife died 3 months ago; he requests a prescription for sleep medication. Discuss the age-related changes in the gastrointestinal system that must be considered before an appropriate hypnotic can be prescribed.
- ❑ X. M. has come for a follow-up visit for contact dermatitis. While the dermatitis has responded well to the prescribed treatment, X. M. complains of constipation and asks your opinion regarding the use of Milk of Magnesia for this problem. Is this an appropriate solution for this concern? If not, describe additional information that must be obtained before the problem can be addressed.
- ❑ L. D., age 16, has come in for a high school sports physical. The practitioner notes a 15-pound weight loss since last year. Menses are absent.
- ❑ P. D. has brought her daughter, age 18 months, to the family health center for routine immunizations. She expresses concern stating that "she just picks at her food."
- ❑ A. N. is brought to the Emergency Department by family members. Patient is alert and oriented and states that he just vomited a large quantity of frank blood. History includes complaints of decreased appetite, back pain, and recent weight loss. He has a history of fractured vertebrae 5 years ago, and use of two packs of cigarettes a day for 20 years. He is a welder by occupation. Past history also includes colon resection 18 months ago for cancer.
- ❑ M. M. has come to the health clinic complaining of fatigue, anorexia, and recent weight loss. He states that he completed an alcohol rehabilitation program 4 years ago after 35 years of alcohol abuse. Upon examination, sclera appear jaundiced.
- ❑ B. D. has just returned to the medical/surgical unit following a gastric resection. A nasogastric tube and an IV are in place. The patient is complaining of pain in the incisional area. Morphine sulfate is ordered for pain, and it has been within the prescribed time since the patient was last medicated.

WEB SITES OF INTEREST

American Liver Foundation- Hepatitis Hotline- ***www.liverfoundation.org***

Crohn's and Colitis Foundation of America- ***www.ccfa.org***

Healthy Weight- ***www.healthyweight.com***

National Institute of Diabetes and Digestive and Kidney Disease- ***www.niddk.nih.gov***

PERFORMANCE CHECKLIST

ABDOMEN—Essential Behaviors

	Yes	No	Comments
Wash hands			
Provide privacy			
Explain procedure to client			
Use a systematic approach			
Obtain or review history			
Obtain proper lighting			
Position the patient			
Inspect the abdomen for:			
Symmetry			
Contour			
Umbilicus			
Condition of skin			
Presence or absence of pulsations or movements			
Hair distribution			
Lesions			
Auscultate the abdomen in all four quadrants for:			
Presence or absence of bowel sounds			
Bowel sounds: per minute			
Vascular sounds			
Percuss the abdomen for:			
General tympany			
Liver span			
Splenic dullness			
Costovertebral angle tenderness			
Presence of a fluid wave, if indicated			

(Continued)

PERFORMANCE CHECKLIST

ABDOMEN—Essential Behaviors (cont'd)

	Yes	No	Comments
Palpation of the abdomen—light and deep			
Bend the knees to increase relaxation			
Instruct client to breathe slowly			
Perform light palpation (about 1 cm) in all four quadrants, noting areas of guarding			
Perform deep palpation (5-8 cm) in all four quadrants, noting areas of guarding			
Palpate:			
Liver			
Spleen			
Kidneys			
Complete special procedures—check for:			
Rebound tenderness (Blumberg Sign)			
Inspiratory arrest (Murphy's Sign)			
Iliopsoas muscle test			
Obturator test			
Special considerations			
Transcultural			
Developmental			
Document findings			

Chapter 20

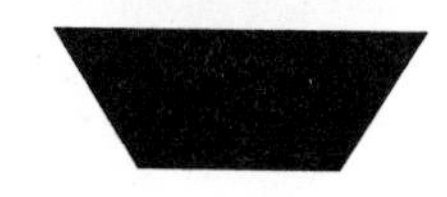

Musculoskeletal System

ANNOTATED LEARNING OBJECTIVES

At the completion of this chapter the student will:

List the functions of the musculoskeletal system.

The primary function of the musculoskeletal system is to provide support and movement of the body. The system also provides protection of vital inner organs, produces red blood cells, and provides for storage of minerals.

Differentiate between synovial and nonsynovial joints.

Nonsynovial joints consist of bones united by fibrous tissue or cartilage and are immovable. Synovial joints are freely movable. The bones are separated from each other and enclosed in a joint cavity that is filled with lubricant known as synovial fluid.

List the motions allowed by the temporomandibular joint.

The temporomandibular joint, felt in the depression anterior to the tragus of the ear, allows the opening and closing of the jaws, the gliding action needed for protrusion and retraction of the jaw, and the side-to-side movement of the lower jaw.

Describe the shape and surface landmarks of the spine.

The spine has four curves, giving it a double S shape when viewed from the side. Surface landmarks that help to orient the examiner to the levels of the spine include the following: the spinous processes of C7 and T1 are at the base of the neck; the inferior angle of the scapula is at the level of the interspace between T7 and T8; the iliac crest is at the level of L4; and an imaginary line drawn to join the symmetric dimples over the posterior superior iliac spines crosses S2.

KEY TERMS

Bursa

Tendon

Ligament

Sprain

Synovial joint

Intervertebral discs

Nucleus pulposus

Rotator cuff

Osteoporosis

Myalgia

Crepitation

TEACHING STRATEGIES

- Have students create flash cards with the movements of the body on one side and the definition of the term on the other. Each word needs to become part of the working vocabulary of the health care provider.

- ▼ Assign students to draw stick figures in positions representing the above movements.
- ▼ Create a matching quiz, listing the movable joints in one column and the possible movements of the joints in the other.
- ▼ Obtain a picture of a skeleton. Assign students to label the anatomical landmarks of each joint.
- ▼ Assign students to work in groups of three: one to follow the checklist and textbook, one to perform the examination, and one to act as client. Allow sufficient time for students to rotate roles so that each has an opportunity to be the examiner.
- ▼ Instruct students to document the results of the above examination, using appropriate descriptions for the location of any unusual findings.
- ▼ Have the students search the Internet for community resources available to patients with musculoskeletal disorders and design a resource book.
- ▼ Assign students to complete a musculoskeletal assessment on a client in the clinical area.
- ▼ Have students document the results of the musculoskeletal assessment.
- ▼ Assign students to develop or locate exercises that would be appropriate for various age groups.

CRITICAL THINKING EXERCISES

Application to Clinical Practice

For each individual described in the situations below, have students discuss the developmental, age, socioeconomic, and transcultural considerations that should be considered during the gathering of subjective and objective data and the provision of health care.

In addition, have students relate expected (normal) findings to those described, discuss any additional assessments that might be needed before a judgment/diagnosis can be made, and identify at least one relevant nursing diagnosis for any actual or potential problem identified. Have the student identify community resources available to the patient.

- ❑ M. G., a 61-year-old female, comes to the nurse practitioner with complaints of pain and stiffness in both lower extremities. When asked, she indicates that the stiffness is greater in the right thigh and that she has pain on weight bearing of the right leg. A limp was observed as she entered the examining room. When questioned about recent injuries, she is unaware of any. Further questioning reveals that she spent a greater than usual period working in her yard the preceding day. She also states that she had been doing heavier work with a spade than usual and that this is only the second day she has been able to garden since the winter.
- ❑ C. D., age 20, has come to the sports medicine clinic with a complaint of pain in the right shoulder. Although range of motion is within normal limits, the client complains of pain during circumduction. History includes swimming since age 4, with event of choice being the 20-meter freestyle.
- ❑ P. G., a petite, 65-year-old Irish American female has come to the health center complaining of back pain. She has been taking prednisone for rheumatoid arthritis and is post menopausal.
- ❑ J. M. has come for her monthly prenatal visit. When asked how she is feeling, she complains of low back pain and aching, numbness and weakness in the upper extremities.
- ❑ M. C. was admitted through the Emergency Department during the night. The health care provider is completing the initial assessment. M. C. is 70 years of age. She states that she heard a snap and then fell. She states she does not take estrogen or calcium supplements. Her right leg was observed to be abducted and externally rotated before the application of Buck's traction.
- ❑ P. A. has come for a routine physical. Examination of the left shoulder reveals separation of the joint. P. A. has full ROM and muscle strength and no complaints of pain.
- ❑ Chart review of A. M. yields the following notation: Widowed, white female, age 78, lengthening of the arm-trunk axis, kyphosis, backward head tilt and slight flexion of the hips and knees.

WEB SITES OF INTEREST

Ankylosing Spondylitis Association- ***www.spondylitis.org***

Arthritis Foundation- ***www.arthritis.org***

Backpain Hotline- ***www.texasback.com***

National Institute of Arthritis and Musculoskeletal and Skin Diseases- ***www.nih.gov/niams***

National Association of Orthopaedic Nurses- ***www.naon.nurses.com***

PERFORMANCE CHECKLIST

MUSCULOSKELETAL SYSTEM

	Yes	No	Comments
Obtain relevant history, functional and self care assessments			
Gather equipment			
Tape measure			
Goniometer			
Skin-marking pen			
Light if needed			
Provide privacy			
Wash hands			
Observe for symmetry			
Inspect each joint for:			
Size			
Contour			
Range of motion/limitation			
Inspect skin and tissue over joints for:			
Color			
Swelling			
Masses			
Deformity			
Palpate each joint for:			
Temperature			
Muscle			
Articulation			
Joint capsule			
Muscle strength			
Test			
Grade			

(Continued)

PERFORMANCE CHECKLIST

MUSCULOSKELETAL SYSTEM (cont'd)

	Yes	No	Comments
Record findings including notations regarding specific joints			
Temporomandibular			
Cervical spine			
Shoulders			
Elbow			
Wrist			
Phalen's test			
Tinel's test			
Hand			
Hip			
Knee			
Ballottement test			
McMurray's test			
Bulge sign			
Ankle			
Foot			
Special considerations			
Developmental			
Document findings			

Chapter 21

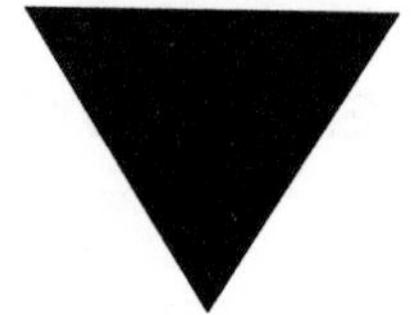

Neurologic System

ANNOTATED LEARNING OBJECTIVES

At the completion of this chapter the student will:

Name the two parts of the nervous system.

The central nervous system (CNS) includes the brain and spinal cord. The peripheral nervous system includes the 12 pairs of cranial nerves, the 31 pairs of spinal nerves, and their branches.

Describe the various functions of the central nervous system.

The cerebral cortex is the cerebrum's outer layer of nerve cell bodies. The cerebral cortex is the center for humans' highest functions, governing thought, memory, reasoning, sensation, and voluntary movement. Each half of the cerebrum is a hemisphere, and each hemisphere is divided into four lobes: frontal, parietal, temporal, and occipital.

Lobe	Function
Cerebral cortex	
Frontal lobe	Personality Behavior Emotions Intellectual function Ability to write words Speech motor (Broca's area)
Parietal lobe	Primary center for sensation Ability to recognize body parts Left versus right
Temporal lobe	Primary auditory reception center Language comprehension (Wernicke's area)
Occipital	Primary visual reception center Understanding of written material
Diencephalon	
Thalamus	Main relay station for the nervous system. Pain threshold

Component	Function
Hypothalamus	Center for temperature control, sleep, pituitary regulation, heart rate, blood pressure, emotional regulation, and autonomic nervous system activity.
Cerebellum	Blending and coordinating of motion of the various muscles involved in voluntary movements
Brain stem	
Midbrain	Contains nerve pathways between the cerebral hemispheres and the medulla Center for visual reflexes Origin of righting and postural reflex
Pons	Connects medulla oblongotta and midbrain, ventral to the cerebellum
Medulla oblongata	Continuation of the spinal cord in the brain Controls quality of respirations and heart rate as well as swallowing and hiccoughing; gag and cough reflex

Describe the function of the peripheral nervous system.

The peripheral nervous system carries messages to the CNS from sensory receptors and from the CNS to muscles and glands.

Relate the name and function of each of the 12 cranial nerves to its assessment.

Cranial Nerve	Name	Assessment
CN I	Olfactory	Sensory Smell—coffee, cloves, peppermint
CN II	Optic	Sensory Visual acuity—Snellen chart (cover eye not being examined) Test for visual fields Examination with opthalmoscope
CN III	Oculomotor	Motor Move eye up, down and peripherally Test for accommodation Pupillary constriction Observe for ptosis of the upper eyelid
CN IV	Trochlear	Motor Inferior lateral movement of the eye
CN V	Trigeminal	Sensory Corneal reflex Sensation of skin of the face (eyebrow, cheeks and chin) using a wisp of cotton Motor Chewing, biting, lateral jaw movements (move jaw side to side)
CN IV	Abducens	Motor Inferior lateral eye movements
CN VII	Facial	Sensory Taste—anterior 2/3 of tongue sweet—sugar; salt; sour—vinegar; and bitter—quinine, rinse mouth between applications Motor Movement of forehead and mouth Raise eyebrows, show teeth, smile and puff out cheeks
CN VIII	Acoustic	Sensory Hearing, balance Weber and Rinne tests Otoscope
CN IX	Glosso-pharyngeal	Motor Swallowing and phonation Sensory Taste—posterior 1/3 of tongue See CN VII
CN X	Vagus	Sensory Sensations of posterior 1/3 of tongue, throat Motor Gag reflex (stimulate back of pharynx with a tongue blade) Swallowing and phonation
CN XI	Spinal accessory	Motor Shoulder movement, shoulder shrug, head rotation—push against examiner's hand
CN XII	Hypoglossal	Motor Tongue movement—protrude tongue, push tongue into the cheek

Relate the term "dermatome" to the spinal nerves.

A dermatome is an area of skin supplied with afferent nerve fibers by a single posterior spinal root. The areas supplied by each nerve are shown graphically in the text. There are 31 pairs of spinal nerves: 12 thoracic, 5 lumbar, 5 sacral, and 1 coccygeal. The spinal nerves are "mixed" nerves because they contain both sensory and motor fibers.

Describe the term "reflex arc."

A reflex arc is a response below the level of consciousness where sensory afferent fibers carry a message from a receptor, travel through the dorsal root into the spinal card, synapse in the cord, and send a message through motor efferent fibers to cause a response in the innervated muscle. Reflexes control and permit quick reaction to potentially painful or damaging situations. Reflexes also help the body maintain balance and appropriate muscle tone. There are four types of reflexes: deep tendon reflexes (myotatic), superficial, visceral, and pathologic (abnormal).

Describe the autonomic nervous system.

The part of the nervous system that governs the glands, cardiac muscle, and the smooth muscles such as the digestive system, respiratory system, and the skin. The autonomic nervous system is divided into two subsidiary systems: the sympathetic system and the parasympathetic system. Its function is to maintain homeostasis of the body.

List developmental considerations for infants and older adults.

Infants

- Neurologic system not completely developed at birth
- Neurons are not yet myelinated
- Movements are directed primarily by primitive reflexes
- Sensory and motor development proceeds along with the gradual acquisition of myelin following a cephalocaudal and proximodistal order

Aging Adult

- Steady loss of neurons evidenced by:
  - General loss of muscle bulk
  - Loss of muscle tone in the face, neck and around the spine
  - Decreased muscle strength
  - Impaired fine coordination and ability
  - Loss of vibratory sense at the ankle
  - Decreased or absent Achilles reflex
  - Loss of position sense at the great toe
  - Loss of ankle jerk
  - Irregular pupil shape
- Decrease in nerve conduction velocity between 5 and 10 percent—may affect reaction time
- Increase delay at the synapse— impulse takes longer to travel
- Sensation of pain and touch may be diminished
- Diminished sense of taste and smell
- Slowing of motor system
- Decrease in muscle strength and agility
- Possible dyskinesias
- Progressive decrease in cerebral blood flow—dizziness and loss of balance with position change

Differentiate among the three types of neurologic examinations.

A screening examination is performed on well persons who have no significant subjective findings revealed in the history. A complete examination is performed on individuals who present with neurologic concerns identified through the neurologic history. A neurologic recheck is performed on individuals who have had a complete neurologic examination and are being seen for follow-up care. See the textbook for areas included in a screening and a complete examination.

KEY TERMS

Proprioception

Stereognosis

Graphesthesia

Cremasteric reflex

Dyskinesia

TEACHING STRATEGIES

- ▼ Have students develop flash cards with areas of the brain on one side and related behavior/sensation/function on the back.
- ▼ Using the behaviors/functions that must be assessed in a neuro examination, have students develop a game of "Challenge and Response." In this game, one student states the name of the behavior/function and the other student must provide the correct information within 30 seconds.
- ▼ Administer a matching test for the cranial nerves and their related functions.
- ▼ Assign students to develop visual materials that depict primitive reflexes routinely assessed in infants.
- ▼ Assign specific neurologic disorders to small groups. Have each group describe the relevant neuro examinations and expected findings.
- ▼ Working in pairs, have students perform a complete neurologic assessment on one another.
- ▼ Using chart forms from clinical facilities used by the school, have students complete documentation of the examination completed on a peer.
- ▼ Observe each student for performance of reflex examination. Students frequently do not stretch the tendon or relax the client well enough.
- ▼ Assign students to complete appropriate parts of the neurologic examination in the clinical area.
- ▼ When possible, have students work with an experienced preceptor.
- ▼ Have students compile a list of resources available to patients with neurological disorders. This list should include resources from the Internet.

CRITICAL THINKING EXERCISES

Application to Clinical Practice

For each individual described in the situations below, have students discuss the developmental, age, socioeconomic, and transcultural considerations that should be considered during the gathering of subjective and objective data and the provision of health care.

In addition, have students relate the anatomic area (body part) of injury/physiologic alteration to the neurologic source of injury/physiologic alteration, discuss any additional assessments that might be needed before a judgment/diagnosis can be made, identify at least one relevant nursing diagnosis for any actual or potential problem identified, and list available resources available to the patient.

❑ D. L. experienced a cerebrovascular accident (CVA) 1 week ago. His left side is paralyzed. While his speech is clear, he confabulates, reads aloud without comprehension, displays poor judgment, and overestimates his ability to perform simple tasks. He has a short attention span and has difficulty with the concept of time. Behavior is frequently impulsive and impatient.

❑ J. L. also experienced a CVA within the past week. J. L. is easily frustrated, anxious, and fearful; speech is slurred. She needs verbal cuing for any task she is asked to carry out. Only food on the left side of the tray is eaten and she only responds when approached from the left side.

❑ S. C. comes to the health clinic with complaints of vision changes, difficulty walking, easy fatigability, and extremity stiffness. Examination reveals hyperactive deep tendon reflexes, clonus, positive Babinski reflex, and absent abdominal reflexes. Romberg's test is positive. The client's family report recent change in emotional status. Tentative diagnosis is multiple sclerosis.

❑ C. C., age 55, has come for a follow-up visit following an ankle fusion to improve her gait. She has a benign tumor in the spinal cord at T 10 that has gradually impaired her gait over a period of 15 years. She reports occasional urinary incontinence. Sensation and mobility are decreased, especially in the right extremity and atrophy of the right lower extremity is noted.

❑ P. D. has come to the health care practitioner with complaints of facial weakness, difficulty walking, and incontinence. History includes an acute illness 1 week before symptoms began. Examination reveals symmetrical loss of deep tendon reflexes. Tentative diagnosis, Guillain-Barré syndrome.

❑ C. M. has been diagnosed with myasthenia gravis and is being followed as an outpatient. Describe an appropriate follow-up neurologic examination.

❑ R. R has been referred to the neurologic clinic for evaluation. History provided by his wife includes confusion, loss of short-term memory, poor judgment, ritualistic and repetitive behaviors. Tentative diagnosis—Alzheimer's disease.

WEB SITES OF INTEREST

American Association of Neuroscience Nurses- ***www.aann.org***

American Association of Spinal Cord Injury Nurses- ***www.epva.org***

American Paralysis Association- ***www.apacure.com***

National Headache Foundation- ***www.headaches.org***

National Stroke Organization- ***www.stroke.org***

Parkinson's Disease Foundation- ***www.parkinsons-foundation.org***

PERFORMANCE CHECKLIST

NEUROLOGIC SYSTEM

NOTE: The neurological examination may be integrated with each part of the body; findings should be recorded as a functional unit.

	Yes	No	Comments
Sequence of exam			
Mental status—may be assessed during history			
Cranial nerves			
Motor system			
Sensory system			
Reflexes			
Maintain patient privacy			
Provide for proper lighting			
Assess mental status			
Level of consciousness			
Thought processes			
Appearance and behavior			
Speech			
Obtain history—ask questions regarding:			
Headache			
Pain			
Head injury			
Dizziness/vertigo			
Seizures			
Tremors			
Weakness			
Incoordination			
Numbness or tingling			
Difficulty swallowing			
Difficulty speaking			

(Continued)

PERFORMANCE CHECKLIST

NEUROLOGIC SYSTEM (cont'd)

	Yes	No	Comments
Significant past history			
Environmental/occupational hazards			
Additional history for infants and children—Obtain information regarding:			
Prenatal care			
Delivery			
Apgar scores			
Congenital defects			
Reflexes			
Balance			
Achievement of developmental milestones			
Exposure to lead			
Problems in school			
Family history of neurologic problems			
Additional history for the aging adult—Ask questions regarding:			
Dizziness			
Change in mental function			
Tremors			
Sudden vision change			
Provide for exposure of areas to be examined			
Test the cranial nerves * See chart with objective 4 and notes in chapter regarding which nerves are routinely tested			
Cranial nerve I			
Cranial nerve II			
Cranial nerve III			
Cranial nerve IV			

(Continued)

PERFORMANCE CHECKLIST

NEUROLOGIC SYSTEM (cont'd)

	Yes	No	Comments
Cranial nerve V			
Cranial nerve VI			
Cranial nerve VII			
Cranial nerve VIII			
Cranial nerve IX			
Cranial nerve X			
Cranial nerve XI			
Cranial nerve XII			
The motor system			
Muscles			
Size			
Strength			
Tone			
Involuntary movements			
Cerebellar function			
Balance tests			
Gait			
Romberg's test			
Check coordination			
Rapid alternating movements (RAM)			
Rapid finger to thumb			
Finger to finger			
Finger to nose			
Heel to shin			
Examine the sensory system			
Stereognosis			
Pain—sharp and dull			

(Continued)

PERFORMANCE CHECKLIST

NEUROLOGIC SYSTEM (cont'd)

	Yes	No	Comments
Light touch			
Vibration			
Temperature (only when pain sensation is abnormal)			
Position			
Tactile discrimination			
Graphesthesia			
Two-point discrimination			
Extinction			
Point location			
Reflexes			
Deep tendon reflexes (DTRs)			
Scale			
4+—very brisk, hyperactive			
3+—brisker than average			
2+—average, normal			
1+—diminished, low normal			
0—no response			
Biceps			
Triceps			
Brachioradialis			
Quadriceps			
Achilles			
Clonus			
Superficial reflexes			
Abdominal			
Cremasteric			
Plantar			
Document findings			

Chapter 22

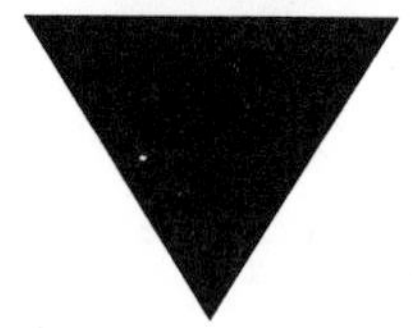

Male Genitalia

ANNOTATED LEARNING OBJECTIVES

At the completion of this chapter the student will:

List the structures of the male genital.

The structures of the male genital include the penis and scrotum externally and the testis, epididymis and vas deferens internally. The left testis is lower than the right because the left spermatic cord is longer.

Name the major structures of the penis.

The penis consists of three cylindrical columns of erectile tissue—the two corpora cavernosa and the corpus spongiosum. The glans, corona, urethra, foreskin or prepuce, and frenulum are the other major structures. A description is found in the text.

Describe the function of the cremaster muscle.

The cremaster muscle elevates the testis toward the body when the ambient temperature is cool, bringing the testes closer to the body to absorb the heat necessary for sperm viability. The muscle relaxes and the scrotum lowers when the temperature is warmer. This keeps the testes at 3 degrees Celcius below the abdominal temperature. A temperature of less than 98.6° is necessary for the development of sperm.

Identify the structures that provide transport of sperm.

The epididymis, the vas deferens, and ejaculatory duct provide for the transport of sperm.

Relate the significance of the inguinal canal and the femoral canal.

The inguinal canal, the oblique passage in the lower anterior abdominal wall though which the spermatic cord passes, is the frequent site of hernias. The femoral canal, a potential space located 3 cm medial to and parallel with the femoral artery, is also a site of hernias.

KEY TERMS

Corona
Frenulum
Glans penis
Corpus cavernosum
Spongiosum penis

TEACHING STRATEGIES

- Discuss infection control precautions.
- Assign students to debate the pros and cons of circumcision of the newborn.
- Discuss developmental considerations for the male genital exam.
- Use mannequins to provide students the opportunity to palpate normal testes and those with nodules.
- Discuss ways of creating an environment that will provide psychological comfort for both client and practitioner.

- Assign students to prepare or obtain teaching materials for the teaching of self testicular exam.
- Assign students to instruct a client or group of clients on self testicular exam.
- Have students prepare or obtain information on sexually transmitted diseases and their prevention.
- Assign the students to search the Internet for resources available to men with sexual dysfunctions such as erectile disorder and prepare resource packets for clients.
- Have the students conduct a sexual history on a client
- Discuss the feelings that may be experienced by both the client and the examiner and approaches to increase the comfort of both.
- Assign students to a health care provider who will serve as preceptor for each student to have experience with this examination.
- Review documentation of examinations performed by students.
- Assign students to keep a log during their experience with a preceptor. Encourage them to record both successes and questions.

CRITICAL THINKING EXERCISES

Application to Clinical Practice

For each individual described in the situations below, have students discuss the developmental, age, socioeconomic, and transcultural considerations that should be considered during the gathering of subjective and objective data and the provision of health care.

In addition, have students relate expected (normal) findings to those described, discuss any additional information that might be needed before a judgment/diagnosis can be made, and identify at least one relevant nursing diagnosis for any actual or potential problem identified.

- ❑ T.J. has come to the health care provider complaining of recently noticing a "bulge" in his lower abdomen. He is 35 years old and works for a trucking company.
- ❑ P. H., age 12, has been brought to the health care center by his mother for a school physical. In private, she relates her concern about sometimes finding his bed wet in the morning over the last 3 months.
- ❑ A. D. has come to the health care provider complaining of pain and discomfort in his scrotum. Examination reveals dilated, tortuous veins.
- ❑ M. J. has been referred for an examination for a possible problem of infertility. Interview reveals the use of "Jockey" type underwear both day and night.
- ❑ M.O., recently discharged with an above-the-knee amputation, is being interviewed by the home health nurse during the initial visit for the home health agency. The amputation was necessitated by DM-related peripheral vascular disease. Discussion reveals that the client is impotent and has not sought help for the problem. His wife is alive and well.
- ❑ During the examination of E. H., age 5 months, the examiner notes that the urethral meatus is on the underside of the penis.
- ❑ During an examination, R. R expresses concern for yellowish nodules on the scrotum. The nodules are firm, nontender, and measure 0.75 to 1 cm in diameter.
- ❑ L. D. has come for an evaluation of a firm nodule he noticed about 6 months ago attached to his testicles. He states he had not been concerned because he was hit in the testicles with a baseball shortly before he noticed the nodule.

WEB SITES OF INTEREST

American Urological Society- ***http://auanet.org/***

Taking a sexual history-
www.wellweb.com/impotent/chris/disease.htm

Impotence Center-
www.wellweb.com/impotent/chris/contents.htm

The Safe Sex Page- ***www.safesex.org***

American Cancer Society- ***www.cancer.org***

PERFORMANCE CHECKLIST

MALE GENITALIA—Essential Behaviors

	Yes	No	Comments
Obtain relevant history			
Gather equipment			
Provide privacy			
Explain procedure to client			
Use appropriate client positions			
Wash hands			
Don gloves			
Inspect:			
Penis			
Glans			
Urethral meatus			
Culture any discharge			
Base of penis			
Scrotum			
Rugae			
Posterior surface			
Transilluminate as indicated			
For hernia			
Palpate:			
Penis			
Shaft			
Compress the glans			
Scrotum			
Spermatic cord			
Testes			
For hernia			
Document findings			

Chapter 23

Anus, Rectum, and Prostate

ANNOTATED LEARNING OBJECTIVES

At the completion of this chapter the student will:

Summarize the anatomy of the anus and rectum.

The anal canal is a 3.8-cm outlet of the gastrointestinal tract. It is lined with modified skin that merges with the rectal mucosa. In addition to autonomic nerves, numerous somatic sensory nerves are present and make the area sensitive to pain. Internal and external sphincters surround the canal. The external sphincter provides voluntary control for the expulsion of feces and gas.

Anal columns in the rectum end at the anorectal junction contain an artery and a vein. Enlargement of these veins form hemorrhoids. The anal valve is at the lower end of each column, and the anal crypt is a small recess above the anal valve and between the columns.

The rectum, a 12-cm long portion of the distal large intestine, extends from the sigmoid colon to the anal canal. The valves of Houston are semilunar transverse folds in the rectal interior. The peritoneum covers only the upper 2/3 of the rectum.

Describe the prostate gland.

The prostate gland is 2.5 cm long by 4 cm in diameter. The gland lies in front of the anterior wall of the rectum and 2 cm behind the symphysis pubis. It secretes a fluid that contributes to the seminal fluid and consists of a median lobe and two lateral lobes, separated by a shallow groove called the medial sulcus. The seminal vesicles, which project like rabbit ears above the prostate, secrete a fluid that nourishes the sperm. Two bulbourethral glands the size of a pea are located inferior to the prostate on either side of the urethra.

Outline structures that can be examined via the rectum.

In addition to the prostate, the uterine cervix may be palpated through the anterior rectal wall. The sigmoid colon, extending from the iliac flexure of the descending colon to the rectum, is 40 cm long. The sigmoid is accessible to examination via the colonoscopy.

Describe age-related considerations for examination of anal, rectal, and prostate structures.

Passage of the first stool of a newborn indicates patency of the rectum. The nerves of the rectal area become myelinated between 1 1/2 to 2 years of age. Toilet training cannot start until this occurs.

At puberty, the prostate doubles to reach adult size.

Benign prostatic hypertrophy is evident in males at the age of 40 and increases with age.

KEY TERMS

Meconium

TEACHING STRATEGIES

- Obtain anatomic models for students to practice the rectal examination.
- Assign students to work with a preceptor who performs frequent rectal exams in his/her practice so that students can have experience with a variety of clients.

- ▼ Instruct students to document the results of the above examination using appropriate descriptions for the location of any unusual findings.
- ▼ Assign students to obtain a rectal history in the clinical setting.
- ▼ Discuss the above history in post conference. Have students identify their comfort level during the interview. Did the client seem at ease?
- ▼ Have students prepare teaching materials related to the rectal examination and the prostate examination.
- ▼ Have students conduct classes on colorectal and prostate cancer screening.

CRITICAL THINKING EXERCISES

Application to Clinical Practice

For each individual described in the situations below, have students discuss the developmental, age, socioeconomic, and transcultural considerations that should be considered during the gathering of subjective and objective data and the provision of health care.

In addition, have students relate expected (normal) findings to those described, discuss any additional information that might be needed before a judgment/diagnosis can be made, and identify at least one relevant nursing diagnosis for any actual or potential problem identified.

- ❑ C. D. suffers from colitis. During the interview, she relates that stool seems to be coming from her vagina.
- ❑ P.A., a fighter pilot, has come to the flight surgeon complaining of bright red blood in her stools. Chart review indicates identification of external hemorrhoids on previous examinations.
- ❑ This is the first home visit to L. J. During the initial history, L. J. indicates that stools have become black and tarry in appearance since hospitalization. Medications include the addition of an iron preparation to the regimen.
- ❑ During the first visit for M. K., age 4 weeks, the health care provider notes a generalized reddened area with papules, vesicles, and pustules in the diaper area.
- ❑ A. W., age 50, has come for an annual physical. During the interview he states that he has begun to get up during the night to empty his bladder. Rectal exam reveals enlargement of the prostate.
- ❑ H. H. has come for a follow-up visit for a urinary infection. Review of her medical record reveals that she has not had a rectal examination in 6 years and that her family history includes colorectal cancer in her father. When the exam is suggested, she declines, stating that she is not having any problems.
- ❑ M. C., age 70, is being visited for the first time by the home health nurse following discharge from the hospital for removal of her gall bladder. During the interview, she indicates that she frequently has problems with constipation.
- ❑ M. H., age 21, has come to the health care provider complaining of a recent episode of "sudden wetness" in her underwear that was not urine. Examination reveals a few tufts of hair over the coccyx. A sinus tract is visible.

WEB SITES OF INTEREST

American Cancer Society- ***www.cancer.org***

National Cancer Institute- ***www.nih.gov/nci***

American Urological Association- ***www.aua.org***

PERFORMANCE CHECKLIST

ANUS, RECTUM, AND PROSTATE

	Yes	No	Comments
Obtain relevant history			
Gather equipment			
Provide privacy			
Explain procedure to client			
Position appropriately			
Wash hands			
Don gloves			
Inspect:			
Perianal area without pressure while client performs a Valsalva maneuver			
Sacrococcygeal area			
Palpate:			
Anus (with examining finger and bidigitally)			
Rectum (with examining finger and bidigitally)			
Prostate or cervix			
Examine:			
Stool visually			
Perform guaiac test			
Document findings			

Chapter 24

Female Genitalia

ANNOTATED LEARNING OBJECTIVES

At the completion of this chapter the student will:

List the external structures of the female genitalia.

The external female genitalia consists of the vulva, the mons pubis, the labia majora and minora, the clitoris, the urethral meatus, paraurethral or Skene's glands, vaginal orifice, hymen, and vestibular or Bartholin's glands. The space between the labia minora into which the urethra and vagina open is termed the vestibule.

Describe the structures of the internal female genitalia.

The vagina is a tubular canal, 9 cm in length. It extends from the vestibule to the cervix. The walls are thick and have transverse folds referred to as *rugae*. The rugae enable the vagina to dilate during intercourse and childbirth. The uterus is a pear-shaped, muscular organ divided in three segments anatomically. The fundus or top of the uterus, the corpus or body, and the cervix, which projects into the vagina. The opening of the cervix is referred to as the *os*. The two pliable tubes, 10 cm in length, extending from the fundus of the uterus to the brim of the pelvis are the fallopian tubes. Close to the distal end of each fallopian tube is an oval-shaped, glandular structure called the *ovary*. The recess around the cervix is referred to as the *fornix*, anterior and posterior.

Describe the functions of the female reproductive system.

The female reproductive system manufactures ova for fertilization, transports the fertilized ovum for implantation, protects the fertilized embryo during development, regulates hormone production, and serves as the female organ of copulation, the birth canal, and a channel for the exit of menstrual flow.

Cite changes noted during pregnancy.

Weeks gestation	Physical change	Name of sign
2	absent menstruation	Amenorrhea
4–6	cervix softens mucus plug forms vaginal secretions—thick, white and >acid	Goodell's sign
6–8	isthmus of uterus softens	Hegar's sign
8–12	cyanosis of vaginal mucosa and cervix	Chadwick's sign
10–12	uterus globular in shape too large for pelvis palpable just above symphysis pubis	
20–24	uterus oval in shape rises almost to the liver intestines displaced	
term	mucus plug dislodges	Bloody show

Outline the changes observed during the perimenopausal period.

The cessation of the menses occurs between the ages of 35 and 60 years. Ovarian function declines, the menses become farther apart and produce a lighter flow than usual. The uterus shrinks in size, the ovaries atrophy to 1 to 2 cm and are not palpable after menopause. The sacral ligaments relax, the pelvic musculature weakens, and the uterus droops. The cervix shrinks and looks paler. The vagina becomes shorter, narrower, and less elastic. The vaginal epithelium atrophies, resulting in a fragile mucosal surface that is at risk for bleeding and vaginitis. Vaginal pH becomes more alkaline. Externally, the mons pubis fat pad atrophies and the labia and clitoris gradually decrease in size. Pubic hair becomes thin and sparse.

KEY TERMS

Bloody show
Dysuria
Nocturia
Hematuria
Menopause
Dyspareunia
Amenorrhea
Menses
Menorrhagia
Dysmenorrhea

TEACHING STRATEGIES

- ▼ Discuss infection control precautions.
- ▼ Discuss developmental considerations of the female genital examination.
- ▼ Use mannequins to provide students the opportunity to learn the anatomy of the female genitalia.
- ▼ Discuss ways of creating an environment that will provide psychological comfort for both client and practitioner.
- ▼ Assign students to prepare or obtain teaching materials for young girls to prepare them for the onset of menses and another set for women to prepare them for menopause.
- ▼ Discuss the above materials and their applicability for use in presenting the information to males.
- ▼ Have students prepare or obtain information on sexually transmitted diseases and their prevention.
- ▼ Assign students to a health care provider who will serve as preceptor for each student to have experience with this examination.
- ▼ Assign students to keep a log during their experience with a preceptor. Encourage them to record both successes and questions.
- ▼ Assign students to obtain a sexual history from a client.
- ▼ Live models may be hired for students to learn to perform this examination.
- ▼ Review documentation of examinations performed by students.

CRITICAL THINKING EXERCISES

Application to Clinical Practice

For each individual described in the situations below, have students discuss the developmental, age, socioeconomic, and transcultural considerations that should be considered during the gathering of subjective and objective data and the provision of health care.

In addition, have students relate expected (normal) findings to those described, discuss any additional information that might be needed before a judgment/diagnosis can be made, and identify at least one relevant nursing diagnosis for any actual or potential problem identified.

- ❑ B. G. has come for a yearly examination. During the interview she appears depressed and relates symptoms of headache, mood swings, intermittent low grade temperatures, and lethargy.
- ❑ M. N. has come for relief of the symptoms of extreme perineal itching and burning. She states she has a white, curdlike, foul-smelling vaginal discharge. Record review indicates she was placed on antibiotics for a URI 5 days ago.
- ❑ B.W., age 7, has been brought to the health care provider because the child is complaining of painful urination. Interview reveals that the use of bubble bath was begun about 2 weeks ago.
- ❑ D. S. has come for a visit to the clinic because of painful ulcerations in the genital area. She also complains of dysuria and malaise, fever, and anorexia.

- ❑ S. M., age 72, has come for a yearly physical examination. Findings are as follows: Mons pubis decreased in size, pubic hair thin and gray, labia atrophied with dry, pale appearance, Bartholin's glands atrophied, vaginal wall appears dry, ovaries nonpalpable.
- ❑ J. W. is being treated with radiation for ovarian cancer. During interview, she relates that urine seems to be coming from her vagina.
- ❑ Interview with V. D. has elicited the following complaints: menstrual irregularities for 6 months, dull pain in the left lower quadrant of the abdomen, and a feeling of general fatigue and heaviness in the pelvis.

WEB SITES OF INTEREST

American Urogynecologic Society- ***www.augs.org***

All About Menopause- ***www.menopause.org***

Center for Human Reproduction- ***www.centerforhumanreprod.com***

Planned Parenthood Federation of America, Inc. ***www.ppfa.org***

The Safe Sex Page- ***www.safesex.org***

PERFORMANCE CHECKLIST

FEMALE GENITALIA

	Yes	No	Comments
Obtain relevant history			
Gather equipment			
Provide privacy			
Wash hands			
Discuss measures to increase client comfort			
Position client for vaginal exam			
Don gloves			
Inspect external genitalia for:			
Color			
Hair distribution			
Symmetry			
Clitoris			
Labia			
Urethral opening			
Vaginal opening			
Perineum			
Palpate:			
Glands			
Skene's			
Bartholin's			
Special maneuvers			
Palpate the perineum			
Assess vaginal tone			
Assess for vaginal wall bulging or urinary incontinence			

(Continued)

PERFORMANCE CHECKLIST

FEMALE GENITALIA (cont'd)

	Yes	No	Comments
Internal genitalia—Speculum exam			
Inspect cervix os for:			
Color			
Position			
Size			
Obtain			
Smears			
Cultures			
Complete 5% acetic acid wash			
Inspect vaginal wall as speculum is removed			
Perform			
Bimanual examination			
Rectovaginal examination			
Document findings:			
Hair distribution			
Venous pattern			

Chapter 25

The Pregnant Woman

ANNOTATED LEARNING OBJECTIVES

At the completion of this chapter the student will:

Discuss pregnancy and the endocrine placenta.

One follicle ruptures and ovulation occurs. If the ovum meets a viable sperm, fertilization occurs. Progesterone helps to maintain a rich vascular endometrial wall where the fertized ovum will implant. A specialized layer of cells becomes the placenta that functions as an endocrine organ and produces several hormones. These hormones help in the growth and maintenance of the fetus and direct changes in the woman's body to prepare for birth and lactation. The average length of pregnancy is 280 days.

Discuss the changes associated with each trimester of pregnancy.

Pregnancy is divided into three trimesters: (1) the first 12 weeks, (2) from 13 to 27 weeks, and (3) from 28 weeks to delivery. Recommendations for weight gain are outlined in the chapter.

First trimester (First 12 weeks)

Blastocyst implants in uterus
Breast tingling and tenderness begin
More than half of women experience nausea and vomiting
Uterus becomes globular in shape, softens, and flexes easily over the cervix
Urinary frequency increases
Blood pressure may drop because of falling peripheral vascular resistance.

Second trimester (Weeks 13-27)

Colostrum may be expressed from nipples
Skin changes—areolas and nipples darken, abdominal skin becomes pigmented, and stretch marks may be noted on the breast, abdomen, and areas of weight gain
Stomach displacement occurs
Altered esophageal spincter and gastric tone often cause heartburn
Constipation is more likely to occur
Increased tidal volume is observed
"Quickening," or fetal movement is felt

3rd trimester (Weeks 28-delivery)

Increased blood volume may cause a functional systolic murmur
Uterine enlargement causes diaphragm to rise, causing decreased lung expansion space
Pulse rate rises 15 to 20 beats per minute
Hemorrhoids occur
Lordosis frequently occurs

State methods of determining weeks of gestation.

Weeks of gestation may be calculated using the Naegel's rule. That is the first day of the last normal menstrual period; add seven days and subtract three months. The number of weeks gestation also can be estimated by abdominal exam, by measuring the maternal serum human choriogonadotropin, and by signs such as "quickening," the first perceived fetal movement.

Discuss developmental considerations associated with pregnancy.

The risks for the adolescent who is pregnant are largely psychosocial. Young mothers are at risk for the downward cycle of poverty because of incomplete education, lack of support from family and significant others, and failure to limit family size. The adolescent is also at risk for preeclampsia and for bearing a low birthweight infant.

Primigravidae pregnant after age 35 years are at risk to be infertile. Women 35 years and older are offered genetic counseling and prenatal testing. The older woman is at risk for congenital anomalies. Because the incidence of chronic diseases increases with age, old women who are pregnant more often suffer medical complication such as diabetes and hypertension. They experience more spontaneous abortions.

KEY TERMS

Gravida
- Primigravida
- Multigravida

Presumptive sign
Probable sign
Positive sign
Quickening
Colostrum
Linear nigra
Striae gravidarum
Expected date of confinement (EDC)

TEACHING STRATEGIES

- ▼ Assign the students to attend a prenatal class.
- ▼ Assign students to rotate through a perinatal clinic with a practitioner. This assignment should include a pre- and post-natal home visit. Have the students design a teaching plan for each patient.
- ▼ Give the students a series of dates for last menstrual cycle, and have them calculate the expected date of confinement (EDC).
- ▼ Have a student interview a patient from a different culture in order to understand the patient's cultural beliefs and practices associated with pregnancy.

CRITICAL THINKING EXERCISES

Application to Clinical Practice

For each individual described in the situations below, have students discuss the developmental, age, socioeconomic, and transcultural considerations that should be considered during the gathering of subjective and objective data and the provision of health care.

In addition, have students relate expected (normal) findings to those described, discuss any additional information that might be needed before a judgment/diagnosis can be made, and identify at least one relevant nursing diagnosis for any actual or potential problem identified. For each situation, design a teaching plan.

- ❑ A. M. is a 40-year-old executive primigravida. She is currently in her first trimester and comes to the clinic for a prenatal visit. She complains of urinary frequency, heartburn, and leg pain. She has also noticed a small amount of vaginal discharge.
- ❑ R. G. is a 25-year-old Arabic gravida 3 who presents with her husband and 2 children. She is a full-time student beginning her third trimester.
- ❑ B. D. is a 16-year-old high school student who presents to the neighborhood nursing clinic. Her last menstrual period was 3 months before her visit, and she admits to being sexual active and occasionally using condoms.
- ❑ D. G., 2nd trimester primigravida 1, calls the neighborhood nursing center complaining of inability to perform exercises as she did prior to pregnancy. She also states, " I feel weird movement in my stomach."
- ❑ K. Y. is a 36-year-old gravida 2. She has a family history of hypertension and is borderline hypertensive. You receive her call, and she complains of hand swelling, headache, blurring vision, and epigastric pain.

WEB SITES OF INTEREST

Association of Women's Health, Obstetric, and Neonatal Nurses- ***www.awhonn.org***

American College of Nurse Midwives- ***www.acnw.org***

Midwifery Services, Inc.- ***www.midwife-ny.com***

Parenthood Web's Pregnancy and Labor Corner- ***www.parenthoodweb.com***

Abiding Hearts Support Group- ***www.imt.net***

PERFORMANCE CHECKLIST

THE PREGNANT WOMAN

	Yes	No	Comments
Wash hands			
Obtain relevant history			
Determine EDC and present number of weeks gestation			
Gather equipment			
Provide privacy			
Explain procedure to client			
Instruct woman to undress, empty bladder			
Save urine to dip for protein and glucose			
Position appropriately			
Inspect skin for pigment changes and scars			
Oral mucous membranes			
Neck			
Palpate thyroid gland			
Breast			
Inspect and palpate			
Heart			
Auscultate heart sounds			
Heart rate			
Peripheral vasculature			
Edema			
Varicosities			
Thrombophlebitis			
Homan's sign			
Neurologic			
Deep tendon reflexes			
Abdomen			
Measure fundus height			

(Continued)

PERFORMANCE CHECKLIST

THE PREGNANT WOMAN (cont'd)

	Yes	No	Comments
Perform Leopold's maneuvers			
Auscultate fetal heart tones			
Pelvic examination			
Note signs of pregnancy			
Condition of the cervix			
Size and position of the uterus			
Pelvimetry			
Measure blood pressure			
Obtain routine laboratory studies			
Equipment needed			
Stethoscope			
Sphygmomanometer			
Centimeter measuring tape			
Fetoscope or Doppler			
Reflex hammer			
Urine collection container			
Chemostix			
Pelvic exam equipment from Chapter 24			

Chapter 26

The Complete Health Assessment: Putting It All Together

ANNOTATED LEARNING OBJECTIVES

At the completion of this chapter the student will:

Use recommended techniques to perform a complete history and physical examination.

The examiner needs to develop a sequence that is comfortable for both client and practitioner. Depth of history and extent of physical examination will be dictated by the history provided by the client and/or significant other, the circumstances surrounding the need for health care, and the clinical judgment of the practitioner. Please refer to Chapter 8 for developmental considerations.

TEACHING STRATEGIES

- ▼ Use the problems presented throughout this text or develop others that reflect the patient population seen by students, and schedule a time for students to perform a complete examination on a partner under faculty supervision.
- ▼ Observe students while they are performing the examination. The examination of various body systems should be integrated; for example, while the chest is exposed, the breast can be examined, heart sounds evaluated and lungs sounds auscultated.
- ▼ Have students submit appropriate documentation for the above examination. Assigning a pass-fail grade stresses the importance of the assignment.
- ▼ Assign students to work with a preceptor to perform a number of both complete and focused or follow-up examinations.
- ▼ Have students review a history and physical completed by another practitioner and critique the examination for its completeness and clarity.
- ▼ Assign students to complete admission assessments on clients in the clinical setting.

CRITICAL THINKING EXERCISES

Application to Clinical Practice

At this time, have the student being the client role play one of the situations below or one of the situations provided throughout the text. Instruct the student acting as practitioner to discuss the developmental, age, socioeconomic, and transcultural considerations that should be considered during the gathering of subjective and objective data and the provision of health care. Have the student practitioner describe the type of examination that will be conducted, relate expected (normal) findings to those described or found, discuss any additional information needed before a judgment/diagnosis can be made, identify at least one relevant nursing diagnosis for any actual or potential problem identified, and identify health promotion education needed.

- ❑ R. D., age 72, has come to the health center at the request of her son, whom she recently visited in a neighboring state. Interview reveals increasing fatigue, weakness, anorexia, and constipation. History includes a vaginal hysterectomy at age 40, a vein ligation at age 35, and two full-term pregnancies that resulted in live births. R. D. has been widowed for 12 years and currently lives alone. Both children live in another state. On examination, her abdomen is distended and hard.

- ❑ F. N., age 48, has been referred to the home health psychiatric nurse because of difficulties with recent changes in behavior. One month prior to the visit, the son of the patient died from an apparent drug overdose. The client's wife states that for the past 3 years, F. N. has been accusing her of inviting sexual overtures from various men, including her son and son-in-law. F. N. would make frequent accusations, and one time he interpreted the adjustment of the rear view mirror by his son-in-law to be for the purpose of getting a better look at his wife. Morning breakfast with other retirees at a local restaurant has been discontinued because F. N. began to be suspicious of the other men in the group. Sleep is about 1 to 2 hours a night and brief naps during the day. F. N. is restless and paces in the house or goes into the neighborhood for frequent walks. Weight lost has been 50 pounds in the last 2 years. History includes a colon resection for cancer 6 years ago and Parkinson's disease that is controlled with medication.
- ❑ M. M. has come to the health care provider complaining that 5 months ago her feet began to bother her more and more until she could barely walk. Her podiatrist referred her for further evaluation. Within the past 2 weeks she has experienced generalized exhaustion and "stiffness" in the morning.
- ❑ M. G., a 50-year-old type II diabetic, has come to the health center for a periodic evaluation. Interview and subsequent examination reveal a small ulcer on the plantar surface of her right great toe and another small ulcer on the inner aspect of the right ankle.
- ❑ B. N. has come to the health center with the following symptoms: epigastric fullness both before and after meals; loud, intense belching; occasional epigastric pain; and pain after eating a fatty meal.
- ❑ C. K. has come to the emergency room complaining of pain over the precordium that is also felt in the neck and left arm, and beneath the clavicle
- ❑ E. P., age 70, has come to the health center accompanied by her daughter. The client, with the assistance of the daughter, provides the following information: a rash on the lower left leg which on first sight appears to be a bruise; chronic fatigue beginning 3 weeks ago; headaches; low grade temperature; pain and swelling in several joints; depression; and some memory loss.

EQUIPMENT NEEDED FOR PHYSICAL EXAMINATION

Platform scale with height attachment
Skinfold calipers
Sphygmomanometer—appropriate size
Stethoscope with bell and diaphragm—adult or pediatric
Thermometer
Penlight
Tangential lighting
Otoscope/ophthalmoscope
Tuning fork
Nasal speculum
Tongue depressor
Disposable sharp object or split tongue blade
Pocket vision screener
Skin-marking pen
Flexible tape measure
Ruler marked in centimeters
Reflex hammer
Cotton balls
Vaginal speculum
Examination gloves
Materials to check taste and smell if needed
Materials for cytologic study
Water-soluble lubricant
Guaiac test equipment

PERFORMANCE CHECKLIST

COMPLETE HEALTH ASSESSMENT—Long Outline

	Yes	No	Comments
Obtain relevant history			
Gather equipment			
Provide privacy			
Obtain proper lighting			
Wash hands			
Ensure visualization of each part as it is examined			
Observe general appearance of client			
Appearance in relation to stated age			
Obvious physical deformities			
Mobility			
Gait			
Assistive devices			
ROM			
Involuntary movements			
Personal hygiene			
Clothing			
Appropriate for season			
Clean and neat or disheaveled			
Skin color—note throughout exam			
Examine both hands			
Inspect nails			
Posture and position			
Facial expression & symmetry (cranial nerve VII)			
Affect			
Mood			
Speech			
Articulation			

(Continued)

PERFORMANCE CHECKLIST

COMPLETE HEALTH ASSESSMENT—Long Outline (cont'd)

	Yes	No	Comments
Pattern			
Content appropriate			
Native language			
Hearing			
Vital signs			
Radial pulse			
Respirations			
Blood pressure			
Temperature			
Nutritional status			
Weight			
Height			
Skinfold thickness			
Head and face			
Observe for:			
Eye contact			
Level of consciousness			
Orientation			
Inspect and palpate:			
Scalp			
Hair			
Cranium			
Symmetry			
Temporal artery			
Maxillary and frontal sinuses			

(Continued)

PERFORMANCE CHECKLIST

COMPLETE HEALTH ASSESSMENT—Long Outline (cont'd)

	Yes	No	Comments
Eyes			
Test:			
Visual fields by confrontation (cranial nerve II)			
Extraocular muscles			
Corneal light reflexes			
Six cardinal positions of gaze (cranial nerves III, IV, VI)			
Vision with Snellen eye chart			
Pupil			
Size			
Response to:			
Light			
Accommodation			
Inspect:			
External structures			
Conjunctiva			
Sclerae			
Corneas			
Irides			
With ophthalmoscope inspect:			
Ocular fundus			
Red reflex			
Disc			
Vessels			
Retinal background			

(Continued)

PERFORMANCE CHECKLIST

COMPLETE HEALTH ASSESSMENT—Long Outline (cont'd)

	Yes	No	Comments
Ears			
Inspect external ear			
With otoscope inspect:			
Canal			
Tympanic membrane			
Test hearing:			
Voice			
Rinne test			
Weber test			
Nose			
Inspect for:			
Symmetry			
Lesions			
Test patency of each nostril			
With speculum inspect:			
Nasal mucosa			
Septum			
Turbinates			
Mouth and throat			
Inspect:			
Mouth			
Buccal mucosa			
Teeth			
Gums			
Tongue			
Floor of mouth			
Palate			

(Continued)

PERFORMANCE CHECKLIST

COMPLETE HEALTH ASSESSMENT—Long Outline (cont'd)

	Yes	No	Comments
Uvula—condition and mobility			
Grade tonsils			
Test:			
Gag reflex (cranial nerves IX, X)			
Cranial nerve XII (stick out tongue)			
Palpate mouth, if indicated			
Neck			
Inspect for:			
Symmetry			
Lumps			
Pulsations			
Palpate:			
Cervical lymph nodes			
Carotid pulse			
Trachea			
Test:			
ROM			
Muscle strength			
Chest			
Inspect:			
Configuration of thoracic cage			
Anteroposterior diameter			
Skin characteristics			
Symmetry			
Palpate for:			
Symmetric expansion			
Tactile fremitus			

(Continued)

PERFORMANCE CHECKLIST

COMPLETE HEALTH ASSESSMENT—Long Outline (cont'd)

	Yes	No	Comments
Lumps			
Tenderness			
Spinous processes			
Percussion			
Lung fields			
Diaphragmatic excursion			
Costovertebral angle			
Auscultate			
Breath sounds			
Heart			
Inspect precordium			
Pulsations			
Heave (lift)			
Palpate:			
Apical impulse-note location			
Precordium			
Auscultate:			
Base for murmurs			
Heart sounds with bell and diaphragm			
Apical rate			
Apical rhythm			
Apex with bell			
Upper extremities			
Test			
ROM			
Muscle strength of:			
Hands			

(Continued)

PERFORMANCE CHECKLIST

COMPLETE HEALTH ASSESSMENT—Long Outline (cont'd)

	Yes	No	Comments
Arms			
Shoulders			
Palpate epitrochlear nodes			
Female breasts			
Inspect:			
For symmetry			
For mobility			
For dimpling			
Supraclavicular area			
Infraclavicular area			
Palpate:			
Each breast			
Tail of Spence			
Axilla			
Areola			
Lymph nodes			
Instruct in breast self exam			
Male breasts			
Inspect			
Palpate			
Neck vessels			
Inspect for jugular venous pulse			
Estimate jugular venous pressure			
Abdomen			
Inspect:			
Contour			
Symmetry			

(Continued)

PERFORMANCE CHECKLIST

COMPLETE HEALTH ASSESSMENT—Long Outline (cont'd)

	Yes	No	Comments
Skin characteristics			
Umbilicus			
Pulsation			
Auscultate for:			
Bowel sounds			
Vascular sounds			
Percussion			
Liver span			
Location of spleen			
Palpate all four quadrants, light and deep for:			
Liver			
Spleen			
Kidneys			
Aorta			
Test abdominal reflexes			
Inguinal area			
Palpate each groin for:			
Femoral pulse			
Inguinal nodes			
Lower extremities			
Inspect for:			
Symmetry			
Skin characteristics			
Hair distribution			
Varicose veins			
Palpate pulses			
Popliteal			

(Continued)

PERFORMANCE CHECKLIST

COMPLETE HEALTH ASSESSMENT—Long Outline (cont'd)

	Yes	No	Comments
Posterior tibial			
Dorsalis pedis			
Temperature			
Pretibial edema			
Inspect spaces between toes			
Test ROM and muscle strength of:			
Hips			
Knees			
Ankles			
Feet			
Musculoskeletal			
Note strength during movement			
Observe:			
Joints			
Deep knee bends			
Spine as person touches toes			
ROM of spine			
Gait			
Normal			
On toes			
On heels			
Perform Romberg test			
Neurologic			
Test:			
Babinski reflex			
Position sense of finger			
One hand			

(Continued)

PERFORMANCE CHECKLIST

COMPLETE HEALTH ASSESSMENT—Long Outline (cont'd)

	Yes	No	Comments
Stereognosis			
Cerebellar function			
Finger-to-nose			
Rapid-alternating movements			
Heel down opposite shin			
Sensation in selected area on:			
Face			
Hands			
Legs			
Feet			
Superficial pain			
Light touch			
Vibration			
Elicit deep tendon reflexes in:			
Biceps			
Triceps			
Brachioradialis			
Patellar			
Achilles			
Male genitalia			
Inspect:			
Penis			
Scrotum—transilluminate if indicated			
Palpate:			
Scrotal contents			
For inguinal hernia			
Instruct in self testicular exam			

(Continued)

PERFORMANCE CHECKLIST

COMPLETE HEALTH ASSESSMENT—Long Outline (cont'd)

	Yes	No	Comments
Male rectum			
Inspect the perianal area			
Palpate:			
Rectal walls			
Prostate gland			
Perform Guaiac test			
Female genitalia			
Inspect:			
Perineal area			
Perianal area			
With a speculum			
Cervix			
Uterus			
Adnexa			
Perform bimanual examination of:			
Cervix			
Uterus			
Adnexa			
Rectum			
Rectovaginal walls			
Guiac test			
Make age-appropriate modifications when indicated			
Inform patient that the exam is finished			
Answer questions; discuss further plans after patient is dressed			
Document findings			
Develop a problem list			
Return equipment			

Chapter 27

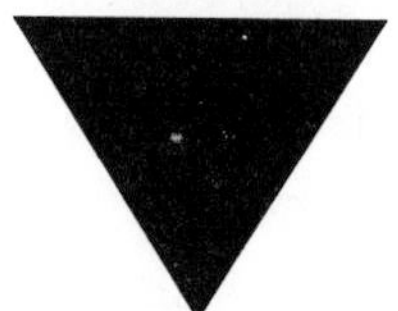

Critical Thinking in Health Assessment

ANNOTATED LEARNING OBJECTIVES

At the completion of this chapter the student will:

Analyze the client's data base, obtained through the collection of subjective and objective data, to develop a problem list and make a judgment or diagnosis regarding the health state of the individual.

The purpose of developing a data base is to provide a means of identifying health problems that need to be addressed. Some of the problems identified are completely within the realm of nursing, others require collaboration with other health care providers. The practitioner needs to develop the ability to identify all problems presented and differentiate between those solely within the purview of nursing and those requiring collaboration with other care providers.

Rank the problems identified in order of priority from the point of view of health risk and importance to the client.

Usually, the health care provider ranks problems according to their effect on the health status of the individual. Values and other socioeconomic considerations may cause the client to rank problems in a different order than the health care provider. Inclusion of the client in the development of the problem list will help the development of mutual goals and increase the acceptance of and participation in the health regimen recommended.

Differentiate between an expert and novice practitioner.

The nursing process alone does not explain the dynamic and interactive processes that occur with diagnosis and planning treatment. Although the nursing process is a logical problem-solving approach to clinical judgments, it seems that expert nurses vault over steps and arrive at a judgment in one leap. The expert has well-developed physical assessment skills and trusts these skills. The use of critical thinking occurs at a different level for expert and novice nurses. The expert thinker learns to assess and modify, if indicated, before acting. The novice thinker needs the familiarity of clear-cut rules to guide action. The expert practitioner uses intuitive links in solving problems, but the novice practitioner operates more from a set of defined, structured rules.

TEACHING STRATEGIES

- ▼ Assign students to develop collaborative problem lists based on the situations presented in the clinical judgment sections of each chapter.
- ▼ For various situations presented in the text, have students identify independent and interdependent nursing interventions.
- ▼ Using existing problems, have students identify the steps of the nursing process for each problem.
- ▼ Using available problems, have students identify the four major components of diagnostic reasoning followed for each problem.

- Using patient records at clinical agencies used by the school of nursing, have students review the available data base as part of the evaluation step of the nursing process.
- Discuss nursing process as a linear versus circular process.
- Apply various nursing theories to the clinical situations in the workbook. Discuss how each theory affects the direction of the interview and the interventions planned.
- Have students conduct a health fair at one of the school's clinical agencies or at a local educational institution. Both the skills developed and the materials obtained or developed for each chapter can be used for the fair.

Assessment Video Series

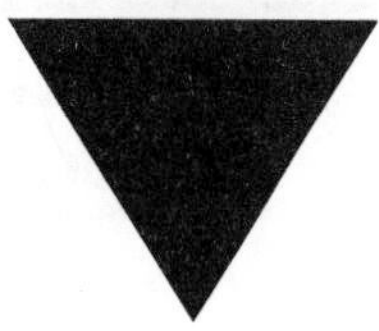

Head, Eyes, and Ears

VIDEO OUTLINE

- Anatomy review
  - Head
  - Eyes
  - Ears
- Health history
  - Head
  - Eyes
  - Ears
- Head examination
  - Skull
  - Face
- Eye examination
  - Visual acuity
  - Visual fields
  - Extraocular muscles
  - External eye
  - Anterior eyeball
  - Ocular fundus
- Ear examination
  - External ear
  - Internal ear
  - Eardrum
  - Hearing acuity

EQUIPMENT FOR ASSESSING THE HEAD, EYES, AND EARS

Snellen chart
handheld visual screener
opaque card or occluder
penlight
applicator stick
ophthalmoscope
otoscope with bright light
pneumatic bulb attachment (for infant or young child)
tuning forks in 512 Hz

CRITICAL THINKING QUESTIONS: HEAD, EYES, AND EARS

1. How do examination techniques and findings differ when palpating the head of an adult and the head of an infant?

2. What additional vision tests may you use and why would you use them?

3. Describe the following abnormal findings, which may be found during inspection of the eyelids: exophthalmos, ptosis, ectropion, hordeolum, chalazion, and carcinoma.

4. Describe the following lumps or lesions that may occur on the external ear: sebaceous cyst, keloid, carcinoma, and otitis externa.

5. Contrast the way you would move the pinna to straighten the ear canal of an adult and of a very young child.

CRITICAL THINKING ANSWERS

1. For an adult, assess shape by placing your fingers in the person's hair and palpating the scalp. Normally, it should be symmetric and smooth. The cranial bones that have normal protrusions are the forehead, the lateral edge of each parietal bone, the occipital bone, and the mastoid process behind each ear. You should detect no tenderness, lumps, depressions, or abnormal protrusions.

   Then, palpate the temporal artery above the cheek bone between the eye and the top of the ear. Palpate the temporomandibular joint as the person opens the mouth. Note normally smooth movement with no limitation or tenderness.

   For an infant, gently palpate the skull and fontanels while the infant is somewhat in a sitting position. The skull should feel smooth and fused except at the fontanels. The fontanels feel firm, slightly concave, and well defined against the edges of the cranial bones. A slight arterial pulsation may be visible in the anterior fontanel. The suture lines feel like ridges.

   By 5 to 6 months, they are smooth and not palpable. The newborn's head may feel asymmetric.

2. Test near vision using a Jaeger card in a person who is over age 40 or reports increasing difficulty reading. Use the cover test to detect small degrees of deviated alignment.

3. *Exophthalmos* (protruding eyes) is a forward displacement of the eyeballs and widened palpebral fissures. "Lid lag" is present, meaning that the upper lid rests well above the limbus and white sclera is visible.

   Ptosis (drooping upper lid) occurs from neuromuscular weakness, oculomotor cranial nerve III damage, or sympathetic nerve damage. It is a positional defect that gives the person a sleepy appearance and impairs vision.

   In *ectropion*, the lower lid is loose and rolling out and does not approximate to the eyeball. The puncta cannot siphon tears effectively so excess tearing results. Exposed palpebral conjunctiva increases risk for inflammation.

   Hordeolum (sty) is a localized staphylococcal infection of the hair follicles at the lid margin. It is painful, red, and swollen—a pustule at the lid margin.

   Chalazion is a beady nodule protruding on the lid. It is an infection or retention cyst of a meibomian gland. It is a nontender, firm, discrete swelling with freely moveable skin overlying the nodule. If it becomes inflamed, it points inside and not on the lid margin, in contrast with a sty.

   Carcinoma is rare, but it occurs most often on the lower lid and medial canthus. It looks like a papule with an ulcerated center, and has rolled-out pearly edges.

4. *Sebaceous cyst* is more common behind the lobule in the postauricular fold. A small nodule with central black punctum indicates blocked sebaceous gland. It is painful if it becomes infected. Often are multiple.

   Keloid is an overgrowth of scar tissue, which invades the original site of trauma. It is more common in dark-skinned people, although it also occurs in whites. In the ear, it is most common at the lobule at the site of a pierced earring.

   Carcinoma is an ulcerated, crusted nodule with an indurated base that fails to heal. It bleeds intermittently. It may also occur in the ear canal and show chronic discharge that is either serosanguinous or bloody. Pain and swelling of the canal are present.

   Otitis externa is an infection of the outer ear, with severe painful movement of the pinna and tragus, redness and swelling of the pinna and canal, scanty purulent discharge, scaling, itching, fever, and enlarged tender regional lymph nodes. Hearing is normal or slightly diminished.

5. In an adult, pull the pinna up and back to straighten the ear canal. In a very young child, pull the pinna straight down.

HEALTH HISTORY QUESTIONS

Head

Headache. Any unusually frequent or unusually severe headaches?

Head injury. Any head injury or blow to your head?

Dizziness. Experienced any dizziness?

Lumps or swelling. Any lumps or swelling in the head? Any recent infection? Any tenderness?

Eyes

Vision problems (decreased acuity, blurring, blind spots). Any difficulty seeing or any blurring? Come on suddenly, or progress slowly? In one eye or both?

Eye pain. Any eye pain? Please describe.

Strabismus or diplopia. Any history of crossed eyes? Now or in the past? Does this occur with eye fatigue?

Redness or swelling. Any redness or swelling in the eyes?

Watering or discharge. Any watering or excessive tearing?

History of eye problems. Any history of injury or surgery to eye? Or any history of allergies?

Glaucoma. Ever been tested for glaucoma? Results?

Use of corrective lenses. Do you wear glasses or contact lenses? How do they work for you?

Self-care measures. Last vision test? Who tested it? What medications are you taking? Systemic or topical? Do you take any medication specifically for the eyes?

Ears

Earaches. Any earache or other pain in ears?

Infections. Any ear infections? As an adult, or in childhood?

Ear discharge. Any discharge from your ears?

Hearing loss. Ever had any trouble hearing?

Exposure to environmental noise. Any loud noises at home or on the job? For example, do you live in a noise-polluted area, near an airport or busy traffic area? Now or in the past?

Tinnitus. Ever felt ringing, crackling, or buzzing in your ears? When did this occur?

Vertigo. Ever felt vertigo, that is, the room spinning around or yourself spinning? (Vertigo is a true twirling motion.)

Self-care measures. How do you clean your ears?

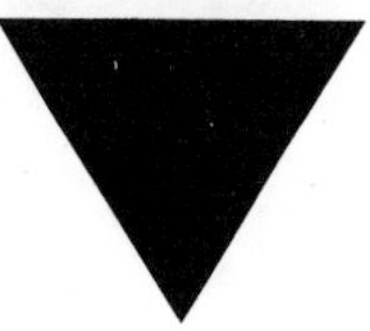

Nose, Mouth, Throat and Neck

VIDEO OUTLINE

- Anatomy review
  - Nose
  - Mouth and throat
  - Neck
- Health history
  - Nose
  - Mouth and throat
  - Neck
- Nose examination
  - External nose
  - Nasal cavity
  - Paranasal sinuses
- Mouth and throat examination
  - Mouth
  - Throat
- Neck examination
  - Neck
  - Lymph nodes
  - Trachea
  - Thyroid gland

EQUIPMENT FOR ASSESSING THE NOSE, MOUTH, THROAT, AND NECK

otoscope with a short, wide-tipped nasal attachment (or a nasal speculum and penlight)
tongue blade
penlight
4 X 4 gauze pad
gloves
stethoscope

CRITICAL THINKING QUESTIONS: NOSE, MOUTH, THROAT, AND NECK

1. How may oral self-care affect mouth examination findings?

2. Describe abnormal findings that may be found during inspection of the internal nose.

3. How do mouth examination findings vary among darkly pigmented people?

4. Describe characteristics of normal and abnormal cervical lymph nodes.

CRITICAL THINKING ANSWERS

1. Poor oral self-care may lead to inadequate oral hygiene and abnormal mouth examination findings. For example, the absence of regular dental care or periodic dental screenings may lead to formation of caries. Ill-fitting dentures may produce lesions or difficulty with speaking or chewing.

2. Inspection of the internal nose may detect rhinitis, in which the nasal mucosa is swollen and bright red, as in an upper respiratory infection. Inspection may also reveal discharge, which is common with rhinitis and sinusitis and may vary from watery and copious to thick, purulent, and green-yellow. In a client with chronic allergy, the nasal mucosa may appear swollen, boggy, pale, and gray.

   Inspection may also detect a deviated septum, which looks like a hump or shelf in one nasal cavity. Or it may uncover a perforated septum, which is a hole in the septum, usually in the cartilaginous part. (It is seen as a spot of light from a penlight shining in the other naris.) In the anterior septum, inspection may commonly reveal epistaxis, which is easily controlled and rarely severe. Less commonly (< 10 percent), it may detect a posterior hemorrhage, which is more profuse, harder to manage, and more serious.

   Finally, inspection may find polyps, which are smooth, pale gray nodules that are avascular, mobile, and nontender. It also may uncover a furuncle (a small boil that is red, swollen, and painful) or a gray-white, nontender lesion associated with carcinoma.

3. Black clients normally may have bluish lips and a dark melanotic line along the gingival margin. In dark-skinned clients, patchy pigmentation of the buccal mucosa is common and normal. Torus palatinus is more common among Native Americans, Inuits, and Asians; a bifid uvula is more common in Native Americans.

4. Cervical lymph nodes often are palpable in healthy clients, although this palpability decreases with age. Normally, they feel movable, discrete, soft, and nontender.

   Abnormal cervical lymph nodes may exhibit lymphadenopathy (enlargement of more than 1 cm) due to infection, allergy, or neoplasm. In acute infection, they may be bilateral, enlarged, warm, tender, and firm, but freely movable. In chronic inflammation, such as tuberculosis, the nodes are clumped. In cancer, they are hard, unilateral, nontender, and fixed. In human immunodeficiency virus (HIV) infection, the nodes are enlarged, firm, nontender, and mobile. Occipital node enlargement is especially common.

HEALTH HISTORY QUESTIONS

Nose

Discharge. Any nasal discharge or runny nose? Continuous?

Frequent colds. Any unusually frequent or severe colds (upper respiratory infections)? How often do these occur?

Sinus pain. Any sinus pain or sinusitis? How is this treated?

Trauma. Ever had any trauma or a blow to the nose?

Epistaxis (nose bleeds). Any nosebleeds? How often?

Allergies. Any allergies or hay fever? To what are you allergic, e.g., pollen, dust, pets?

Altered smell. Experienced any change in sense of smell?

Mouth and Throat

Sores or lesions. Noticed any sores or lesions in the mouth, tongue, or gums?

Sore throat. How about sore throats? How frequently do you get them? Have a sore throat now? When did it start?

Bleeding gums. Any bleeding gums? How long have you had this?

Toothache. Any toothache? Do your teeth seem sensitive to hot or cold? Have you lost any teeth?

Hoarseness. Any hoarseness or voice change? For how long?

Dysphagia. Any difficulty swallowing? How long have you had it?

Altered taste. Any change in sense of taste?

Smoking or alcohol use. Do you smoke? Pipe or cigarettes? Smokeless tobacco? How many packs per day? For how many years? When was your last alcohol drink? How much alcohol did you drink that time? How much alcohol do you usually drink?

Self-care measures. Tell me about your daily dental care. Do you use a toothbrush and floss regularly?

Neck

Neck pain. Any neck pain?

Limited motion. Any limitations to neck range of motion? Any numbness or tingling in shoulders, arms, or hands?

Lumps or swelling. Any lumps or swelling in the neck? Any recent infection? Any tenderness?

History of neck surgery. Ever had surgery of the neck? For what condition? When did the surgery occur? How do you feel about the results?

Breasts and Regional Lymphatics

VIDEO OUTLINE

- Anatomy review
  - Breasts
  - Lymphatics
- Health history
  - Breast symptoms
  - Breast history and self-care
  - Axillary symptoms
- Breast and lymphatic examination
  - Breast inspection
  - Skin
  - Screening for retraction
  - Axillary inspection and palpation
  - Breast palpation
  - Male breast examination
  - Teaching breast self-examination

EQUIPMENT FOR ASSESSING BREASTS AND REGIONAL LYMPHATICS

small pillow
centimeter ruler
teaching aid about breast self-examination

CRITICAL THINKING QUESTIONS: BREASTS AND REGIONAL LYMPHATICS

1. How do breast assessment findings differ between older women and younger adult women?

2. How should you modify breast palpation in a woman with large, pendulous breasts?

3. Which conditions may be associated with a breast lump? Nipple rash? Enlarged axillary lymph nodes?

4. How does breast examination in men differ from that in women?

CRITICAL THINKING ANSWERS

1. On inspection, a younger woman's breasts should be symmetrical in size and shape, although one breast normally may be slightly larger than the other. The skin should be smooth and even colored. The nipples should be symmetrically placed on the same plane on the two breasts. They normally protrude, although some are flat and some are inverted. On palpation, normal breast tissue feels firm, smooth, and elastic, but may feel softer and looser after pregnancy. Normally, you may feel a firm transverse ridge of compressed tissue—the inframammary ridge—in the lower quadrants.

   On inspection, an older woman's breasts look pendulous, flattened, and sagging. Nipples may be retracted, but can be pulled outward. On palpation, the breasts feel more granular, and the terminal ductus around the nipple feels more prominent and stringy. Thickening of the inframammary ridge is normal, and it feels more prominent with age.

2. For a woman with large, pendulous breasts, palpate using a bimanual palpation technique. The woman is in a sitting position, leaning forward. Support the inferior part of the breast with one hand. Use your other hand to palpate the breast tissue against your supporting hand.

3. Benign breast disease, cancer, and fibroadenoma may be associated with a breast lump. Mammary duct ectasia and Paget's disease may result in a nipple rash. A local infection of the breast, arm, or hand, or breast cancer metastases may produce enlarged axillary lymph nodes.

4. The male breast exam is much more abbreviated than the female breast exam. In a male client, inspect the chest wall, noting the skin surface and any lumps or swelling. Palpate the areola area for any lump or tissue enlargement. It should feel even, with no nodules or tissue enlargement. The normal male breast has a flat disc of undeveloped breast tissue beneath the nipple.

HEALTH HISTORY QUESTIONS

Breasts

Pain. Any pain or tenderness in the breasts? When did you first notice it?

Lumps. Ever noticed a lump or thickening in the breast? Where?

Discharge. Any discharge from the nipple?

Rash. Any rash on the breast?

Swelling. Any swelling in the breasts? In one spot or all over?

Injury or surgery. Any trauma or injury to the breasts? Ever had surgery on the breasts? Was this a biopsy? What were the biopsy results?

History of breast disease. Any history of breast disease in yourself? In a family member?

Self-care behaviors. Have you ever been taught breast self-examination? If so, how often do you perform it? What helps you remember? Ever had a mammogram? When was the last one?

Regional Lymphatics

Tenderness. Any tenderness in the underarm area?

Lumps. Any lumps in the underarm area?

Swelling. Any swelling in the underarm area?

Rash. Any axillary rash? Please describe it.

Thorax and Lungs

VIDEO OUTLINE

- Anatomy review
  - Thorax
  - Reference lines
  - Lungs
- Health history
  - Respiratory symptoms
  - Past and current respiratory history
  - Respiratory self-care
- Thorax and lung examination
  - Posterior thorax
  - Anterior thorax

EQUIPMENT FOR ASSESSING THORAX AND LUNGS

stethoscope
small centimeter ruler
skin marking pen

CRITICAL THINKING QUESTIONS: THORAX AND LUNGS

1. Which conditions are associated with a productive cough?

2. Describe the characteristics of the following adventitious sounds: fine crackles, coarse crackles, wheezes, and rhonchi.

3. What assessment findings are normal variations in a pregnant woman?

4. Which nursing diagnoses are most appropriate for a person with wheezes, dyspnea, and tachypnea?

CRITICAL THINKING ANSWERS

1. Chronic bronchitis is characterized by a history of productive cough for 3 months of the year for 2 years in a row. Although sputum production is not diagnostic alone, some conditions have characteristic sputum production:
   - white or clear mucoid—colds, bronchitis, viral infections
   - yellow or green—bacterial infections
   - rust colored—tuberculosis, pneumococcal pneumonia
   - pink, frothy—pulmonary edema, some sympathomimetic medications (a side effect may be pink-tinged mucus).

2. *Fine crackles*, or rales, are discontinuous, high pitched, short, crackling, popping sounds heard during inspiration that are not cleared by coughing.

   Coarse crackles, or coarse rales, are discontinuous, low-pitched, bubbling and gurgling sounds that start in early inspiration and may be present in expiration. They may decrease somewhat by suctioning or coughing but will reappear shortly.

   Sibilant *wheezes* are continuous, high-pitched, musical, squeaking, polyphonic sounds that predominate in expiration, but may occur in expiration and inspiration.

   A second type of wheeze, sonorous *rhonchi*, are continuous, low-pitched, monophonic, musical snoring, moaning sounds. They are heard throughout the respiratory cycle, although they are more prominent on expiration. They may be cleared somewhat by coughing.

3. In a pregnant woman, the thoracic cage may appear wider, and the costal angle may feel wider than in the nonpregnant state. Respirations may be deeper, although this can be quantified only with pulmonary function tests.

4. Nursing diagnoses appropriate for a person with wheezes, dyspnea, and tachypnea are: activity intolerance, ineffective breathing pattern, ineffective airway clearance, fluid volume excess, fatigue, anxiety, and sleep pattern disturbance.

HEALTH HISTORY QUESTIONS

Cough. Do you have a cough? When did it start? Gradual or sudden?

Shortness of breath. Ever had any shortness of breath or hard breathing spells? What brings it on? How severe is it? How long does it last?

Chest pain with breathing. Any chest pain with breathing? Please point to the exact location.

Past history of respiratory infection. Any past history of breathing trouble or lung disease, such as bronchitis, emphysema, asthma, or pneumonia?

Cigarette smoking. Do you smoke cigarettes or cigars? At what age did you start? How many packs per day do you smoke now? For how long?

Environmental exposure to respiratory irritants. Are there any environmental conditions that may affect your breathing? Where do you work? At a factory, chemical plant, coal mine, farm, outdoors in a heavy traffic area?

Self-care behaviors. When was your last tuberculin skin test, pneumonia or influenza immunization, or chest x-ray?

Cardiovascular System: Heart and Neck Vessels

VIDEO OUTLINE

- Anatomy review
  - Neck vessels
  - Heart
- Health history
  - Symptoms
  - Cardiac history and risk factors
- Neck vessel examination
  - Carotid artery
  - Jugular veins
- Heart examination
  - Precordium
  - Heart sounds

EQUIPMENT FOR ASSESSING THE CARDIOVASCULAR SYSTEM: HEART AND NECK VESSELS

small centimeter ruler
straight edge (such as a tongue blade or another ruler)
stethoscope with a diaphragm and bell

CRITICAL THINKING QUESTIONS: CARDIOVASCULAR SYSTEM—HEART AND NECK VESSELS

1. What cardiac risk factors are important to explore during the health history? How do they affect cardiovascular function?

2. How would you modify your technique when assessing an older adult's neck vessels?

3. How do you describe sinus arrhythmia and what does it signify?

4. What heart sounds should you expect to hear in a person with aortic stenosis?

CRITICAL THINKING ANSWERS

1. During the health history, the following cardiac risk factors should be explored: nutrition, smoking, alcohol consumption, exercise, and drug use. These factors affect cardiovascular function in different ways. For example, obesity, cigarette smoking, and low activity level can increase the cholesterol level, which increases the risk of coronary artery disease.

2. In an older adult, use caution in palpating and auscultating the carotid artery. Avoid pressure in the carotid sinus area, which could cause a reflex slowing of the heart rate or could compromise circulation in an artery already narrowed by atherosclerosis.

   When measuring jugular venous pressure, view the right internal jugular vein. The aorta stiffens, dilates, and elongates with aging, which may compress the left neck veins and obscure pulsations on the left side.

3. With sinus arrhythmia, the heart rhythm varies with the client's breathing, increasing at the peak of inspiration and slowing with expiration. Sinus arrhythmia occurs normally in children and young adults. Inspiration momentarily causes a decreased stroke volume from the left side of the heart; to compensate, the heart rate increases.

4. A client with aortic stenosis is likely to have a murmur that is loud, harsh, and midsystolic. Its pattern is crescendo-decrescendo. It is loudest at the second right interspace and radiates widely to the side of the neck, down to the left sternal border, or down to the apex. In addition, auscultation is likely to reveal a normal S1, an ejection click, a paradoxical split S2, and S4 (if left ventricular hypertrophy is present).

HEALTH HISTORY QUESTIONS

Chest pain. Any chest pain or tightness?

Dyspnea. Any shortness of breath?

Orthopnea. How many pillows do you use when sleeping or lying down?

Cough. Do you have a cough?

Fatigue. Do you seem to tire easily? Able to keep up with your family and coworkers?

Cyanosis or pallor. Ever noted your facial skin turn blue or ashen?

Edema. Any swelling of your feet and legs?

Nocturia. Do you awaken at night with an urgent need to urinate? How long has this been occurring? Any recent change?

Personal cardiac history. Any personal history of hypertension, elevated blood cholesterol or triglycerides, heart murmur, congenital heart disease, rheumatic fever or unexplained joint pains as a child or youth, recurrent tonsillitis, or anemia?

Family cardiac history. Any family history of hypertension, obesity, diabetes, coronary artery disease, or sudden death at younger age?

Cardiac risk factors.

- Nutrition. Please describe your daily diet. What is your usual weight? Has there been any recent change?
- Smoking. Do you smoke cigarettes or other tobacco? At what age did you start? How many packs per day? For how many years?
- Alcohol. How much alcohol do you usually drink each week or each day? When was your last drink? What was the number of drinks that episode? Have you ever been told you had a drinking problem?
- Exercise. What is your usual amount of exercise each day or week? What type of exercise? If a sport, what is your usual amount?
- Drugs. Do you take any antihypertensives, beta-blockers, calcium channel blockers, digoxin, diuretics, aspirin, anticoagulants, or over-the-counter or street drugs?

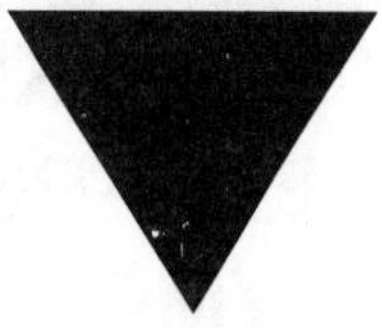

Cardiovascular System: Peripheral Vascular System and Lymphatics

VIDEO OUTLINE

- Anatomy review
  - Arteries
  - Veins
  - Lymphatic vessels
- Health history
  - Symptoms
  - Medications
- Peripheral vascular and lymphatic examination
  - Arms
  - Legs
  - Additional techniques

EQUIPMENT FOR ASSESSING THE CARDIOVASCULAR SYSTEM: PERIPHERAL VASCULAR SYSTEM AND LYMPHATICS

tape measure
tourniquet
blood pressure cuff and stethoscope
Doppler ultrasonic stethoscope

CRITICAL THINKING QUESTIONS: CARDIOVASCULAR SYSTEM—PERIPHERAL VASCULAR SYSTEM AND LYMPHATICS

1. Which assessment findings are you likely to see in a client who seeks care because of leg pain or cramps?

2. How do ulcers caused by chronic arterial insufficiency compare to those of chronic venous insufficiency?

3. How may aging affect your findings when examining an older adult's peripheral vascular and lymphatic systems?

4. What nursing diagnoses commonly are related to abnormal findings in the peripheral vascular system?

CRITICAL THINKING ANSWERS

1. Leg pain or cramps may be an indication of peripheral vascular disease. If the pain is caused by chronic arterial disease, assessment findings may include deep muscle pain with intermittent claudication and cool, pale skin. On the other hand, if the pain is caused by acute arterial disease, findings may include throbbing pain distal to the occlusion, as well as pallor, pulselessness, paresthesia, poikilothermia (coldness), and paralysis (if severe).

   If the pain results from chronic venous disease, assessment may reveal aching, tired lower legs with pain that increases at the end of the day, along with edema, varicosities, and weeping ulcers at the ankles. However, if the cause is acute venous disease, assessment may detect intense, sharp, deep muscle pain that increases with sharp dorsiflexion and is accompanied by redness, warmth, and swelling.

2. Ulcers caused by chronic arterial insufficiency occur at the toes, metatarsal heads, heels, and lateral malleolus. These ulcers are characterized by a pale ischemic base, well-defined edges, and no bleeding. They are associated with deep muscle pain in the calf or foot, coolness, pallor, elevational pallor, dependent rubor, diminished pulses, and signs of malnutrition.

   Ulcers caused by chronic venous insufficiency occur at the medial malleolus and are characterized by bleeding, uneven edges. They are associated with aching pain in the calf or lower leg; firm brawny edema; coarse, thickened skin; brown discoloration; petechiae; and dermatitis.

3. In an aging adult, the dorsalis pedis and posterior tibial pulses may become more difficult to find. Trophic changes associated with arterial insufficiency (thin shiny skin, thick-ridged nails, loss of hair on lower legs) also occur normally with aging.

4. Nursing diagnoses commonly related to the abnormal findings in the peripheral vascular system include altered tissue perfusion (peripheral), sensory/perceptual alteration (tactile), activity intolerance, body image disturbance, fatigue, impaired tissue integrity, pain, risk for peripheral neurovascular dysfunction, sleep pattern disturbance, and sexual dysfunction.

HEALTH HISTORY QUESTIONS

Leg pain or cramps. Any leg pain or cramps? Where?

Skin changes on arms or legs. Any skin changes on arms or legs? Redness, pallor, blueness, brown discolorations?

Leg swelling. Any swelling in one or both legs? When did this swelling start?

Lymph node enlargement. Any "swollen glands" (lumps, kernels)? Where in body? How long have you had them?

Medications. What medications are you taking? For example, are you taking oral contraceptives or antihypertensives?

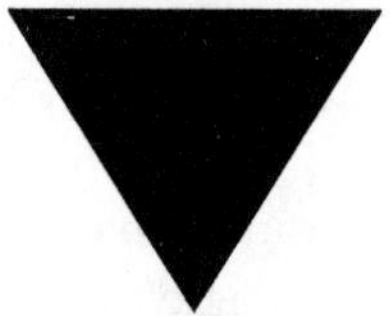

Abdomen

VIDEO OUTLINE

- Anatomy review
  - Surface landmarks
  - Internal anatomy
- Health history
  - Gastrointestinal symptoms
  - Abdominal and medication history and nutrition
- Abdomen examination
  - Inspection
  - Auscultation
  - Percussion
  - Palpation
  - Special procedures

EQUIPMENT FOR ASSESSING THE ABDOMEN

skin-marking pen
small centimeter ruler
stethoscope

CRITICAL THINKING QUESTIONS: ABDOMEN

1. Describe common sites of referred abdominal pain.

2. What bowel sounds would you expect to hear in a client with diarrhea?

3. What abnormal findings can be detected by light palpation of the abdomen?

4. What should you suspect if your palpation detects an enlarged spleen? What should you do next?

CRITICAL THINKING ANSWERS

1. When a person gives a history of abdominal pain, the pain's location may not necessarily be directly over the involved organ. That is because the human brain has no felt image for internal organs. Rather, pain is referred to a site where the organ was located in fetal development. Although the organ migrates during fetal development, its nerves persist in referring sensations from the former location.

   For example, a liver disorder or perforated duodenal ulcer may cause pain on top of the right shoulder. Biliary colic, cholecystitis, pancreatitis, or a duodenal ulcer may produce pain in the right upper quadrant. Appendicitis or a colon disorder may cause pain in the right lower quadrant. Small intestine pain may occur around the umbilicus. Ureteral colic may cause pain along the right or left groin; renal colic may cause pain in the upper right or left quadrant. Heart problems may produce pain on the left side of the chest and left arm. Pancreatitis sometimes results in pain on top of the left shoulder. A penetrating duodenal ulcer may cause pain under the bottom edge of the left scapula or around T9. Cholecystitis may result in pain at the midscapular line around the level of T10. Pancreatitis and renal colic may trigger pain at L1 to L3, which spreads for several inches to the right and left. Rectal lesions may cause pain around S2.

2. Hyperactive bowel sounds may be heard in a client with brisk diarrhea. These loud, gurgling sounds indicate increased motility.

3. Light palpation of the abdomen can detect voluntary muscle guarding, involuntary rigidity, large masses, and tenderness.

   Voluntary muscle guarding occurs when the client is cold, tense, or ticklish. It is bilateral and you will feel the muscles relax slightly during exhalation.

   Involuntary rigidity is a constant boardlike hardness of the muscles. It is a protective mechanism accompanying acute inflammation of the peritoneum. It may be unilateral and the same area usually becomes painful when the person increases intraabdominal pressure by attempting a sit-up.

4. An enlarged spleen may indicate mononucleosis, infection, or trauma. If you feel an enlarged spleen, refer the client but do not continue to palpate it. An enlarged spleen is friable and can rupture easily with overpalpation. Describe the number of centimeters it extends below the left costal margin.

HEALTH HISTORY QUESTIONS

Changes in appetite. Any change in appetite? Is this a loss of appetite?

Dysphagia. Any difficulty swallowing? When did you first notice this?

Food intolerance. Are there any foods you cannot eat? What happens if you do eat them: allergic reaction, heartburn, belching, bloating, indigestion?

Abdominal pain. Any abdominal pain? Please point to it.

Nausea or vomiting. Any nausea or vomiting? How often? How much comes up? What is the color? Is there an odor?

Changes in usual bowel habits. How often do you have a bowel movement?

Abdominal history. Any history of gastrointestinal problems: ulcer, gallbladder disease, hepatitis/jaundice, appendicitis, colitis, hernia?

Medications. What medications are you currently taking? What about alcohol? Cigarettes?

Nutrition. Now I would like to ask you about your diet. Please tell me all the food you ate yesterday, starting with breakfast.

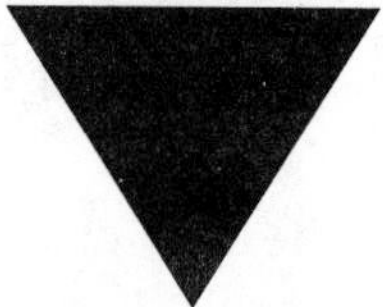

Musculoskeletal System

VIDEO OUTLINE

- Anatomy review
  - Bones
  - Joints
- Muscles
- Health history
  - Joint symptoms
  - Muscle complaints
  - Bone problems
  - Functional assessment and self-care
- Musculoskeletal system examination
  - Examination order
  - Temporomandibular joint
  - Cervical spine
  - Shoulders
  - Elbows
  - Wrists and hands
  - Hips
  - Knees
  - Ankles and feet
  - Spine

EQUIPMENT FOR ASSESSING THE MUSCULOSKELETAL SYSTEM

- tape measure
- goniometer
- skin-marking pen

CRITICAL THINKING QUESTIONS: MUSCULOSKELETAL SYSTEM

1. What other assessment findings can you expect to see in a client who reports joint pain?

2. What abnormal findings may commonly be detected during assessment of the wrists and hands?

3. When are genu varum and genu valgum considered normal? What abnormal conditions may also cause them?

4. How does musculoskeletal assessment of an adolescent differ from that of an adult?

CRITICAL THINKING ANSWERS

1. When caused by rheumatoid arthritis, joint pain may be associated with joint stiffness. When caused by acute inflammation, it may be accompanied by joint swelling, heat, and redness. When joint pain is due to joint injury or muscle contracture, it may also cause limited range of motion. When due to rheumatic fever, joint pain may be associated with chills, fever, and recent sore throat.

2. Assessment of the wrists and hands may reveal subluxation of the wrist, ulnar deviation, ankylosis, Dupuytren's contracture, swan neck or boutonniere deformity in the fingers, atrophy of the thenar eminence, ganglion in the wrist, synovial swelling on the dorsum, generalized swelling, tenderness, Heberden's and Bouchard's nodules, loss of range of motion, limited motion, pain on movement, and Tinel's sign.

3. Genu varum (bow-legged stance) normally occurs for 1 year after a child begins walking. Genu valgum (knock knees) normally occurs between ages 2 and 31/2. Genu varum also occurs with rickets. Genu valgum also occurs with rickets, poliomyelitis, and syphilis.

4. For musculoskeletal assessment of an adolescent, proceed as with the adult, except pay special note to spinal posture. Kyphosis is common during adolescence because of chronic poor posture.

   Screen for scoliosis starting at age 12. Seat yourself behind the standing child, and ask the child to bend forward to touch the toes. Expect a straight vertical spine while standing and also while bending forward. Posterior ribs should be symmetric, with equal elevation of shoulders, scapulae, and iliac crests. You may wish to mark each spinous process with a felt marker. The line-up of ink dots highlights even a subtle curve.

HEALTH HISTORY QUESTIONS

Joints. Any problems with your joints? Any pain, stiffness, limited movement, swelling, heat, or redness?

Muscles. Any problems in the muscles, such as any pain or cramping? Which muscles? Any weakness in muscles?

Bones. Any bone pain? Is the pain affected by movement? Any deformity of any bone or joint? Any accidents or trauma ever affected the bones or joints, such as fractures, joint strain, sprain, or dislocation? Which ones?

Functional assessment. Do your joint, muscle, or bone problems create any limits on your usual activities of daily living? Which ones?

Self-care behaviors. Any occupational hazards that could affect the muscles and joints? Does your work involve heavy lifting? Or any repetitive motion or chronic stress to joints? Any efforts to alleviate these?

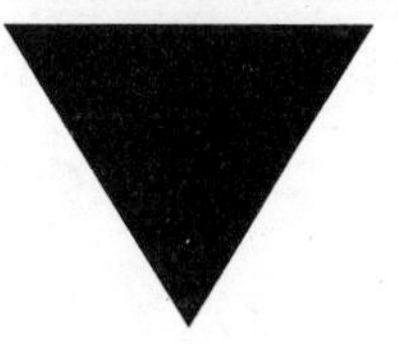

Neurologic System: Cranial Nerves and Sensory System

VIDEO OUTLINE

- Anatomy review
  - Central nervous system
  - Peripheral nervous system
    - Cranial nerves
    - Spinal nerves
    - Sensory pathways
- Health history
  - Neurologic symptoms
  - Neurologic history
- Cranial nerve examination
  - CN I—Olfactory nerve
  - CN II—Optic nerve
  - CN III, IV, and VI—Oculomotor, trochlear, and abducens nerves
  - CN V—Trigeminal nerve
  - CN VII—Facial nerve
  - CN VIII—Acoustic nerve
  - CN IX and X—Glossopharyngeal and vagus nerves
  - CN XI—Spinal accessory nerve
  - CN XII—Hypoglossal nerve
- Sensory system examination
  - Spinothalamic tract
    - Pain
    - Temperature
    - Light touch
  - Dorsal columns
    - Vibration
    - Position
    - Tactile discrimination

EQUIPMENT FOR ASSESSING THE NEUROLOGIC SYSTEM—CRANIAL NERVES AND SENSORY SYSTEM

Cranial Nerves

familiar aromatic substances
hand-held vision screener
opaque cards
ophthalmoscope
penlight
cotton wisp
cotton swab
substances to taste
128-Hertz tuning fork
tongue blade

Sensory System

tongue blade
two test tubes
cotton wisp
tuning fork
familiar small objects, such as a key
paper clip

CRITICAL THINKING QUESTIONS: NEUROLOGIC SYSTEM—CRANIAL NERVES AND SENSORY SYSTEM

1. Which cranial nerve and sensory system assessments would you include in a neurologic screening examination?

2. Describe abnormal assessment findings that occur with lower motor neuron dysfunction of cranial nerve VII.

3. How would you modify your techniques when assessing an older adult's sensory system?

4. Which nursing diagnoses are appropriate for individuals with cranial nerve or sensory deficits?

CRITICAL THINKING ANSWERS

1. In a neurologic screening examination, observe mental status during the health history. Then during the examination, test cranial nerves II (optic); III, IV, and VI (extraocular muscles); V (trigeminal); and VII (facial mobility). To screen the sensory system, assess superficial pain, light touch, and vibration in the arms and legs.

2. When the client tries to wrinkle the forehead or close the eyes tightly, you will see absent or asymmetrical facial movement in Bell's palsy, a lower motor neuron disease that causes paralysis of half of the face. If other lower motor neuron dysfunctions (such as swelling from ear or meningeal infections) cause paralysis, loss of taste also occurs.

3. When assessing an older adult's sensory system, use the same examination as for the younger adult. But be aware that some aging adults show a slower response to your requests, especially to those calling for coordination of movements.

4. Nursing diagnoses appropriate for individuals with cranial nerve or sensory deficits include sensory perceptual alteration (kinesthetic), impaired verbal communication, reflex incontinence, and unilateral neglect.

   Related nursing diagnoses may include activity intolerance, anxiety, risk for aspiration, body image disturbance, risk for caregiver role strain, diversional activity deficit, dysreflexia, fear, impaired home maintenance management, hopelessness, impaired physical mobility, risk for trauma, sensory perceptual alteration (tactile, visual), sexual dysfunction, risk for impaired skin integrity, social isolation, altered thought processes, total incontinence, and altered urinary elimination.

HEALTH HISTORY QUESTIONS

Headache. Any unusually frequent or severe headaches?

Dizziness or vertigo. Ever feel lightheaded, a swimming sensation, or like feeling faint?

Seizures. Ever had any convulsions? When did they start? How often do they occur?

Tremors. Any shakes or tremors in the hands or face? When did these start?

Weakness. Any weakness or problem moving any body part? Is this generalized or local? Does it occur with anything?

Incoordination. Any problem with coordination? Any problem with balance when walking? Do you list to one side? Any falling? Which way? Do your legs seem to give way? Any clumsy movement?

Numbness or tingling. Any numbness or tingling in any body part? Does it feel like pins and needles? When did this start? Where do you feel it? Does it occur with activity?

Difficulty swallowing. Any problem swallowing? Does this occur with solids or liquids? Have you experienced excessive saliva or drooling?

Head injury. Ever had any head injury? Please describe.

History of significant neurologic problems. Any history of stroke (cerebrovascular accident), spinal cord injury, meningitis, encephalitis, congenital defect, or alcoholism?

Exposure to environmental or occupational hazards. Are you exposed to any environmental or occupational hazards, such as insecticides, organic solvents, or lead?

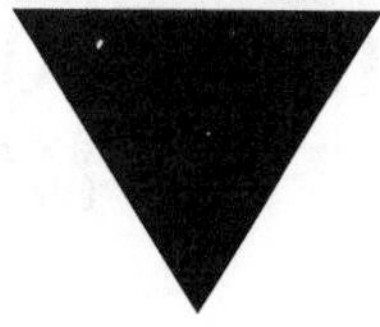

Neurologic System: Motor System and Reflexes

VIDEO OUTLINE

- Anatomy review
  - Central nervous system
    - Corticospinal tract
    - Extrapyramidal tract
    - Cerebellar system
  - Reflex arc
- Health history
  - Neurologic symptoms
  - Neurologic history
- Motor system examination
  - Muscles
  - Cerebellar function
    - Balance
    - Coordination and skilled movements
- Reflex examination
  - Deep tendon reflexes
    - Biceps reflex
    - Triceps reflex
    - Brachioradialis reflex
    - Quadriceps reflex
    - Achilles reflex
    - Clonus
  - Superficial reflexes
    - Abdominal reflexes
    - Cremasteric reflex
    - Plantar reflex

EQUIPMENT FOR ASSESSING THE NEUROLOGIC SYSTEM: MOTOR SYSTEM AND REFLEXES

tongue blade

reflex hammer

CRITICAL THINKING QUESTIONS: NEUROLOGIC SYSTEM—MOTOR SYSTEM AND REFLEXES

1. Which motor system and reflex assessments would you include in a neurologic screening examination?

2. What abnormal findings may commonly be detected when assessing a child's gait?

3. What findings would you expect to see when assessing gait and balance in an older adult?

4. What techniques can you use to elicit deep tendon reflexes?

CRITICAL THINKING ANSWERS

1. In a neurologic screening examination, assess the client's gait, balance, and knee flexion, and test the client's biceps, triceps, patellar, and Achilles reflexes.

2. When assessing a child's gait, abnormal findings include staggering, falling, weakness in climbing up or down stairs, broadbased gait beyond toddlerhood, scissor gait, and failure to hop after age 5.

3. In an older adult, the gait may be slower and more deliberate than in a younger adult, and it may deviate slightly from a midline path.

4. To stimulate a deep tendon reflex, make sure the client's limb is relaxed and the muscle is partially stretched. Direct a short snappy blow of the reflex hammer onto the muscle's insertion tendon.

   If the reflex does not appear, encourage further relaxation, vary the client's position, or increase the strength of the blow.

   Also try reinforcement to relax the muscles and enhance the response. Ask the client to perform an isometric exercise in a muscle group somewhat away from the one being tested. For example, to enhance a patellar reflex, ask the client to lock the hands over the wrists and pull. To enhance a biceps response, ask the client to clench the teeth or grasp the thigh with the opposite hand.

HEALTH HISTORY QUESTIONS

Headache. Any unusually frequent or severe headaches?

Dizziness or vertigo. Ever feel lightheaded, a swimming sensation, or like feeling faint?

Seizures. Ever had any convulsions? When did they start? How often do they occur?

Tremors. Any shakes or tremors in the hands or face? When did these start?

Weakness. Any weakness or problem moving any body part? Is this generalized or local? Does it occur with anything?

Incoordination. Any problem with coordination? Any problem with balance when walking? Do you list to one side? Any falling? Which way? Do your legs seem to give way? Any clumsy movement?

Numbness or tingling. Any numbness or tingling in any body part? Does it feel like pins and needles? When did this start? Where do you feel it? Does it occur with activity?

Difficulty swallowing. Any problem swallowing? Does this occur with solids or liquids? Have you experienced excessive saliva or drooling?

Head injury. Ever had any head injury? Please describe.

History of significant neurologic problems. Any history of stroke (cerebrovascular accident), spinal cord injury, meningitis, encephalitis, congenital defect, or alcoholism?

Exposure to environmental or occupational hazards. Are you exposed to any environmental or occupational hazards, such as insecticides, organic solvents, or lead?

Male Genitalia, Anus, Rectum, and Prostate

VIDEO OUTLINE

- Anatomy review
  - Penis
  - Scrotum
  - Inguinal area
  - Anus and rectum
  - Prostate
- Health history
  - Genitourinary symptoms
  - Genitourinary history
  - Lower GI symptoms
  - Lower GI history
- Male genitalia examination
  - Penis
  - Scrotum
  - Hernia
  - Inguinal lymph nodes
- Anus, rectum, and prostate examination
  - Anus
  - Rectum
  - Prostate gland
- Testicular self-examination

EQUIPMENT FOR ASSESSING MALE GENITALIA, ANUS, RECTUM, AND PROSTATE

- gloves
- materials for collection of urethral specimens
- lubricating jelly
- fecal occult blood test supplies
- teaching aid about testicular self-examination

CRITICAL THINKING QUESTIONS: MALE GENITALIA, ANUS, RECTUM, AND PROSTATE

1. Which presenting symptoms are associated with abnormalities of the male genitalia?

2. What abnormal findings may be detected during inspection of the penis?

3. How do genitalia assessment findings in a male infant compare to those in a male adolescent?

4. Describe abnormal findings that may be noted on inspection of the perianal canal of an infant or child.

CRITICAL THINKING ANSWERS

1. Presenting symptoms associated with abnormalities of the male genitalia include urinary frequency, urgency, hesitancy, or straining; nocturia; dysuria; cloudy, discolored, or foul-smelling urine; hematuria; penile pain, lesions, or discharge; and scrotal pain, lumps, or swelling.

2. Abnormal findings that may be detected during inspection of the penis include inflammation and lesions, such as nodules, a solitary ulcer (chancre), grouped vesicles or superficial ulcers, and wartlike papules. Other abnormalities may include phimosis, paraphimosis, hypospadias, epispadias, pubic lice or nits, and urethral stricture, inflammation, or discharge.

3. In a male infant, the penis is usually 2 to 3 cm long. In a circumcised infant, the glans looks smooth with the meatus centered at the tip. In an uncircumcised infant, the foreskin is normally tight during the first 3 months and should not be retracted. After age 3 months, the infant's foreskin returns to its original position easily after retraction. The scrotum looks large in relation to the penis. The cremasteric reflex is strong. The testes are 1.5 to 2 cm in size.

   In a male adolescent, the penis, testes, and scrotum are larger. Pubic and axillary hair is present. The scrotum color is darker, and the scrotal skin is rougher.

4. Diaper rash is common in children younger than age 1 year and is exhibited as a generalized reddened area with papules or vesicles. Less common abnormal findings include imperforate anus, pustules (caused by secondary infection of diaper rash), signs of physical or sexual abuse, and fissure.

HEALTH HISTORY QUESTIONS

Genitourinary Tract

Frequency, urgency, and nocturia. Urinating more often than usual? Feel as if you cannot wait to urinate? Awaken during the night because you need to urinate?

Dysuria. Any pain or burning with urinating?

Hesitancy and straining. Any trouble starting the urine stream?

Urine discoloration. Is the usual urine clear, discolored, cloudy, foul-smelling, or bloody?

Penis. Any penile pain, lesions, tension, or discharge?

Scrotum, self-care behaviors. Any problem with the scrotum or testicles, such as pain or lumps? Do you perform testicular self-examination?

Genitourinary history. Any difficulty controlling your urine? Any history of kidney disorder, flank pain, urinary tract infection, or prostate trouble?

Sexual activity and contraceptive use. Are you in a relationship involving sexual intercourse now? Do you and your partner use a contraceptive?

STD contact. Any sexual contact with a partner having a sexually transmitted disease, such as gonorrhea, herpes, AIDS, chlamydia, venereal warts, or syphilis?

Lower GI Tract

Usual bowel routine. Do your bowels move regularly? How often? Usual color? Hard or soft? Pain while passing a bowel movement?

Changes in bowel habits. Any change in usual bowel habits? Loose stools or diarrhea? When did this start? Is the diarrhea associated with nausea and vomiting, abdominal pain, or something you ate recently?

Rectal bleeding or blood in the stool. Ever had black or bloody stools? When did you first notice blood in the stools? Is the color bright red or dark red-black? How much blood? Spotting on the toilet paper or outright passage of blood with the stool? Do the bloody stools have a particular smell?

Medications. What prescription and over-the-counter medications do you take, including laxatives, stool softeners, and iron pills? Which ones? How often? Do you ever use enemas to move your bowels? How often?

Rectal conditions. Any problems in rectal area, such as itching, pain, burning, or hemorrhoids? How do you treat these? Any hemorrhoid preparations? Ever had a fissure or fistula? How was this treated?

Family history of bowel disorders. Any family history of polyps or cancer in colon or rectum, inflammatory bowel disease, or prostate cancer?

Self-care behaviors. What is the usual amount of high-fiber foods in your daily diet, including cereals, apples and other fruits, vegetables, and whole-grain breads? How many glasses of water do you drink each day?

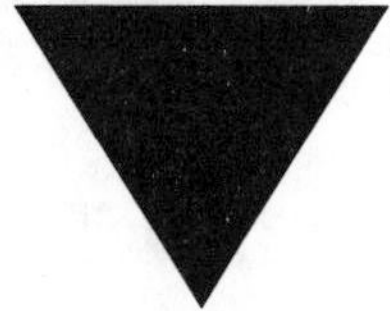

Female Genitalia, Anus, and Rectum

VIDEO OUTLINE

- Anatomy review
  - External genitalia
  - Internal genitalia
  - Anus and rectum
- Health history
  - Genitourinary symptoms
  - Genitourinary history
  - Lower GI symptoms
  - Lower GI history
- Female genitalia examination
  - External genitalia
  - Internal genitalia
  - Cervical smears and cultures
  - Bimanual examination
- Anus and rectum examination
  - Rectovaginal examination
  - Anus
  - Rectum

EQUIPMENT FOR ASSESSING FEMALE GENITALIA, ANUS, AND RECTUM

handheld mirror
gloves
protective clothing and eyewear
basin of warm water
proper-size vaginal speculum
large cotton-tipped applicators
materials for cytologic studies
fixative
water-soluble lubricant
fecal occult blood test supplies
gooseneck lamp

CRITICAL THINKING QUESTIONS: FEMALE GENITALIA, ANUS, AND RECTUM

1. What presenting complaint would lead you to assess the female genitalia?

2. How may you adapt the female genitalia assessment to allow for health education?

3. How do normal genitalia assessment findings differ between nulliparous women and parous women who gave birth vaginally?

4. What normal and abnormal assessment findings may commonly be detected by a rectovaginal examination?

CRITICAL THINKING ANSWERS

1. A presenting complaint of urinary symptoms or vaginal discharge would lead you to assess the female genitalia.

2. To allow for health education during the female genitalia assessment, use the mirror pelvic examination. In this examination, the client props herself up on one elbow (or rests as the head of the table is raised) and holds a mirror between her legs during the examination. The client can see all that the examiner is doing and has a full view of her genitalia. The mirror works well for teaching normal anatomy and its relation to sexual behavior.

3. In a nulliparous woman, the labia meet in the midline. The perineum feels thick, smooth, and muscular. As the woman squeezes the vaginal opening, it feels tight around the examiner's fingers. The cervical opening is small and round.

4. Normal assessment findings are a smooth, thin, firm, and pliable rectovaginal septum; a firm, smooth uterine wall and fundus; a nonpalpable rectovaginal pouch; a small, round cervix; a smooth, even, muscular anal canal; even anal sphincter tone; a smooth rectal wall with no nodularity; and soft, brown stool (if any) on your gloved finger when it is removed.

   Abnormal findings are nodularity or thickening of the rectovaginal septum; decreased or increased anal sphincter tone; perianal tenderness; hemorrhoids; polyps; mass; jelly-like mucus shreds mixed with stool; bright red blood on stool surface or mixed with stool; black, tarry stool; grey, tan stool; pale yellow, greasy stool; or occult bleeding.

HEALTH HISTORY QUESTIONS

Genitourinary Tract

Urinary symptoms. Any problems with urinating? Frequently and small amounts? Cannot wait to urinate?

Vaginal discharge. Any unusual vaginal discharge? Increased amount?

Menstrual history. Tell me about your menstrual periods.

Obstetric history. Have you ever been pregnant?

Menopause. Have your periods slowed down or stopped?

Genitourinary history and self-care. Any other problems in the genital area? Sores or lesions now or in the past? How were these treated? How often do you have a gynecologic checkup?

Sexual activity. Often women have a question about their sexual relationship and how it affects their health. Do you?

Contraceptive use. Are you currently planning a pregnancy, or avoiding pregnancy?

Sexually transmitted disease (STD) contact. Any sexual contact with a partner having a sexually transmitted disease, such as gonorrhea, herpes, AIDS, chlamydial infection, venereal warts, or syphilis? When? How was this treated? Were there any complications? Any precautions to reduce the risk of STDs? Use condoms at each episode of sexual intercourse?

Lower GI Tract

Usual bowel routine. Do your bowels move regularly? How often? Usual color? Hard or soft? Pain while passing a bowel movement?

Changes in bowel habits. Any change in usual bowel habits? Loose stools or diarrhea? When did this start? Is the diarrhea associated with nausea and vomiting, abdominal pain, or something you ate recently?

Rectal bleeding or blood in the stool. Ever had black or bloody stools? When did you first notice blood in the stools? Is the color bright red or dark red-black? How much blood? Spotting on the toilet paper or outright passage of blood with the stool? Do the bloody stools have a particular smell?

Medications. What prescription and over-the-counter medications do you take, including laxatives, stool softeners, and iron pills? Which ones? How often? Do you ever use enemas to move your bowels? How often?

Rectal conditions. Any problems in rectal area, such as itching, pain, burning, or hemorrhoids? How do you treat these? Any hemorrhoid preparations? Ever had a fissure or fistula? How was this treated?

Family history of bowel disorders. Any family history of polyps or cancer in colon or rectum, inflammatory bowel disease, or prostate cancer?

Self-care behaviors. What is the usual amount of high-fiber foods in your daily diet, including cereals, apples and other fruits, vegetables, and whole-grain breads? How many glasses of water do you drink each day?

Head-to-Toe Examination of the Pregnant Woman

VIDEO OUTLINE

- First trimester assessment
  - Health history
  - Measurement
  - Vital signs
  - Musculoskeletal system
  - Head and face
  - Eyes
  - Ears
  - Nose
  - Mouth and throat
  - Neck
  - Extremities
  - Thorax and lungs
  - Heart
  - Breasts
  - Abdomen
  - Genitalia
- Third trimester assessment
  - Measurement, vital signs
  - Musculoskeletal system
  - Thorax and lungs
  - Heart
  - Breasts
  - Abdomen
  - Fundal height
  - Leopold's maneuvers
  - Fetal heart tones

EQUIPMENT FOR ASSESSING THE PREGNANT WOMAN

standing scale with height attachment
thermometer
sphygmomanometer
stethoscope
urine specimen cup
gown
drape
eye chart, opaque card, and ophthalmoscope
otoscope (with ear and nose speculum attachments)
tongue blade
penlight
glass of water
reflex hammer
wedge or small pillow
gloves
gooseneck lamp
vaginal speculum
specimen-collection supplies
lubricant
marking pen
tape measure marked in centimeters
pelvimeter
tissues
Doppler ultrasound device

CRITICAL THINKING QUESTIONS: HEAD-TO-TOE EXAMINATION OF THE PREGNANT WOMAN

1. What information does an obstetric history provide and how is it used?

2. Why should you document the client's position when taking her blood pressure?

3. When is edema in the legs a danger sign in a pregnant client?

4. Why are the external genitalia examined?

5. Why are pelvic measurements important to a prenatal assessment?

6. What is the significance of a fundal height that is higher or lower than expected for the client's weeks of gestation?

CRITICAL THINKING ANSWERS

1. The obstetric history provides information about the number, dates, and outcomes of previous pregnancies. To obtain key data, the examiner may use the G/TPAL method, which gathers information about:
   - **G**ravidity — number of pregnancies
   - **T**erm births — number of neonates born at term (after 37 weeks' gestation), alive or stillborn
   - **P**reterm births — number of neonates born preterm (before 37 weeks' gestation), alive or stillborn
   - **A**bortions — number of pregnancies that ended in spontaneous or therapeutic abortion
   - **L**iving children — number of children who are now alive

   The obstetric history also provides information about each neonate's birth weight and length of gestation; the mother's labor experience, including type of delivery, location of birth, name of obstetrician or nurse-midwife, type of anesthesia, and any labor-related difficulties; maternal complications, such as hypertension, diabetes, infection, or bleeding; neonatal complications; planned infant-feeding method; and special concerns.

   Not only does the client's obstetric history provide vital data about previous pregnancies, but it also alerts the examiner to potential problems in this one.

2. During pregnancy, the client's position can affect her blood pressure. The lateral recumbent position produces the lowest pressure. A seated position creates a higher pressure; a standing position causes a significantly higher pressure. Holding the arm in a dependent position further increases the systolic and diastolic blood pressures.

3. In a pregnant client, edema in the legs may be benign, reflecting blood pooling in the extremities. This naturally occurs as some intravascular fluid shifts into interstitial spaces. However, edema—especially pitting edema—may be a sign of pregnancy-induced hypertension (a potentially life-threatening hypertensive disorder) when accompanied by high blood pressure and proteinuria.

4. The examiner should inspect the skin and mucous membranes of the perineum and vulva to detect excoriations, growths, ulcerations, lesions, varicosities, warts, chancres, and perineal scars. Through inspection and palpation, the examiner should assess for enlargement, tenderness, redness, or discharge of Bartholin's or Skene's glands. These may signal gonorrhea or a chlamydia infection. If the examination reveals a discharge from lesions or inflamed glands, the examiner should obtain a culture specimen to identify the infecting organism and to guide treatment. By providing prompt, effective treatment, the examiner can help prevent the infection from harming the fetus.

5. Pelvic measurements, which include estimations of the subpubic angle, transverse diameter, interspinous diameter, and diagonal conjugate, help evaluate pelvic capacity. They are measured to determine whether the pelvis is large enough to permit vaginal delivery.

6. If the fundal height is higher than expected for the client's weeks of gestation, the examiner should assess further to determine the cause of the unexpected uterine size. The client's estimated date of delivery (EDD) may be incorrect, and the pregnancy may be further advanced than was thought. Or the client's EDD may be correct, but she may be carrying more than one fetus or may have a condition that makes the fetus large for gestational age, such as diabetes mellitus.

   If the fundal height is less than expected for the client's weeks of gestation, the examiner should try to confirm the EDD. If the EDD is correct, the examiner should assess further to determine the cause of the unexpected uterine size because the fetus may be experiencing inadequate growth.

HEALTH HISTORY QUESTIONS

Biographical data. What is your name, address, phone number, age, birthdate, birthplace, marital status, race, religion, cultural origin, and occupation? (Note the client's sex.)

Menstrual history. What is the date of your last menstrual period? (Use this to calculate the EDD.) Was your last menstrual period different from earlier ones? Do you have an idea of when conception occurred?

Current pregnancy. What makes you think that you're pregnant now? Is this a planned pregnancy? If so, what contraceptives had you been using? Do you anticipate any problems with this pregnancy? Do you know your blood type and Rh factor? Are you planning to breastfeed your baby?

Obstetric history. Have you ever been pregnant before? If so, when did each pregnancy occur and how long did each one last? What were the outcomes of each pregnancy? Did you have any problems during previous pregnancies? Did you have vaginal or cesarean deliveries? What was the birth weight and condition of each newborn?

Medical history. Have you ever had a vaginal infection or sexually transmitted disease? Have you had any viral infections, dental treatment, surgery, or X-rays since your last period? What diseases did you have as a child (measles, mumps, etc.)? Do you have any chronic disorders, such as heart disease, diabetes mellitus, or hypertension? Have you ever had abdominal surgery? If so, what type? Do you have any new health concerns now?

Family history. Does anyone in your family or your partner's family have: allergies, bleeding disorders, diabetes, heart disease, hypertension, or kidney problems? Has anyone in either family undergone cesarean delivery, had children born with congenital diseases or deformities, had twins (or other multiple births), or had pregnancy-induced hypertension?

Nutrition. Can you tell me what you ate yesterday? Is this typical for you? What foods do you avoid? Do you crave any particular foods?

Health habits. Have you taken any prescription or over-the-counter drugs since you became pregnant? Do you have any drug allergies? How much caffeine do you consume? Do you use tobacco, alcohol, or illicit drugs? If so, what type and how often?

Psychosocial needs. How do you feel about this pregnancy? How does your partner feel about it? What about your family, friends, and other members of your usual support system? Have you ever attended childbirth education classes? Would you like to know more about them?

Head-to-Toe Examination of the Neonate

VIDEO OUTLINE

- Health history and preparation
- Head-to-toe examination
    - General appearance
    - Vital signs and measurements
    - Skin
    - Head
    - Eyes
    - Ears
    - Nose
    - Mouth
    - Neck
    - Chest
    - Abdomen
    - Arms
    - Legs
    - Genitalia
    - Neurologic system
    - Spine
    - Rectum
    - Final procedures

EQUIPMENT FOR ASSESSING THE NEONATE

- gestational age assessment form
- radiant warmer or examination table with overhead heating element
- neonatal stethoscope
- axillary or other approved thermometer
- platform balance scale
- tape measure
- ophthalmoscope
- small piece of cold metal
- gloves
- Doppler ultrasound device with appropriate-sized blood pressure cuff
- otoscope

CRITICAL THINKING QUESTIONS: HEAD-TO-TOE EXAMINATION OF THE NEONATE

1. What vital information about a neonate can the nurse obtain from the maternal history?

2. What information can the nurse gain from the gestational age assessment? Why is it important to know the neonate's age at the time of the examination?

3. Why is nasal patency so important to the neonate's health? What other techniques may the nurse use to assess it?

4. What effects can maternal hormone levels have on a neonate's assessment findings?

5. What is an innocent murmur and why is it common in neonates?

6. Which developmental reflexes are commonly present in neonates? Why are they tested?

CRITICAL THINKING ANSWERS

1. The maternal history can provide clues to potential or current neonatal health problems. For example, the mother's prenatal history could uncover use of fetal teratogens (such as alcohol, street drugs, and cigarettes) during pregnancy, which could affect the neonate's health. The maternal obstetric history could reveal preterm delivery or low-birth-weight, which could determine the neonate's gestational age. The mother's postnatal history could detect such problems as postpartum depression or infection, which could affect the neonate's care.

2. During the gestational age assessment, you examine the neonate to estimate the amount of time spent in the uterus (number of weeks from the first day of the mother's last menstrual period to the neonate's date of birth). The assessment is based on physical and neurologic characteristics, and requires you to compare the neonate's growth against standardized norms. Gestational age assessment is important because it helps assess the ability of the neonate's organ systems to adapt to extrauterine life and to identify neonates who have a higher risk of complications (those born before or after term or who are small-for-gestational age or are large-for-gestational age).

   You need to know the neonate's age to determine whether development is appropriate for his or her age. Many health and developmental problems may be detected early—and managed—if you know the neonate's age at the time of the examination.

3. You must determine the patency of the neonate's nares because most neonates are obligate nose-breathers. Other ways to assess for nasal patency are to pass a small-lumen catheter down each naris or to observe the neonate breathe with the mouth shut and one nostril occluded at a time. If the nares are blocked, you may suction them gently with a bulb syringe.

4. Maternal production of the hormone estrogen can cause transient breast engorgement, nipple secretion ("witch's milk"), genital engorgement, and a serosanguineous vaginal discharge or leukorrhea (mucoid discharge) in the neonate. These effects should resolve within the first few weeks after birth.

5. Innocent murmurs are heart murmurs that have no valvular or other pathologic cause. They are relatively common in the first 2 to 3 days after birth because the fetal shunts close during this time, marking the transition from fetal to pulmonic circulation. These murmurs are usually grade i or ii, systolic, accompany no other signs of cardiac disease, and disappear in 2 to 3 days. Innocent murmurs may also occur in children because the contractile force of the heart is greater in children, which increases blood flow velocity. This increased velocity plus a smaller chest measurement make an audible murmur.

6. The rooting, sucking, palmar grasp, plantar, Babinski, tonic neck, Moro, placing, and stepping reflexes are commonly present in neonates. They are tested to assess neurologic function. The presence of these reflexes in the neonate and their disappearance at predictable times during the first year or so after birth indicate normal neurologic system function.

HEALTH HISTORY QUESTIONS

Antepartal history. How was this pregnancy spaced? Was it planned? What were the mother's and father's attitudes toward the pregnancy? Was the mother medically supervised? If so, beginning at what month? What was the mother's health during the pregnancy? Were there any complications? During what month were diet and medications prescribed and or taken? How frequently did the mother use alcohol, street drugs, or cigarettes or have x-rays taken during the pregnancy?

Obstetric history. What is the mother's parity? If there were previous pregnancies, what were their outcomes? Were there any complications?

Maternal and paternal medical histories. What is the age and health of each parent? Does either parent have any chronic or acute illness, disorder, or disability?

Family's socioeconomic and demographic factors. What is the place of birth of each family member? Where does the family live? Are all utilities present and working? Is the family's income sufficient for its needs? Who else lives with the parents and neonate? What religion and race, nationality, or culture do the family belong to? How much education have the family members received? What are the family members' current and previous occupations?

Intrapartal history. What was the duration of the pregnancy, name of the hospital, course and duration of labor, and type of delivery? Was anesthesia or any other medication used? What was the neonate's birth weight, Apgar scores, and overall condition? When was the onset of breathing? Was there any cyanosis, need for resuscitation, or use of special equipment or procedures?

Postpartal history. Were there any problems in the nursery, such as neonatal jaundice? How long was the mother's and neonate's hospital stay? Was the neonate discharged with the mother? Was the baby breast fed or bottle fed? How much weight has the neonate gained? Did the neonate have any feeding problems, "blue spells," colic, diarrhea, or patterns of crying and sleeping? How is the mother's postpartum health and reaction to the neonate?

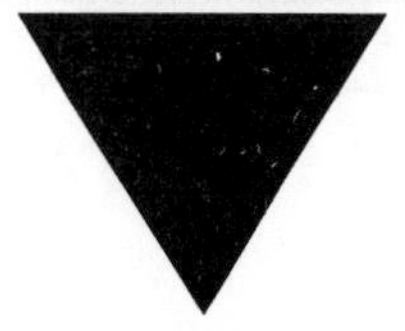

Head-to-Toe Examination of the Child

VIDEO OUTLINE

- Preparation
- Health history and general appearance
- Head-to-toe examination
  - Measurement
  - Head
  - Eyes
  - Ears
  - Nose and sinuses
  - Mouth and throat
  - Neck
  - Chest and heart
  - Abdomen
  - Arms
  - Legs
  - Genitalia

EQUIPMENT FOR ASSESSING THE CHILD

- Snellen E chart
- opaque cards
- wall marked in centimeters or inches
- ruler
- balance scale
- tape measure
- standard growth chart
- thermometer
- sphygmomanometer
- stethoscope with pediatric endpiece
- penlight
- ophthalmoscope
- otoscope
- tuning fork
- tongue blade
- reflex hammer
- gloves

CRITICAL THINKING QUESTIONS: HEAD-TO-TOE EXAMINATION OF THE CHILD

1. When assessing the child's general appearance, what findings would cause concern?

2. What mistakes may commonly occur when assessing a child's height and weight?

3. What condition should an examiner expect if pain results from pulling on the auricle?

4. What abnormal findings may be found when assessing respirations?

5. Name one common illness in which the spleen typically is enlarged.

6. What is the difference between pigeon toes (pes varus) and metatarsus adductus?

CRITICAL THINKING ANSWERS

1. You may note alterations in physical appearance, body structure, mobility, or behavior, which suggest similar health concerns in children and adults. In addition, you may detect poor parental bonding, which may indicate deprivation of physical or emotional care. You also may find signs of child abuse, such as the child's avoidance of eye contact or lack of separation anxiety (if age-appropriate), or the parent's disgust at the child's odor, sounds, drooling, or stools.

2. Use of a narrow measuring pole on the platform scale to measure a child's height may result in a false-low reading because the child may not stand erect. To avoid this problem, measure height by standing the child with the back against a flat ruler taped to the wall, and encourage the child to stand straight and tall and to look straight ahead without tilting the head. Make sure that the shoulders, buttocks, and heels touch the wall. Hold a book or flat board on the child's head at a right angle to the wall. Mark just under the book, noting the measure to the nearest 1 mm.

   When plotting height and weight, use of standard growth charts for all ethnic groups may lead to inaccurate assessment of the child's growth. For example, Asian children (especially girls) typically are shorter and lighter than their white counterparts, who are reflected in the standard growth charts. To avoid inaccurate assessment, use your judgment and consider genetic background of the small-for-age child.

3. Severe painful movement of the auricle (pinna) and tragus may indicate otitis externa, an infection of the outer ear. Other symptoms include redness and swelling of the auricle and canal, scanty purulent discharge, scaling, itching, fever, and enlarged tender regional lymph nodes. Hearing is normal or slightly diminished.

4. In children, a rapid respiratory rate commonly may accompany pneumonia, fever, pain, heart disease, or anemia. Asymmetric expansion may occur with diaphragmatic hernia or pneumothorax. In children under age 7, the absence of abdominal respirations occurs with inflammation of the peritoneum.

5. In a child, the spleen normally is easily palpable with a soft, sharp, movable edge. However, the spleen typically is enlarged in an acute infection, such as mononucleosis, or trauma. An enlarged spleen is tender only if the peritoneum is inflamed.

6. In pigeon toes, or toeing in, the child tends to walk on the lateral side of the foot, and the longitudinal arch looks higher than normal. It often starts as a forefoot adduction, which usually corrects spontaneously by age 3, as long as the foot is flexible. In metatarsus adductus, the hindfoot aligns with the lower leg and just the forefoot angles inward. It usually is present at birth and resolves spontaneously by age 3.

HEALTH HISTORY QUESTIONS

Biographical data. What is the child's name, nickname, address, phone number, parents' names and work phone numbers, child's age, birthdate, birthplace, sex, race, and ethnic origin. What other children and family members live at home?

Source of history. Who is furnishing the information and what is his or her relationship to the child? How reliable is the informant? Are there any special circumstances, such as the need for an interpreter?

Reason for seeking care. What is the reason for the visit?

Present health or history of present illness. What is the usual health of the child? Are there any common health problems or major health concerns? If the child is ill, what are the symptoms' location, character or quality, quantity or severity, timing, setting, aggravating or relieving factors, and associated factors. How does the parent know the child is in pain? Assess the parent's coping ability and other family members' reactions to the child's symptoms and illness.

Past health. What was the child's prenatal status, labor, delivery, and postnatal status. Has the child had any illnesses, serious accidents or injuries, serious or chronic illnesses, hospitalizations, operations, or allergies? Has the child had the necessary immunizations? Is the child currently taking any medications?

Developmental history. What was the child's height and weight at birth and at ages 1, 2, 5, and 10? Has the child had any rapid gain or loss? What is the child's process of dentition? At what ages did milestones occur, such as holding the head erect, walking, speaking words with meaning, and toilet training? What is the child's current state of development?

Nutritional history. How is the child's appetite? What has the child eaten in the past 24 hours and the past week?

Family history. What is the age and health or cause of death of the child's blood relatives, such as parents, grandparents, and siblings?

Review of systems. What is the state of the child's overall health, skin, head, eyes, ears, nose and sinuses, mouth and throat, neck, breasts, respiratory system, cardiovascular system, gastrointestinal system, urinary system, genital system, sexual health, musculoskeletal system, neurologic system, hematologic system, and endocrine system?

Functional assessment. How would you characterize the child's interpersonal relationships, activity and rest patterns, home environment, exposure to environmental hazards, coping and stress management, and habits. What is the parent's economic status? How do the parents promote the child's health?

Head-to-Toe Examination of the Adult

VIDEO OUTLINE

- Health history
- Head-to-toe examination
  - Measurement
  - Skin
  - Vital signs
  - Head and face
  - Eyes
  - Ears
  - Nose
  - Mouth and throat
  - Neck
  - Posterior and lateral chest
  - Anterior chest
  - Heart
  - Upper extremities
  - Breasts
  - Neck vessels
  - Heart
  - Abdomen
  - Inguinal area
  - Lower extremities
  - Musculoskeletal system
  - Neurologic system
  - Lower extremities
  - Neurologic/musculoskeletal
  - Male genitalia
  - Male rectum
  - Female genitalia

EQUIPMENT FOR ASSESSING THE ADULT

platform scale with height attachment
skinfold calipers
Snellen eye chart
urine collection device
sphygmomanometer
stethoscope with bell and diaphragm endpieces
thermometer
opaque cards
penlight
ophthalmoscope
otoscope
tuning forks (high-pitched or low-pitched)
nasal speculum (for attachment to otoscope)
tongue blades
gloves
glass of water
rulers marked in centimeters
skin-marking pen
small pillow
teaching aid about breast self-examination
tangential lighting
reflex hammer
cotton wisps
key or other familiar-feeling object
teaching aid about testicular self-examination
lubricant
fecal occult blood test materials
vaginal speculum
material for cytologic studies
tissues

CRITICAL THINKING QUESTIONS: HEAD-TO-TOE EXAMINATION OF THE ADULT

1. What information can be gained about the client's mental status during the health history interview?

2. How would you adapt breast inspection for a woman with pendulous breasts?

3. If you detect a heart murmur during auscultation, what should you do?

4. If the client were to have abdominal distention, how would you assess his liver span?

5. What alternative techniques might you use to palpate the liver and spleen?

6. If the popliteal pulse is difficult to find, what technique might you use to palpate it?

7. What techniques can you use to elicit a deep tendon reflex, if it does not appear at first?

CRITICAL THINKING ANSWERS

1. By talking with and observing the client during the health history interview, you obtain information about the client's mental status, which is inferred through such behaviors as consciousness, language, mood, affect, orientation, attention, memory, abstract reasoning, thought processes, thought content, and perceptions.

2. For a client with pendulous breasts, screen for retraction with one additional technique. To do this, have the woman lean forward while you support her forearms and observe for breast movement. Normally, the breasts move forward freely and symmetrically.

3. If you hear a murmur during auscultation, describe it by indicating these characteristics:
   - *timing* in relation to S1 and S2
   - *loudness* from grade i to grade vi
   - *pitch*, which may be high, medium, or low
   - *pattern*, which may be crescendo, decrescendo, or crescendo-decrescendo
   - *quality*, which may be musical, blowing, harsh, or rumbling
   - *location* in which the murmur is heard best
   - *radiation*, or areas where the sound is transmitted
   - *posture*, if the murmur is affected by a change in the client's position.

   In addition to characterizing the murmur, request an order for the client to have an ECG, phonocardiogram, and echocardiogram to determine whether the murmur is innocent or pathologic.

4. In a client with abdominal distention or tense abdominal muscles, you can use the scratch test to define the liver border. To do this, place your stethoscope over the liver. With one finger, scratch short strokes over the abdomen, starting in the right lower quadrant and moving progressively up toward the liver. When the scratching sound in the stethoscope becomes magnified, you have crossed the border between a hollow organ and a solid one, which is the liver.

5. As an alternative liver palpation technique, you may use the hooking technique. To do this, stand up at the client's shoulder and swivel your body to the right so that you face the client's feet. Hook your fingers over the costal margin from above. As the client takes a deep breath, try to feel the liver edge bump your fingertips.

   As an alternative spleen palpation technique, roll the client onto his or her right side to displace the spleen more forward and downward. Then palpate for the spleen as you would with the client supine.

6. Typically, you would palpate the popliteal pulse with the supine client's leg extended but relaxed, your thumbs anchored on the client's knee, and your fingers curled around into the popliteal fossa. Then you would press your fingers forward hard to compress the artery against the bone (the lower edge of the femur or the upper edge of the tibia). Often, the popliteal pulse is just lateral to the medial tendon. If the pulse remains difficult to find, turn the client prone and lift up the lower leg. Let the leg relax against your arm and press in deeply with both thumbs.

7. If a deep tendon reflex does not appear, try encouraging the client to relax, changing his or her position, or increasing the strength of the reflex hammer's blow. Also try reinforcement to relax the muscles and enhance the response. To do this, ask the client to perform an isometric exercise in a muscle group somewhat away from the one being tested. For example, to enhance a patellar reflex, ask the client to lock the fingers together and "try to pull them apart." To enhance a biceps reflex, ask the client to clench the teeth or to grasp the thigh with the opposite hand.

HEALTH HISTORY QUESTIONS

Biographical data. What is the client's name, address, phone number, age, birthdate, birthplace, sex, marital status, race, ethnic origin, and occupation (usual and present)?

Source of history. Who is furnishing the information? How reliable is the informant? Are there any special circumstances, such as the need for an interpreter?

Reason for seeking care. What is the reason for the visit?

Present health or history of present illness. What is the client's general state of health? If the client is ill, what are the symptoms' location, character or quality, quantity or severity, timing, setting, aggravating or relieving factors, and associated factors. What is the client's perception of the symptom?

Past health. Has the client had any childhood illnesses, accidents, injuries, serious or chronic illnesses, hospitalizations, operations, or allergies? If the client is female, what is her obstetric history? Which immunizations has the client had and when? When was the last examination date? Is the client currently taking any medications?

Family history. What is the age and health or cause of death of the client's blood relatives, such as parents, grandparents, and siblings? Is there any family history of heart disease, high blood pressure, stroke, diabetes, blood disorders, cancer, sickle cell anemia, arthritis, allergies, obesity, alcoholism, mental illness, seizure disorder, kidney disease, or tuberculosis?

Review of systems. What is the state of the client's overall health, skin, hair, head, eyes, ears, nose and sinuses, mouth and throat, neck, breasts, axillae, respiratory system, cardiovascular system, peripheral vascular system, gastrointestinal system, urinary system, genital system, sexual history, musculoskeletal system, neurologic system, hematologic system, and endocrine system?

Functional assessment. Can the client perform activities of daily living? What is the client's self-esteem level, self-concept, daily activity and exercise profile, sleep and rest patterns, nutritional and elimination patterns, interpersonal relationships and resources, coping and stress management, personal habits, alcohol consumption, and exposure to environment hazards.

Perception of health. How does the client define health? How does the client view his or her current health? What are the client's concerns? What does he or she think will happen in the future? What are the client's health goals? What does he or she expect from health care providers?

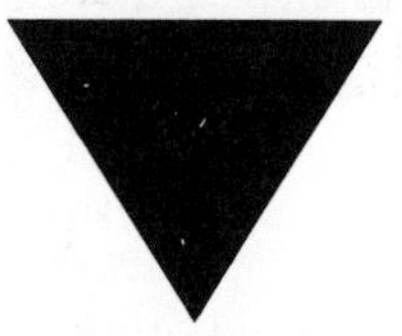

Head-to-Toe Examination of the Older Adult

VIDEO OUTLINE

- Health history
- Head-to-toe examination
    - Measurement
    - Skin
    - Vital signs
    - Head and face
    - Eyes
    - Ears
    - Nose
    - Mouth and throat
    - Neck
    - Posterior and lateral chest
    - Anterior chest
    - Heart
    - Upper extremities
    - Breasts
    - Neck vessels
    - Heart
    - Abdomen
    - Inguinal area
    - Lower extremities
    - Musculoskeletal system
    - Neurologic system
    - Lower extremities
    - Neurologic/musculoskeletal
    - Male genitalia
    - Male rectum
    - Female genitalia

EQUIPMENT FOR ASSESSING THE OLDER ADULT

standing scale with height attachment
lighted Snellen eye chart
near vision (reading) chart
central vision chart, such as Amsler grid
opaque card
urine specimen cup
gooseneck lamp
gloves
drape
sphygmomanometer
stethoscope
thermometer
penlight
ophthalmoscope
otoscope with ear and nose speculum attachments
high-pitched tuning fork
bottle of vanilla or other substance with recognizable smell
tongue blades
glass of water
marking pen
ruler
small pillow
reflex hammer
cotton wisp
low-pitched tuning fork
key or other familiar-feeling object
lubricant
vaginal speculum
specimen-collection supplies
tissues

CRITICAL THINKING QUESTIONS: HEAD-TO-TOE EXAMINATION OF THE OLDER ADULT

1. During the health history, how would you assess a geriatric client's risk factors and functional status?

2. What strategies can you use to assess a geriatric client's understanding of prescribed medications, medication use, and compliance with the prescribed regimen?

3. During a geriatric client's physical examination, how would you screen for risk factors?

4. How could you adapt the physical examination for a geriatric client with arthritis?

5. Which assessment findings may indicate a prostate disorder?

6. What physiologic changes occur in the female genitalia as a result of menopause?

CRITICAL THINKING ANSWERS

1. To assess a geriatric client's risk factors, the examiner should ask about the status of each body system. For example, a client who reports vision changes may be at risk for glaucoma. A client who complains of joint stiffness may be at risk for arthritis and a subsequent decrease in functioning. The examiner also should inquire about socioeconomic factors that may increase his risk. For example, a client with poor vision and little social support may find it difficult to travel to the health care provider's office, which can increase his risk of complications. Or a client with limited finances may be at risk for various disorders because he cannot afford housing, good nutrition, or medications. In addition, the examiner should ask about health habits and beliefs that can raise the client's risk. For example, a client who regularly eats a high-fat, high-sodium diet is at increased risk for developing cardiac disease or hypertension.

   To assess functional status, the examiner may use a standardized instrument that assesses the geriatric client's ability to perform activities of daily living (ADLs), such as using the telephone, getting to places out of walking distance, shopping, doing housework, handling money, eating, dressing, undressing, grooming, getting in and out of bed, bathing or showering, preparing meals, and using the bathroom. Or the examiner can ask detailed questions about the client's ADLs as well as his past and present self-concept, occupation, activity and exercise levels, sleep and rest patterns, nutrition and elimination patterns, interpersonal relationships, resources, coping and stress management, and environment (including any hazards).

2. For each medication the geriatric client takes, the examiner should have him identify its name, prescribed dose, and therapeutic and adverse effects. (If the client is unsure of this information, ask him to bring all the medications in with him.)

   To assess the client's medication use, the examiner can ask if he has a system to remember to take the medication, such as a multi-compartment pill box, egg carton, or alarm and drug information cards. (If he does not have a system, help him create one.) The examiner also may ask the following questions: Does your medicine seem to work well? Does it cause side effects? Do you ever feel like skipping your medication because of them?

   To evaluate the client's compliance further, inquire about factors that may affect his ability to get or use medications. The following questions may help uncover this information: Is cost a problem? Do you ever decrease or skip a dose or postpone refilling a prescription because you can't afford it? Do you have any problems in traveling to the pharmacy to refill a prescription? Do you take any over-the-counter medications, instead of prescription ones? Do you ever share medications with neighbors, friends, or family members?

3. During the physical examination, the examiner should assess each body system, noting any abnormal signs and risk factors. For example, the examiner should note obesity, which increases the client's risk of diabetes and heart disease and can affect his ability to perform ADLs; decreased sense of smell, which can lead to reduced appetite and poor nutrition; and impaired mobility, which can reflect a musculoskeletal disorder and increase the risk of falls and other problems.

   If joint, range-of-motion (ROM), and muscle strength assessments suggest limitations, the examiner should assess the client's risk for reduced functioning by performing a functional assessment for ADLs. This applies the ROM and muscle strength assessments to the accomplishment of specific activities. The examiner uses them to determine whether the client can adequately and safely perform functions essential to independent home life.

4. Before the appointment, the examiner can advise an arthritic geriatric client to take a mild analgesic or anti-inflammatory medication to ease joint pain during positioning. Also the examiner can schedule the appointment for a time when the client's joint pain is at its least.

   During the examination, the examiner should minimize the number of position changes, allow extra time for positioning and repositioning, and allow rest periods if the client needs them. When assessing a joint, the examiner should use firm support, gentle movement, and gentle return to a relaxed state.

5. An abnormal prostate gland may be enlarged or atrophied; flat with no groove; nodular; hard, boggy, soft, or fluctuant; fixed; or tender. An enlarged, smooth, rubbery or firm gland with an obliterated central groove suggests benign prostatic hypertrophy. A swollen, exquisitely tender, slightly asymmetrical gland may indicate acute prostatitis. An enlarged, boggy gland with isolated firm areas suggests chronic prostatitis. One or more hard, irregular, fixed nodules on the gland may be a sign of carcinoma.

6. In their late forties and early fifties, women experience menopause, the decreasing frequency and eventual cessation of menstruation. This causes a decrease in the female hormones, estrogen and progesterone, which produces various changes, including reproductive organ atrophy.

   In a postmenopausal client, the pubic hair is decreased; it may become thin and sparse in later years. As fat deposits decrease, the mons pubis appears smaller and the labia become flatter. In a client over age 60, the size of the clitoris is decreased.

   The internal genitalia also change after menopause. The rugae of the vaginal walls decrease, and the walls look pale pink because of the thinned epithelium. The cervix shrinks and looks pale and glistening. It may retract, appearing to be flush with the vaginal wall. In some clients, the cervix may be difficult to distinguish from the surrounding vaginal mucosa. In others, the cervix may protrude into the vagina if the uterus has prolapsed.

   Upon bimanual examination, the uterus typically feels smaller and firmer, and the ovaries are not palpable.

HEALTH HISTORY QUESTIONS

Biographical data. What is your name, address, phone number, age, birthdate, birthplace, marital status, race, religion, cultural origin, and occupation? (Note the client's sex.)

Social support. Who lives with you? Have you talked to any friends or relatives by phone during the last week? How satisfied are you about how often you see your relatives and friends? Is there someone who would take care of you for a short time or a long time, if needed? Who do you rely on for emotional support or help with problems? Who meets your need for affection?

Economic status. Do you own your own home? Are you covered by private medical insurance, Medicare, Medicaid, or some disability plan? How well do your finances cover your housing, nutrition, and medications? Do you feel that you need any financial assistance?

Psychological health status. Is your daily life full of things that keep you interested? Have you ever very much wanted to leave home? Does it seem that no one understands you? Are you happy most of the time? Do you feel weak all over much of the time? Is your sleep fitful and disturbed? How would you describe your satisfaction with your life in general now? Do you feel you now need help with your mental health? For example, do you feel the need to talk with a counselor or psychiatrist?

Physical health status. During the past month, how many days were you so sick that you couldn't do your usual activities, such as working around the house or visiting with friends? Relative to other people your age, how would you rate your current overall health? Do you use an aid for walking, such as a wheelchair, walker, cane, or anything else? How much do your health problems stand in the way of you doing things you want to do? Have you ever had, or do you currently have, any of the following health problems: arthritis or rheumatism, lung or breathing problem, hypertension, heart trouble, phlebitis or poor circulation in the arms and legs, diabetes or low blood sugar, digestive ulcer, other digestive problem, cancer, anemia, effects of stroke, other neurological problem (specify), thyroid or other glandular problem (specify), skin disorder such as pressure sore or burn, speech problem, hearing problem, vision or eye problem, kidney or bladder problem, problem with falling, problem with eating or your weight (specify), problem with depression or your nerves (specify), problem with behavior (specify), problem with your sexual activity, problem with alcohol, problem with pain, or other health problem (specify).

Health promotion practices. When was the last time you saw your health care provider? What was the reason for that visit? When were your last eye, dental, and hearing exams? What was the date of your most recent mammography, proctoscopy, tonometry, or other test? Do you have any drug allergies? How much caffeine do you consume? Do you use tobacco, alcohol, or illicit drugs? If so, what type and how often?

Cultural beliefs. What culture do you belong to? How do you feel about health care providers who are not of the same cultural background? Does your culture influence how you cook or what you eat? If so, how? How does your culture influence your health-related practices? For example, do you rely on cultural healers or use cultural healing practices, such as using herbal remedies, praying, or wearing talismans? What do you believe promotes health? For example, do you think that eating certain foods, wearing good luck amulets, or performing rituals to ancestors can improve your health?

Activity and sleep patterns. How active are you? How frequently do you walk or get other exercise? What is your usual sleep pattern? Do you feel rested during the day? Do you have enough energy to carry out your daily activities? Do you need naps? If so, how many and how long? Do you have any sleeping problems?

Nutritional habits. Can you tell me what you ate yesterday? Is this typical for you? How does your diet differ from when you were in your 40s and 50s? Why? What factors affect the way you eat? Do you have any food preferences? Do you have any difficulty chewing or swallowing? How many convenience foods and soft foods do you eat? Who shops for food and prepares your meals? Do you eat alone?

Activities of daily living. Of the following activities, tell me which ones you can do without any help and which ones you need help to do: using the telephone, getting to places out of walking distance, shopping for clothes and food, doing your housework, handling your money, feeding yourself, dressing and undressing yourself, taking care of your appearance, getting in and out of bed, taking a bath or shower, preparing your meals, and getting to the bathroom on time. During the past 6 months, have you had any help with such things as shopping, doing housework, bathing, dressing, and getting around?

Medication history. What medications are you taking now or have you taken in the last month? Can you identify the name, dose, therapeutic effects, and adverse effects for each one? How do you take each one? Many people have problems remembering to take their medications, especially ones they need to take regularly. How often do you forget to take your medications? Do you ever skip a dose? If so, how often?

(Adapted from Pearlmen R.: Development of a functional assessment questionnaire for geriatric patients: COPE. *J Chronic Dis* 40:85S–94S, 1987. Elsevier Science Ltd., Pergamon Imprint, Oxford, England.)

Test Manual

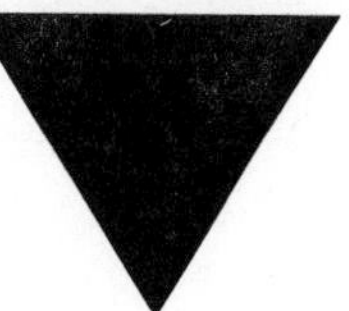

Chapter 1

Assessment for Health and Illness

1. The biomedical model of Western tradition views:
   A. health as the absence of disease.
   B. health and disease as a cyclical process.
   C. the treatment of disease as nursing's primary focus.
   D. optimal health as high-level wellness.

Correct Answer: A

Rationale: The biomedical model of Western tradition views health as the absence of disease.

Cognitive Level: Knowledge

2. Which of the following best describes the role of the nurse when providing holistic care?
   A. Accurately diagnosing and treating an illness
   B. Following the physician's orders when planning the patient's care
   C. Expanding assessment factors to include things such as culture and values, family and social roles, and self care behaviors
   D. Assessing biophysical signs and symptoms in patient care

Correct Answer: C

Rationale: Consideration of the whole person is the essence of holistic health. The holistic model includes such things as culture and values, family and social roles, health self-care behaviors, job-related stress, developmental tasks, and failures and frustrations of life. All are significant to health.

Cognitive Level: Comprehension

3. The public's concept of health has changed since the 1950s. Which of the following statements most accurately describes this change?
   A. Accurate diagnosis and treatment by a physician are essential for all health care.
   B. Lifestyle, personal habits, exercise, and nutrition are essential to health.
   C. An individual is considered healthy when signs and symptoms of disease have been eliminated.
   D. Assessment of health is critical to identifying disease-causing pathogens.

Correct Answer: B

Rationale: The accurate diagnosis and treatment of illness are an important part of health care. But the public's concept of health has expanded since the 1950s. We have an increasing interest in lifestyle, personal habits, exercise and nutrition, and the social and natural environment.

Cognitive Level: Comprehension

4. Why is the concept of prevention essential when describing health?
   A. The majority of deaths among Americans under age 65 are not preventable.
   B. The means to prevention is through treatment provided by primary health care practitioners.
   C. Prevention places emphasis on the link between health and personal behavior.
   D. Disease can be prevented by treating the external environment.

Correct Answer: C

Rationale: A natural progression to prevention now rounds out our concept of health. Guidelines to prevention place emphasis on the link between health and personal behavior.

Cognitive Level: Comprehension

5. Nursing diagnosis:
   A. is used to evaluate the etiology of disease.
   B. is used to evaluate the response of the whole person to actual or potential health problems.
   C. focuses on the function and malfunction of a specific organ system.
   D. is a process based on the medical diagnosis.

Correct Answer: B

Rationale: The nursing diagnosis is used to evaluate the response of the whole person to actual or potential health problems.

Cognitive Level: Knowledge

6. Which of the following statements should be included in the patient's history?
   A. Blood pressure is 170/80.
   B. Patient states that he has a rash.
   C. Patient appears anxious.
   D. Patient has diminished reflexes in legs.

Correct Answer: B

Rationale: Subjective data are information obtained from the patient, what the person says about himself or herself during history taking.

Cognitive Level: Application

7. An example of objective information obtained during the physical assessment includes:
   A. last menstrual period one month ago.
   B. patient history of allergies.
   C. patient use of medications.
   D. 2x5 cm scar present on the right lower forearm.

Correct Answer: D

Rationale: Objective data are information that the health professional observes by inspecting, percussing, palpating, and auscultating during the physical examination; and the patient's record and laboratory studies.

Cognitive Level: Comprehension

8. The nursing assessment database consists of:
   A. making a judgment or diagnosis.
   B. subjective and objective data; and the patient's record and laboratory studies.
   C. nursing and medical diagnoses.
   D. primarily subjective information related to the most recent visit.

Correct Answer: B

Rationale: The database consists of subjective and objective data; and the patient's record and laboratory studies.

Cognitive Level: Comprehension

9. Mr. H., a 40-year-old male, is one-week post hernia repair. He comes to the clinic with complaints of "difficulty getting around the house; I can't even do the dishes without getting tired and sore." When charting the nursing diagnosis most appropriate for Mr. H., you would document:
   A. shortness of breath due to surgery.
   B. dyspnea on exertion.
   C. altered tissue perfusion.
   D. activity intolerance.

Correct Answer: D

Rationale: Nursing diagnoses are used to evaluate the response of the whole person to actual or potential health problems. Medical diagnoses focus on the etiology of the disease.

Cognitive Level: Analysis

10. You are a visiting nurse making an initial home visit for a patient who has many chronic medical problems. Which type of database is most appropriate to collect in this setting?
    A. An episodic database because of the ongoing, complex medical problems of this patient
    B. A follow-up database to evaluate changes at appropriate intervals
    C. An emergency database because of the need to rapidly collect information and make accurate diagnoses
    D. A complete health database because of the nurse's primary responsibility for monitoring the patient's health care

Correct Answer: D

Rationale: The complete database is collected in a primary care setting, such as a pediatric or family practice clinic, independent or group private practice, college health service, women's health care agency, visiting nurse agency, or community health agency. In these settings the nurse is the first health professional to see the patient and has primary responsibility for monitoring the person's health care.

Cognitive Level: Application

11. You are most likely to perform an episodic history:
    A. in an outpatient clinic for the patient who presents with a cold and flu-like symptoms.
    B. while admitting a patient to the hospital for surgery the following day.
    C. on a patient who is experiencing sudden, severe shortness of breath.
    D. upon a patient's admission to a long-term care facility.

Correct Answer: A

Rationale: In an episodic or problem-centered database the nurse collects a "mini" database, smaller in scope than the completed database. It concerns mainly one problem, one cue complex, or one body system.

Cognitive Level: Application

12. Mrs. J. is at the clinic to have her blood pressure checked. She has been coming to your clinic weekly since she changed medications two months ago. You would:
    A. check only her blood pressure since her complete health history was documented two months ago.
    B. collect a follow-up database then check her blood pressure.
    C. obtain a complete health history before checking her blood pressure since much of her history information may have changed.
    D. ask her to read her health record and indicate any changes since her last visit.

Correct Answer: B

Rationale: A follow-up database is used in all settings to follow-up short-term or chronic health problems.

Cognitive Level: Application

13. A.J. is brought by ambulance to the Emergency Room suffering from multiple traumas received in an automobile accident. He is alert and cooperative, but his injuries are quite severe. How would you proceed with the data collection?
    A. Collect all information on the history form including social support patterns, strengths, and coping patterns.
    B. Perform lifesaving measures and not ask any history questions until he is transferred to the Intensive Care Unit.
    C. Collect history information first, then perform the physical examination and institute lifesaving measures.
    D. Simultaneously ask history questions while performing the examination and initiating lifesaving measures.

Correct Answer: D

Rationale: The emergency database call for a rapid collection of the database, often compiled concurrently with lifesaving measures.

Cognitive Level: Analysis

14. The age-specific charts for the periodic health examination:
    A. list a frequency schedule for periodic health visits and preventive services for a specific age group.
    B. recommend that every individual receive an annual physical exam.
    C. are used to help identify the diagnosis of an illness.
    D. are helpful in identifying developmental delays in children.

Correct Answer: A

Rationale: The age-specific charts for the periodic health examination define a lifetime schedule of health care, organized into packages for eight specific age groups.

Cognitive Level: Knowledge

15. A 42-year-old Asian patient is being seen at the clinic for an initial examination. You know that it is important to include cultural information in his health assessment:
    A. to provide cultural health rights for the individual.
    B. to identify the cause of his illness.
    C. to make accurate disease diagnoses.
    D. to provide culturally sensitive and appropriate care.

Correct Answer: D

Rationale: The inclusion of cultural considerations in health assessment is of paramount importance to gather data that are accurate and meaningful and to intervene with culturally sensitive and appropriate care.

Cognitive Level: Comprehension

16. Which of the following statements best describes cultural diversity in the United States as identified in the 1990 Census Report?
    A. The population of Asians will increase in number to exceed that of Hispanics by the 21st century.
    B. Approximately one-half of the population of the United States consists of people from minority racial, ethnic, and cultural groups.
    C. The Native American population is projected to increase slightly by the year 2000.
    D. African Americans comprise more than 30% of the total population in the United States.

Correct Answer: B

Rationale: According to the United States Census Bureau, 51%, more than one-half of the population of the United States, consists of people from non-Anglo-Saxon racial, ethnic and cultural groups.

Cognitive Level: Knowledge

17. In the health promotion model, the focus of the health professional includes:
    A. identifying negative health acts of the consumer.
    B. helping the consumer choose a healthier lifestyle.
    C. identification of biomedical model interventions.
    D. changing the patient perceptions of disease.

Correct Answer: B

Rationale: In the health promotion model, the focus of the health professional is on helping the consumer choose a healthier lifestyle.

Cognitive Level: Knowledge

18. Which of the following would be included in a holistic model of assessment?
    A. A patient's perception of his or her health status
    B. The nurse's perception of disease related to the patient
    C. Anticipated growth and development patterns
    D. Nursing goals for the patient

Correct Answer: A

Rationale: Holistic health views the mind, body, and spirit as functioning as a whole within the environment. A holistic model includes the patient's perception of his or her health status, not the nurse's perception or goals.

Cognitive Level: Comprehension

19. Objective data in the assessment is obtained:
    A. by what the patient says about himself during the history.
    B. during the initial interview.
    C. from the nursing diagnosis.
    D. by the nurse during the physical assessment.

Correct Answer: D

Rationale: Objective data is obtained by the health care professional during the physical examination through inspection, palpation, percussion, and auscultation.

Cognitive Level: Comprehension

20. Which of the following would be considered a risk diagnosis in the classification of nursing diagnoses?
    A. Focusing on strengths and reflecting an individual's transition to higher levels of wellness
    B. Identifying existing levels of wellness
    C. Evaluating previous problems and goals
    D. Identifying potential problems the individual may develop

Correct Answer: D

Rationale: Risk diagnoses are potential problems that an individual does not currently have but is particularly vulnerable to develop.

Cognitive Level: Application

21. Collaborative problems require:
    A. independent nursing actions.
    B. interdependent management by medicine and nursing.
    C. physician orders.
    D. autonomous nursing practice.

Correct Answer: B

Rationale: Collaborative problems are clinical problems that are amenable to interdependent management by medicine and nursing.

Cognitive Level: Knowledge

22. Mr. Smith, age 65, has been diagnosed with hypertension for 10 years. He is not experiencing any problems at this time and is at the clinic for a bi-monthly check-up. Which type of database is most appropriate to collect in this situation?
    A. Problem-centered database
    B. Follow-up database
    C. Complete total database
    D. Emergency database

Correct Answer: B

Rationale: The status of identified problems are evaluated at regular intervals for short-term or chronic health problems such as hypertension.

Cognitive Level: Comprehension

Chapter 2

Developmental Tasks and Health Promotion Across the Life Cycle

1. Jean Piaget proposed four stages of cognitive development. Which of the following statements is true with regard to these stages?
   A. A child who is "gifted" may actually skip a stage and move on to a higher stage.
   B. Each stage is distinct and clearly separate from the other stages.
   C. Each stage builds on the foundations of the previous stages.
   D. A child's age determines what stage he or she is in.

Correct Answer: C

Rationale: The child's cognitive development proceeds through four definite and sequential stages. Although the ages of reaching the stages are approximate, the sequence of stages never varies. All children move through the same stages in the same order; no stage is skipped.

Cognitive Level: Analysis

2. Sigmund Freud's psychoanalytic theory proposes that:
   A. people experience conflict between their natural instincts and the restrictions society places on them.
   B. people are driven by a need for oral gratification all of their lives.
   C. whether people resolve the conflicts in early childhood doesn't seem to affect their adult personalities.
   D. people generally move back and forth through the stages all of their lives.

Correct Answer: A

Rationale: He believed that people experience conflict between their natural instincts and society's restrictions on them.

Cognitive Level: Knowledge

3. Erik Erikson's theory of psychosocial development proposes eight stages of ego development. Each stage involves a bi-polar "crisis." Which statement is true regarding these crises?
   A. If the crisis cannot be resolved at a certain stage, a person generally skips that stage.
   B. There is always an absolute resolution to each crisis.
   C. An effective resolution would involve a mixture of mostly positive outcomes with some negative outcomes.
   D. Most people never resolve all the crises and therefore never get to all eight stages.

Correct Answer: C

Rationale: The bipolar aspect means that the crisis can have a positive or a negative outcome. The crisis must be resolved for the person to continue into the next stage. When resolution of this crisis is successful, the infant holds relatively more trust than mistrust.

Cognitive Level: Analysis

4. If you hide a block under a baby's blanket and she looks for it you understand that she has begun to develop the concept of:
   A. separation anxiety.
   B. relativism.
   C. object prehension.
   D. object permanence.

Correct Answer: D

Rationale: Gradually, the infant learns the important concept of object permanence, that objects and people continue to exist even when they are no longer in sight. This starts around 7 months when the infant searches for an object that is partially hidden but does not search for one completely out of sight.

Cognitive Level: Application

5. A baby can sit alone before he is able to crawl. This is true because development of gross motor skills:
   A. occurs in a distal to proximal direction.
   B. occurs in a cephalocaudal direction.
   C. is generally the result of a baby's chronological age.
   D. is generally simply the result of the baby's increased desire to move.

Correct Answer: B

Rationale: Gross Motor Skills. Their development of gross motor skills is predictable because it follows the direction of myelinization (laying down of myelin) in the nervous system; cephalocaudal (head to foot direction) and proximodistal (central to peripheral direction, or midline before extremities).

Cognitive Level: Application

6. An 18-month-old child comes to the Well Child Clinic for a well-child visit. You note the following as you observe him: rounded "pot belly" abdomen, marked lordosis "sway back," short slightly bowed legs, and a large head. Your conclusion is:
   A. he is built like a normal toddler.
   B. he probably has delayed physical maturation, especially of the long bones.
   C. he probably has a vitamin deficiency or some form of malnutrition.
   D. he probably has hydrocephalus.

Correct Answer: A

Rationale: Toddler lordosis describes the normal upright posture of the toddler, with the pot belly, sway back, and short, slightly bowed legs.

Cognitive Level: Application

7. Erikson believes toilet training to be representative of which of his stages?
   A. Initiative vs. guilt
   B. Integrity vs. despair
   C. Industry vs. inferiority
   D. Autonomy vs. shame and doubt

Correct Answer: D

Rationale: The quest for autonomy characterizes Erikson's second stage. The toddler wants to be autonomous and to govern his or her own body and experiences. Erikson believed that toilet training symbolizes this stage.

Cognitive Level: Knowledge

8. Being able to think about history and philosophy and analyze and use scientific reasoning corresponds to which of Piaget's stages?
   A. Concrete operations
   B. Sensorimotor skills
   C. Formal operations
   D. Preoperational skills

Correct Answer: C

Rationale: Adolescence corresponds to Piaget's fourth stage, in which the person focuses on formal operations and the ability to develop abstract thinking, deal with hypothetical situations, and make logical conclusions from reviewing evidence. The adolescent is no longer limited to the present but can ponder the lessons of the past and the possibilities of the future. The adolescent now can analyze and use scientific reasoning.

Cognitive Level: Comprehension

9. The developmental crisis of generativity vs. stagnation could be resolved by:
   A. changing jobs frequently to get a feel for what was "missed in their youth."
   B. having and raising a family.
   C. buying a large house and filling it with loved belongings.
   D. travelling around the world.

Correct Answer: B

Rationale: Erikson believed that during the middle years adults have the urge to contribute to the next generation. This need can be fulfilled either by producing the next generation or by producing something to pass on to the next generation.

Cognitive Level: Application

10. Which of the following statements best describes the tasks of late adulthood?
   A. Older adults must quickly try to resolve the conflicts of earlier times.
   B. Older adults must accept that they cannot change the past and make peace with their lives.
   C. Older adults must never feel satisfied with their lives because it gives them goals to achieve in the future.
   D. Older adults generally feel great sadness and worry about death and this allows them to accept their mortality.

Correct Answer: B

Rationale: This period relates to Erikson's last stage,

with its key polarity of integrity vs. despair. A successful resolution to this final conflict occurs when the adult accepts "one's one and only life cycle as something that had to be and that, by necessity, permitted of no substitutions" (1963). The adult feels content with his or her one life on earth, satisfied that if it were possible to do it over again, he or she would live it the same way.

Cognitive Level: Comprehension

11. A 24-month-old child comes to your clinic for a well-child visit. His mother describes him as a child who falls apart if she changes even the smallest thing in his environment. You tell his mother:
    A. this is expected behavior from a toddler because they typically experience ritualism and global thinking.
    B. this indicates that he has been spoiled and she should change things in his environment often, to get him used to it.
    C. this behavior is unusual in a toddler since negativism generally doesn't emerge until age 3.
    D. this indicates that he is insecure and probably hasn't successfully developed trust in infancy.

Correct Answer: A

Rationale: Ritualism emerges with negativity. A 2-year-old wants things done in the same way; any change in schedule is upsetting. Another mark of the toddler's sensitivity to change is global thinking. A change is one small part (such as a minor shift in room arrangement) changes the whole environment, and the 2-year-old child's equanimity disintegrates.

Cognitive Level: Analysis

12. Levinson proposes a series of eras throughout the lifespan. Which statement is true regarding these eras for the adult?
    A. The eras do not overlap.
    B. The eras are about 15 years long.
    C. Each era alternates between structure building and transition.
    D. Each era is marked by a change in personality.

Correct Answer: C

Rationale: Daniel Levinson's (1986) time frame of early adulthood is much broader than Erikson's. It encompasses 22 to 40 years. Levinson believes that an adult's life alternates between periods of structure building, in which a lifestyle is fashioned, and periods of transition, in which this lifestyle is evaluated, appraised, and modified.

Cognitive Level: Comprehension

13. At the well-child clinic you are advising the mother of an 8-month-old child about health and safety. One important thing you must make her aware of is:
    A. children at this age are at risk for choking because they explore the environment with their mouths.
    B. children at this age are at high risk for falls as they learn to walk.
    C. children at this age are likely to go easily to a babysitter.
    D. children at this age are prime candidates for toilet training since they are so receptive to new ideas.

Correct Answer: A

Rationale: According to Freud, an infant's first year is considered the Oral stage. The infant takes pleasure in rooting, sucking, and eating. Most sensory exploration of the world comes through the mouth. The nipple, thumb, fingers, toes, toys—anything that can be reached—all go in the mouth.

Cognitive Level: Comprehension

14. You are teaching a class to daycare providers. Which of the following statements about growth and development should be included?
    A. Preschoolers are still very unaware of gender and sex.
    B. Preschoolers "pretend" in order to reduce anxiety about their sex roles.
    C. Preschoolers are capable of delayed imitation.
    D. Preschoolers are highly egocentric.

Correct Answer: C

Rationale: Piaget's preoperational stage covers age 2 to 7 years, a longer span than the preschool years. It is characterized by symbolic function, because the child now uses symbols to represent people, objects, and events. The symbolic function is revealed in child's play, as in delayed imitation.

Cognitive Level: Application

15. An infant weighs 7 pounds at birth. At the well-child visit 6 months later you would expect the infant to weigh at least:
   A. 14 pounds.
   B. 21 pounds.
   C. 12 pounds.
   D. 17 pounds.

Correct Answer: A

Rationale: Growth spurts double the birth weight by 4 to 6 months and triple the birth weight by 1 year.

Cognitive Level: Application

16. Erikson's stage of integrity vs. despair could be described as:
   A. an adjustment to the tasks of middle age.
   B. cataloging life events to gain a sense of integrity.
   C. being productive and contributing to society.
   D. a time to review career goals and possibly change paths to avoid despair.

Correct Answer: B

Rationale: The Life Review. One important task of late adulthood is performing a life review. The life review is a cataloging of life events, a considering of one's successes and failures with the perspective of age. The objective of the task is to gain a sense of integrity in reviewing one's life as a whole.

Cognitive Level: Comprehension

17. You are advising a father about his 2-year-old daughter's eating habits. He is concerned because she seems "not to eat anything anymore." You tell him:
   A. this is normal due to a decrease in activity.
   B. this is normal due to a decrease in basal metabolic rate that occurs around age 18 months.
   C. this is normal due to a slower period of growth.
   D. this is normal because growth stops for a while at age 2.

Correct Answer: C

Rationale: The rate of growth decelerates during the 2nd year with the child gaining an average of 2.5 kg ($5\frac{1}{2}$ lb) in body weight.

Cognitive Level: Analysis

18. Physical growth is most rapid during which period:
   A. from 16 to 18 years of age.
   B. from 6 to 10 years of age.
   C. from 3 to 5 years of age.
   D. from birth to 1 year of age.

Correct Answer: D

Rationale: The first year is the most dramatic period of growth and development. Height, weight, and head circumference reflect physical growth and are sensitive indicators of an infant's general health.

Cognitive Level: Comprehension

19. You observe a mother with her 2-year-old child. In a period of just a few minutes the child has said "No" to her many times. He even says "No" when he would like to have said yes. Which statement about this child's behavior is true?
   A. He is a toddler and is exhibiting ritualistic behavior.
   B. He is trying to assert his autonomy through negativism.
   C. He is very spoiled and needs to be punished.
   D. He is just trying to "push his mother's buttons."

Correct Answer: B

Rationale: As they test their powers, they sometimes clash with their parents' restrictions, and a battle of wills results. "No" seems to be their favorite word. This negativism is a normal part of the quest for autonomy.

Cognitive Level: Comprehension

20. Which statement correctly characterizes ageism?
   A. Ageism is most common in Asian cultures.
   B. Ageism is the result of true concern about the aged population.
   C. Ageism may result in age discrimination.
   D. Ageism incorporates many theories of aging.

Correct Answer: C

Rationale: Ageism means discrimination based on age. It is a derogatory attitude that characterizes older adults as sickly, senile, and useless, and as a burden on the economy. The attitude stems in part from our cultural emphasis on youth, beauty, and vigor. Other cultures respect and revere their aging members.

Cognitive Level: Comprehension

21. A father describes his adolescent son's "strange new clothes and hair style." He states that he is worried about the frequent changes his son seems to make in his appearance. You explain that his son is:
    A. experimenting with different identities, which is necessary to forming an identity of his own.
    B. probably getting into trouble and should begin counseling.
    C. probably experimenting with drugs or alcohol since such behavior is unusual in an adolescent.
    D. experiencing a loss of self-esteem and may need help to overcome this difficult time.

Correct Answer: A

Rationale: Erikson believes the main conflict of the fifth stage in his theory to be identity vs. role diffusion. Finding one's own identity is stressful. In the search for identity, teens often form cliques, wear fad clothing, and follow rock singers, movie stars, or charismatic heroes in an attempt to siphon identity from them.

Cognitive Level: Analysis

22. Finding a partner (heterosexual or homosexual), or committing one's life to a cause indicates successful resolution of which of Erikson's stages?
    A. generativity vs. stagnation
    B. autonomy vs. shame and doubt
    C. identity vs. role confusion
    D. intimacy vs. isolation

Correct Answer: D

Rationale: Once self-identity is established after adolescence, it can be merged with another's in an intimate relationship. During the early 20s the adult seeks the love, commitment, and intimacy of a lasting relationship.

Cognitive Level: Comprehension

23. The mother of a 2-month-old baby reports that she often lets the baby "cry it out" instead of going to her in the middle of the night. In talking over this practice with her you should make her aware that:
    A. babies can become spoiled if they're picked up in the middle of the night.
    B. 2-month-old babies are old enough to learn to sleep through the night.
    C. babies are just developing the ability to manipulate and should not be picked up if it is unnecessary.
    D. babies are developing a sense of trust and need to be responded to when they cry.

Correct Answer: D

Rationale: Erikson viewed the mother as the primary caregiver. The crucial element in this stage, (trust vs. mistrust) then, is the quality of the mother-child relationship. When the mother is responsive and consistent in her nurturing, the infant learns trust.

Cognitive Level: Analysis

24. An 8-year-old boy's father is very interested in seeing his child succeed in soccer. Your assessment reveals a small boy who expresses a sincere interest in playing chess and feels like a failure at soccer. Which statement is true in regard to this situation?
    A. This child should be encouraged to compete in team sports to develop a sense of competency.
    B. This child obviously has an introverted personality and should be "left alone."
    C. This child should be given opportunities to achieve success and a sense of competency in any area he chooses.
    D. This father needs to decrease his expectations for his son.

Correct Answer: C

Rationale: Real achievement at this stage (industry vs. inferiority) builds a feeling of confidence, competence, and industry. The reality is that no one can master everything. If the child believes that he or she cannot measure up to society's expectations, the child loses confidence and does not take pleasure in the work.

Cognitive Level: Analysis

25. You have decided to test a 10-year-old's ability to understand conservation. Which test would you use?
    A. Ask her to sort blocks by color and by shape.
    B. Ask her to order the blocks from smallest to biggest.
    C. Ask her to make a code using the alphabet and then write you a message in the code she has made up.
    D. Ask her to determine which glass of water has more water in it, the tall, skinny glass or the short, fat glass.

Correct Answer: D

Rationale: Understanding conservation of matter is the ability to tell the difference between how things seem and how they really are. It is the ability to see that mass or quantity stays constant even though shape or position is transformed.

Cognitive Level: Analysis

26. Which topic would be most appropriately stressed to parents of a school age child?
    A. Choking safety
    B. Bicycle safety
    C. Electrical safety
    D. Poison safety

Correct Answer: B

Rationale: Leading causes of death: Motor vehicle crashes and injuries from non-motor vehicles.

Cognitive Level: Comprehension

27. You have decided to perform the Denver II screening test on a 12-month-old infant during a routine well-child visit. You should let his parents know that:
    A. the Denver II is a test to determine intellectual ability and may indicate if there will be problems later in school.
    B. the Denver II will tell you if the child has a speech disorder so that treatment can be begun.
    C. the Denver II tests three areas of development: cognitive, physical, and psychological.
    D. the Denver II is a screening instrument designed to detect children who are slow in development.

Correct Answer: D

Rationale: This (the Denver II) is a screening instrument designed to detect developmental delays in infants and preschoolers. It tests four functions: gross motor, language, fine motor-adaptive, and personal-social. The Denver II is not an intelligence test; it does not predict current or future intellectual ability. It is not diagnostic; it does not suggest treatment regimens.

Cognitive Level: Application

28. A 12-month-old infant is screened using the Denver II and is found to have some delays in gross motor skills. The screening is important because:
    A. it can help diagnose a child with problems.
    B. it provides for early detection, leading to earlier intervention.
    C. it can be used in conjunction with other tests to determine a child's overall intellectual level.
    D. it can be used by a physical therapist to determine the appropriate treatment.

Correct Answer: B

Rationale: This (the Denver II) is a screening instrument designed to detect developmental delays. What the Denver II does do is screen; it helps identify children who may be slow in development. This is important because early detection increases the opportunities for effective treatment.

Cognitive Level: Analysis

29. Levinson describes the period of middle adulthood as beginning with a mid-life transition. Which statement best describes this mid-life transition?
    A. Most people experience a need to change careers around the age of 40.
    B. This is a time when people feel a desire to pursue more youthful activities.
    C. This is a time of major reassessment—"what have I done with my life?"
    D. Most people find that they have basically met all of their goals and experience rejuvenation.

Correct Answer: C

Rationale: Levinson (1986) describes the era of middle adulthood as beginning with a mid-life transition. Roughly between 40 and 45 years, the person starts a major reassessment, "What have I done with my life?"

Cognitive Level: Analysis

30. An 18-month-old who makes the statement, "all done" is using what form of speech?
    A. Telegraphic speech
    B. Holophrasic speech
    C. Pre-operational speech
    D. Complex-interactive speech

Correct Answer: A

Rationale: At 1 year, sentences begin with the one-word holophrase, in which one word represents a complete thought, e.g., "out" for "I want to go out." A 2-year-old uses simple two-word phrases—"all gone," "me up," "baby crying."

This is called telegraphic speech, which is usually a combination of a noun and a verb and includes only words that have concrete meaning.

Cognitive Level: Analysis

31. An adolescent is beginning to develop the ability to deal with hypothetical situations and abstract thinking. You would consider this finding:
    A. abnormal since abstract thinking should begin to take place in early childhood.
    B. a normal finding during this stage of development.
    C. an expected finding only in the elderly.
    D. advanced for this patient's age.

Correct Answer: B

Rationale: In adolescence, thinking is no longer concrete. Adolescents can analyze and use scientific reasoning.

Cognitive Level: Analysis

32. The stage of early adulthood (20-40 years) is concerned with emancipation from parents and building an independent lifestyle. Tasks of this era include:
    A. pursuing activities enjoyed during childhood.
    B. becoming more involved with activities in their family of origin.
    C. forming an intimate bond with another and choosing a mate.
    D. assisting younger siblings with gaining their identity.

Correct Answer: C

Rationale: Tasks of early adulthood include such things as growing independent from the parents' home; establishing a career; forming an intimate bond with another and choosing a mate; managing one's own household; and forming a meaningful philosophy of life.

Cognitive Level: Comprehension

33. Which of the following statements best characterizes resolution of Erikson's last ego stage, integrity versus despair?
    A. The adult feels content with his or her life, satisfied that if it were possible to do it over again, he or she would live it the same way.
    B. The adult feels the need to pursue youthful activities as a culmination of their life experiences.
    C. The individual becomes more interested in society's extrinsic rewards.
    D. The individual experiences a loss of recognition and authority.

Correct Answer: A

Rationale: A successful resolution to Erikson's final stage of integrity versus despair comes when the adult feels content with his or her life on earth, satisfied that if were possible to do it over again, he or she would live it the same way.

Cognitive Level: Analysis

34. Normal physical changes that occur during middle adulthood (40-64 years) include:
    A. deterioration of internal organ systems.
    B. decreased sensory function and visual changes for far vision.
    C. increased abdominal fat deposits from decreased activity.
    D. increased muscle tone and decreased muscle strength.

Correct Answer: C

Rationale: During middle adulthood the hair thins, an abdominal paunch grows from increased fat deposits and decreased activity, most organ systems remain constant, and sensory function remains intact except for some visual changes for near vision.

Cognitive Level: Knowledge

Chapter 3

Transcultural Considerations in Assessment

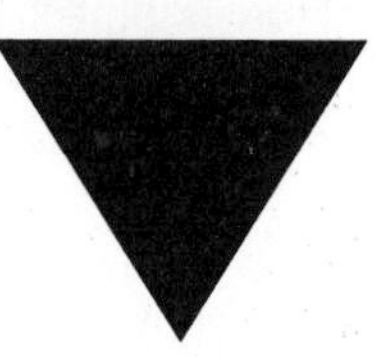

1. Which statement correctly reflects the acquisition of culture?
   A. Culture is genetically determined, based on racial background.
   B. Culture is biologically determined, based on physical characteristics.
   C. Culture is learned through language acquisition and socialization.
   D. Culture is a nonspecific phenomenon and is adaptive but unnecessary.

Correct Answer: C

Rationale: Culture is (1) learned from birth through language acquisition and socialization.

Cognitive Level: Comprehension

2. Culture has four basic characteristics. Which statement correctly reflects one of these characteristics?
   A. A cultural group living in an arid environment will make adaptations to this condition.
   B. Cultures are static and unchanging, despite changes around them.
   C. Cultures are never specific, which makes them hard to identify.
   D. Culture is most clearly reflected in a person's language.

Correct Answer: A

Rationale: Culture has four basic characteristics. Culture is . . . (3) adapted to specific conditions related to environmental and technical factors and to the availability of natural resources; and (4) dynamic and ever-changing.

Cognitive Level: Analysis

3. The specific and distinct knowledge, beliefs, skills, and customs acquired by members of a society are known as:
   A. social learning.
   B. culture.
   C. cultural skills.
   D. mores.

Correct Answer: B

Rationale: The culture that develops in any given society is always specific and distinctive, encompassing all the knowledge, beliefs, customs, and skills acquired by members of the society.

Cognitive Level: Knowledge

4. The term subculture is used:
   A. to define small groups of people that do not want to be identified with the larger culture.
   B. to identify fairly large groups of people with shared characteristics.
   C. to single out groups of people for differential and unequal treatment.
   D. To fit as many people into the majority culture as possible.

Correct Answer: B

Rationale: The term subculture is used for fairly large aggregates of people who have shared characteristics that are not common to all members of the culture and that enable them to be thought of as a distinguishable subgroup.

Cognitive Level: Comprehension

5. The female secretaries employed by a large insurance firm are unhappy to discover that they receive less pay than male secretaries at the same firm. Which statement is true with regard to these female secretaries?
   A. They could be classified as members of a minority group.
   B. They are probably less productive than the male secretaries.
   C. Only the secretaries of African descent are members of a minority group.
   D. The mainstream culture would say that they are being fairly compensated.

Correct Answer: A

Rationale: The term minority refers to "a group of people, who because of their physical or cultural characteristics, are singled out from the others in the society in which they live for differential and unequal treatment, and who therefore regard themselves as objects of collective discrimination" (Wirth, 1945). The concept of minority varies widely and is contextual.

Cognitive Level: Analysis

6. Every society has what is called the dominant value orientation. Which of the following best describe the dominant value orientation of the majority culture in the United States?
   A. Belief in ancestral knowledge and reverence for aged members of the society
   B. Working hard, being self-supporting, and financially independent
   C. Living within a communal group and rejecting personal belongings
   D. Moving away from other people and living in a cabin without heat, lights, or water

Correct Answer: B

Rationale: The dominant value orientations of the United States include individuality, material wealth, comfort, humanitarianism, physical beauty, democracy, newness, cleanliness, education, science, achievement, free enterprise, punctuality, rationality, independence, respectability, self-discipline, effort, and progress (Herberg, 1995).

Cognitive Level: Analysis

7. One aspect of society's value orientation concerns the dimension of time. An example of a person with "present" time value orientation would be:
   A. a newly diagnosed diabetic who seeks a consultation with a medicine man who can contact ancestral spirits for guidance.
   B. a patient with a total hip replacement who has not been able to plan for discharge.
   C. a patient with leukemia who continually seeks the latest medication and treatments.
   D. a patient who feels loss after an amputation but is looking forward to finding out about prosthetic limbs.

Correct Answer: B

Rationale: The focus may be on the present, with little attention being paid to the past or the future. These individuals are concerned with "now" and the future is perceived as vague or unpredictable. You may have difficulty encouraging these individuals to prepare for the future.

Cognitive Level: Application

8. The statement "for the good of the whole, not the good of the one" could be representative of a cultural value orientation with regard to relationships. With which cultural value orientation does this fit most closely?
   A. Lineal
   B. Individual
   C. Group-think
   D. Collateral

Correct Answer: D

Rationale: Collateral relationships focus primarily on group goals and the family orientation is all-important.

Cognitive Level: Analysis

9. M.P., 20, is an Asian-American. She would like to go to college but has an aged, ill father at home. If M.P.'s cultural value orientation regarding relationships is collateral, she will be likely to:
   A. stay home and take care of her father.
   B. go ahead with college since she is young and her needs must come first.
   C. find a nurse to take care of her father so that she can go to college.
   D. ask her minister what she should do and then take her minister's advice.

Correct Answer: A

Rationale: Collateral relationships focus primarily on group goals and the family orientation is all-important. If collateral relationships are valued, decisions about the person may be interrelated with the impact of illness on the entire family or group.

Cognitive Level: Application

10. Which is the predominant value orientation for relationships in the United States?
    A. Lineal
    B. Individual
    C. Group-think
    D. Collateral

Correct Answer: B

Rationale: Perhaps the individual value orientation concerning relationships is predominant among the majority of white Americans.

Cognitive Level: Comprehension

11. The essence of family consists of:
    A. only those people who are related by blood or marriage.
    B. parents, children, and possibly step-children.
    C. people who are living together as a unit.
    D. parents, children, grandparents, aunts, and uncles.

Correct Answer: C

Rationale: The essence of family consists of individuals living together as a unit.

Cognitive Level: Comprehension

12. Mr. J.P. and Mrs. R.P. are married and have two children. Which of the following categories does their family fit into?
    A. Extended
    B. Nuclear
    C. Blended
    D. Cohabitation

Correct Answer: B

Rationale: Six categories of family exist: (1) nuclear (husband, wife, and a child[ren]); (2) single parent (either mother or father and at least one child); (3) extended family (which may include grandparents, aunts, uncles, cousins, and even people who are not biologically related); (4) blended (husband, wife, and child[ren] from previous relationships); (5) cohabitation (unmarried man and woman sharing a household with child[ren]); and (6) gay (same gender couples and child[ren]).

Cognitive Level: Comprehension

13. Mr. A.K. is from an African village and is now living in America with his family. He visits the clinic to seek assistance with a persistent cough and fever. During your interview, he identifies the man with him as his brother. You understand that:
    A. Mr. A.K. and this man have the same mother.
    B. Mr. A.K. and this man have the same father.
    C. Mr. A.K. and this man may be from the same village.
    D. Mr. A.K. and this man were breast-fed by the same woman.

Correct Answer: C

Rationale: Relationships that may seem apparent sometimes warrant further exploration when interviewing people from culturally diverse backgrounds. In some African cultures, anyone from the same village or town may be called "brother" or "sister."

Cognitive Level: Analysis

14. Mrs. T.B. brings her 15-month-old son in for a well-child visit. When asked questions about his pattern of behaviors and appetite she seems at a loss for answers. What is your best response?
    A. Determine whether Mrs. T.B. is the primary provider of care for her son.
    B. Contact social services since she may be neglecting her son.
    C. Assume that she knows her son's habits and may be hiding something unusual.
    D. Discuss with her how important it is to observe growth and development patterns in order to see a delay early.

Correct Answer: A

Rationale: When assessing infants and children, it is important to identify the primary provider of care because this individual may or may not be the biologic parent.

Cognitive Level: Application

15. Dr. T.W. is frequently bothered when patients arrive at the clinic late for appointments. He is so irritated by this behavior that he often finds it hard to provide appropriate care to these individuals. What should Dr. T.W. do first in trying to overcome his difficulty?
    A. Identify the meaning of health to the patient.
    B. Allow the patients to arrive late and build this into his schedule.
    C. Understand that these cultural practices are helpful to the patient.
    D. Examine his own culturally based values, beliefs, attitudes, and practices.

Correct Answer: D

Rationale: The first step is understanding your own culturally based values, beliefs, attitudes, and practices.

Cognitive Level: Comprehension

16. In the majority culture of America, coughing, sweating, and diarrhea are symptoms of an illness. For some individuals of Hispanic origin, however, these symptoms are a normal part of living. This is probably because:
    A. Hispanics are usually in a lower socio-economic group and are more likely to be sick.
    B. Hispanics derive their meaning of health from their cultural group.
    C. Hispanics come from Mexico and coughing is normal and healthy there.
    D. Hispanics have less efficient immune systems and are often ill.

Correct Answer: B

Rationale: Secondly, you need to identify the meaning of health to the patient, remembering that concepts are derived, in part, from the way in which members of their cultural group define health.

Cognitive Level: Comprehension

17. The germ theory, which posits that microscopic organisms such as bacteria and viruses are responsible for specific disease conditions, is a basic belief of which theory of illness?
    A. Biomedical
    B. Naturalistic
    C. Holistic
    D. Magico-religious

Correct Answer: A

Rationale: Among the biomedical explanations for disease is the germ theory, which posits that microscopic organisms such as bacteria and viruses are responsible for specific disease conditions.

Cognitive Level: Comprehension

18. If an Asian-American is experiencing a symptom, such as diarrhea (which is felt to be "yin"), they are likely to try to treat it with:
    A. high doses of medicines thought to be "cold."
    B. no treatment at all, since diarrhea is an expected part of life.
    C. foods that are "hot" or "yang."
    D. readings and eastern medicine meditations.

Correct Answer: C

Rationale: Yin foods are cold and yang foods are hot. Cold foods are eaten with a hot illness, and hot foods are eaten with a cold illness.

Cognitive Level: Application

19. Among many Asians there is a belief in the yin/yang theory, rooted in the ancient Chinese philosophy of Tao. Which statement would most accurately reflect "health" in an Asian with these naturalistic beliefs?
    A. A person is able to work and produce.
    B. A person is able to care for others and function socially.
    C. A person is happy, stable, and feels good.
    D. All aspects of the person are in perfect balance.

Correct Answer: D

Rationale: Many Asians believe in the yin/yang theory, in which health is believed to exist when all aspects of the person are in perfect balance.

Cognitive Level: Analysis

20. Illness is seen as a part of life's rhythmic course and as an outward sign of disharmony within. This statement most accurately reflects the views about illness from the:
    A. biomedical theory.
    B. naturalistic theory.
    C. magico-religious theory.
    D. reductionist theory.

Correct Answer: B

Rationale: The naturalistic perspective posits that the laws of nature create imbalances, chaos, and disease. From the perspective of the Chinese, for example, illness is not seen as an introducing agent but as a part of life's rhythmic course and as an outward sign of disharmony within.

Cognitive Level: Application

21. An individual who takes the magico-religious perspective of illness and disease is likely to believe that:
    A. their illness was caused by supernatural forces.
    B. their illness was caused by germs and viruses that are too small to be seen and thus mysterious.
    C. their illness was caused by an imbalance within their spiritual nature.
    D. their illness was caused by eating foods that were not right to balance their needs.

Correct Answer: A

Rationale: The third major way in which people view the world and explain the causation of illness is from a magico-religious perspective. The basic premise of this explanatory model is that the world is seen as an arena in which supernatural forces dominate. The fate of the world and those in it depends on the action of supernatural forces for good or evil.

Cognitive Level: Comprehension

22. If a Native-American has come to your clinic to seek help with regulating her diabetes it would be safe to assume:
    A. she has obviously given up her beliefs in naturalistic causes of disease.
    B. she will comply with the treatment prescribed.
    C. she may also be seeking the assistance of a shaman or medicine man.
    D. she will need extra help in dealing with her illness and may be experiencing a crisis of faith.

Correct Answer: C

Rationale: When self-treatment is unsuccessful, the individual may turn to the lay or folk healing systems, to spiritual or religious healing, or to scientific biomedicine. In addition to seeking help from you as a biomedical/scientific health care provider, patients may also seek help from folk or religious healers.

Cognitive Level: Analysis

23. You are aware that an elderly Hispanic woman with traditional beliefs has been admitted to your unit. As a culturally sensitive nurse you:
    A. further assess her cultural beliefs and offer the assistance in contacting a curandero or priest if she desires.
    B. automatically get a curandero for her, since it is not culturally appropriate for her to request one.
    C. contact the hospital administrator about your best course of action.
    D. ask the family what they would like you to do, since Hispanics traditionally give control of decisions to their families.

Correct Answer: A

Rationale: In addition to seeking help from you as a biomedical/scientific health care provider, patients may also seek help from folk or religious healers. Some people such as those of Hispanic or Native American origins, may believe that the cure is incomplete unless healing of body, mind, and spirit are all carried out, although the division of the person into parts is itself a Western concept.

Cognitive Level: Analysis

24. Mr. C.Y., age 63, is a Chinese-American. He enters the hospital with complaints about chest pain, shortness of breath, and palpitations. Which statement most accurately reflects the nurse's best course of action?
    A. Mr. C.Y. is obviously having cardiac difficulty and should have a full cardiac assessment.
    B. Mr. C.Y. is obviously having difficulty after learning of his wife's cancer and is expressing psychosomatic complaints.
    C. It is unclear what is happening with Mr. C.Y. and his assessment should include physical and psychosocial realms.
    D. Mr. C.Y. is not in any danger at present and should be sent home with instructions to contact his physician in the morning.

Correct Answer: C

Rationale: Wide cultural variation exists in the manner in which certain symptoms and disease conditions are perceived, diagnosed, labeled, and treated. Chinese-Americans sometimes convert mental experiences or states into bodily symptoms, e.g. complain of cardiac symptoms because the center of emotion in the Chinese culture is the heart.

Cognitive Level: Application

25. Symptoms, such as pain, are often influenced by a person's cultural heritage. Which of the following is a true statement with regard to pain?
    A. Nurses' attitudes toward their patients' pain are unrelated to their own experiences with pain.
    B. A nurse's years of clinical experience and current position are a strong indicator of his/her response to patient pain.
    C. A nurse's area of clinical practice is most likely to determine his/her assessment of a patient's pain.
    D. The ethnic background of a patient is important in a nurse's assessment of that patient's pain.

Correct Answer: D

Rationale: In research studies of nurses' attitudes toward pain, it was discovered that the ethnic background of patients is important in the nurses' assessment of both physical and psychological pain.

Cognitive Level: Comprehension

26. Which of the following statements is true regarding pain?
    A. All patients will behave the same way when in pain.
    B. Just as patients vary in their perception of pain, so will they vary in their expression of it.
    C. A patient's expression of pain is largely dependent on the amount of tissue injury associated with the pain.
    D. Cultural norms have very little to do with pain tolerance—it is always biologically determined.

Correct Answer: B

Rationale: In addition to expecting variations in pain perception and tolerance, you should also expect variations in the expression of pain. It is a well-known fact that individuals turn to their social environment for validation and comparison.

Cognitive Level: Comprehension

27. Which of the following is the best definition of spirituality?
    A. That which arises out of each person's unique life experience and his or her personal effort to find meaning and purpose in life.
    B. An organized system of beliefs concerning the cause, nature, and purpose of the universe.
    C. A personal search to discover a supreme being.
    D. A belief that each person exists forever in some form, such as belief in reincarnation, the afterlife, etc.

Correct Answer: A

Rationale: Spirituality arises out of each person's unique life experience and his or her personal effort to find purpose and meaning in life.

Cognitive Level: Comprehension

28. Working with children with a different cultural perspective can be especially difficult. Why?
    A. Children have spiritual needs that are direct reflection of what is occurring in the home.
    B. Children have spiritual needs that are influenced by the stage of development.
    C. Parents are often the decision makers and have no knowledge of their children's spiritual needs
    D. Parental perceptions about their child's illness are almost always influenced by religious beliefs.

Correct Answer: B

Rationale: Illness during childhood may be an especially difficult clinical situation. Children as well as adults have spiritual needs that vary according to the child's developmental level and the religious climate that exists in the family.

Cognitive Level: Application

29. Mrs. H.L., 30, has recently moved to the United States with her husband. They are living with relatives until they can get a house of their own. When company arrives to visit with Mrs. H.L.'s sister, she feels suddenly shy and retreats to the back bedroom to hide until the company leaves again. She states that this is just because she doesn't know how to speak perfect English. Mrs. H.L. could be experiencing:
    A. culture shock.
    B. cultural unfamiliarity.
    C. cultural taboos.
    D. culture disorientation.

Correct Answer: A

Rationale: These individuals may be in various stages of culture shock, a term used to describe the state of disorientation or inability to respond to the behavior of a different cultural group because of its sudden strangeness, unfamiliarity, and incompatibility to the stranger's perceptions and expectations.

Cognitive Level: Analysis

30. After a symptom is recognized the first effort at treatment is often self-care. Which statement is true with regard to self-care?
    A. Self-care is always less expensive than biomedical alternatives.
    B. Self-care is usually ineffective and may delay more effective treatment.
    C. Self-care is not recognized as valuable by most health care providers.
    D. Self-care is influenced by the accessibility of over-the-counter medicines.

Correct Answer: D

Rationale: After a symptom is identified, the first effort at treatment is often self-care. The availability of over-the-counter medications, relatively high literacy level of Americans, and influence of the mass media in communicating health-related information to the general population have contributed to the high percentage of cases of self-treatment.

Cognitive Level: Comprehension

31. Many individuals embrace the hot/cold theory of health illness. Which of the following best describes the basic tenets of this theory?
    A. The treatment of disease consists of adding or subtracting cold, heat, dryness, or wetness to restore the balance of the humors of the body.
    B. The four humors of the body consist of blood, yellow bile, spiritual connectedness, and social aspects of the individual.
    C. Herbs and medicines are classified on their physical characteristics and humors of the body.
    D. The causation of illness is based on supernatural forces which influence the humors of the body.

Correct Answer: A

Rationale: The hot/cold theory of health and illness is based on the four humors of the body: blood, phlegm, black bile, and yellow bile. These humors regulate the basic bodily functions, described in terms of temperature, dryness, and moisture.

Cognitive Level: Comprehension

32. In the hot/cold theory, illnesses are believed to be caused by hot or cold entering the body. Which of the following patients' conditions is most consist with a "cold" condition?
    A. Child with symptoms of itching and a rash
    B. Elderly male with gastrointestinal discomfort
    C. Diabetic patient with renal failure
    D. Teenager with an abscessed tooth

Correct Answer: B

Rationale: Illnesses believed to be caused by cold entering the body include earache, chest cramps, gastrointestinal discomfort, rheumatism, and tuberculosis. Those illnesses believed to be caused by heat, or over-heating include sore throats, abscessed teeth, rashes, and kidney disorders.

Cognitive Level: Analysis

33. When providing culturally competent care, nurses must incorporate cultural assessment into their health assessment. Which statement is most appropriate to use when initiating an assessment of cultural beliefs with an elderly Native American patient?
    A. "Do you want to see a medicine man?"
    B. "Are you of the Christian faith?"
    C. "How often do you seek help from medical providers?"
    D. "What cultural or spiritual beliefs are important to you?"

Correct Answer: D

Rationale: Native Americans may seek assistance from a medicine man or "shaman," but the nurse should not assume this. An open-ended question regarding cultural and spiritual beliefs is best utilized initially when performing a cultural assessment.

Cognitive Level: Analysis

34. There are a variety of healing beliefs and practices used by numerous subcultural groups in the United States. Which statement best explains why it is important for the nurse to be aware of alternative healing practices?
    A. Many of these practices will interfere with the medical model of treatment.
    B. Western medicines will interact with folk remedies and cause an adverse reaction for the patient.
    C. Many folk remedies are harmless and can be utilized in conjunction with Western medical practices and treatments.
    D. The patient and family can be educated regarding the ineffectiveness of folk healing methods.

Correct Answer: C

Rationale: It is dangerous to assume that all folk healing remedies are harmless; however, the majority are quite harmless and may or may not be effective cures.

Cognitive Level: Comprehension

35. Often, cultural conflict can develop between health care providers and patients regarding the perception of time. Which of the following describes an individual with "past" time value orientation?
    A. Patient inquiring about the "latest treatment"

and most modern equipment available

B. Individual who fails to see the value of childhood immunizations

C. Individual who is chronically late for appointments because "something else came up"

D. Individual who seeks consultation from older family members and ancestors asking for guidance and assistance during an illness

Correct Answer: D

Rationale: In times of crisis, individuals with a "past" time value orientation will offer guidance from ancestors and family elders. Their focus is on the past with traditions and ancestors playing an important role in the person's life.

Cognitive Level: Application

Chapter 4

The Interview

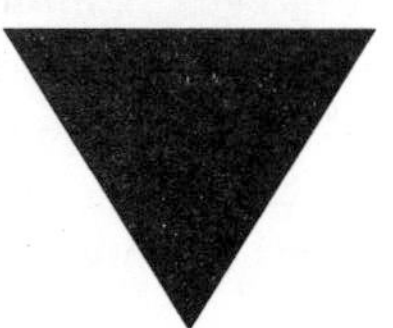

1. You are conducting an interview with Mrs. F.L. She has recently learned that she is pregnant and has come to the clinic today to begin prenatal care. She states that she and her husband are excited about the pregnancy but have a few questions. She looks nervously at her hands during the interview and sighs loudly. With your knowledge of communication which statement is most accurate?
   A. Mrs. F.L. is excited about her pregnancy but nervous about labor.
   B. Mrs. F.L. is excited about her pregnancy but her husband is not and this is upsetting to her.
   C. Mrs. F.L. is exhibiting incongruent verbal and nonverbal behavior.
   D. Mrs. F.L. is not excited about her pregnancy but believes you will respond negatively to her if she states this.

Correct Answer: C

Rationale: Communication is all behavior, conscious and unconscious, verbal and nonverbal. All behavior has meaning.

Cognitive Level: Analysis

2. Receiving is a part of the communication process. Which receiver is most likely to misinterpret a message sent by a health care professional?
   A. A well-adjusted adolescent in for a sports physical
   B. A recovering alcoholic in for a basic physical examination
   C. A hearing-impaired man who uses sign language to communicate and has an interpreter with him
   D. A man whose wife has just been diagnosed with lung cancer

Correct Answer: D

Rationale: The receiver attaches meaning determined by his or her past experiences, culture, self-concept, as well as current physical and emotional state.

Cognitive Level: Analysis

3. Because the physical environment in which an interview takes place is an important consideration for the success of an interview, the interviewer should:
   A. reduce noise by turning off televisions and radios.
   B. place the distance between you and the patient about 2 feet or closer.
   C. arrange seating across a desk or table to allow the patient some personal space.
   D. provide a dim light that makes a room cozier and will help the patient relax.

Correct Answer: A

Rationale: Reduce noise. Multiple stimuli are confusing. Turn off the television, radio, and any unnecessary equipment.

Cognitive Level: Application

4. In an interview, it will sometimes be necessary to take notes to aid your memory later. Which of the following statements is true regarding note-taking?
   A. Taking notes allows you to break eye contact with the patient, which may increase their level of comfort.
   B. Taking notes allows the patient to continue at their own pace as you record what they are saying.
   C. Taking notes allows you to shift your attention away from the patient, which may increase their level of comfort.
   D. Taking notes may impede your observation of the patient's nonverbal behaviors.

Correct Answer: D

Rationale: Some use of history forms and note-taking may be unavoidable. But be aware that note-taking during the interview has disadvantages: It breaks eye contact too often; it shifts your attention away from the patient, diminishing his or her sense of importance; it can interrupt the patient's narrative flow; it impedes your observation of the patient's nonverbal behavior.

Cognitive Level: Comprehension

5. The following statement could be found at which phase of the interview? "Mr. B., I would like to ask you some questions about your health and your usual daily activities so that we can better plan your stay here."
   A. During the body of the interview
   B. Opening/introducing the interview
   C. Closing the interview
   D. During the summary

Correct Answer: B

Rationale: If you are gathering a complete history, give the reason for this interview.

Cognitive Level: Comprehension

6. Mrs. H. has just entered the emergency room after being battered by her husband. The nurse will need to get some information from her in order to begin treatment. What is the best choice for an opening with Mrs. H.?
   A. "Mrs. H., my name is Mrs. C."
   B. "Mrs. H., my name is Mrs. C. It sure is cold today!"
   C. "Mrs. H., my name is Mrs. C. I'll need to ask you a few questions about what happened."
   D. "Mrs. H., my name is Mrs. C. You sure look like you're in pain, can I get you anything?"

Correct Answer: C

Rationale: Address the person, using his or her surname. Introduce yourself and state your role in the agency. You do not need friendly small talk to build rapport.

Cognitive Level: Application

7. For the following statement, identify which verbal skill is used: "You mentioned shortness of breath. Tell me more about that."
   A. Direct question
   B. Open-ended question
   C. Reflection
   D. Facilitation

Correct Answer: B

Rationale: The open-ended question asks for narrative information. It states the topic to be discussed but only in general terms. Use it to begin the interview, to introduce a new section of questions, and whenever the person introduces a new topic.

Cognitive Level: Comprehension

8. Mr. Y has finished giving you information about the reason he is seeking care. You find that you are missing some information about past hospitalizations. Which statement would be most appropriate to gather these data?
   A. "Mr. Y., you mentioned that you have been hospitalized on several occasions. Would you tell me more about that?"
   B. "Mr. Y., I just need to get some additional information about your past hospitalizations. When was the last time you were admitted for chest pain?"
   C. "Mr. Y., at your age, surely you have been hospitalized before!"
   D. "Mr. Y., I just need permission to get your medical records from County Medical."

Correct Answer: B

Rationale: Use direct questions after the person's opening narrative to fill in any details he or she left out. Also use direct questions when you need many specific facts, such as when asking about past health problems or during the review of systems.

Cognitive Level: Application

9. In using verbal responses to assist the patient's narrative, some responses focus on the patient's frame of reference and some focus on the health care provider's perspective. An example of a verbal response that focuses on the health care provider's perspective would be:
   A. facilitation.
   B. reflection.
   C. confrontation.
   D. empathy.

Correct Answer: C

Rationale: Recall that in the last four responses (confrontation, interpretation, explanation, summary), the frame or reference shifts from the patient's perspective to yours.

Cognitive Level: Knowledge

10. When taking a history from Mr. J., you notice that he is pausing often and looking at you expectantly. What would be your best response to this?
    A. Be silent and allow him to continue when he is ready.
    B. Smile at him and say, "Don't worry about all of this, Mr. J. I'm sure we can find out why you're having these pains."
    C. Lean back in your chair and ask, "Mr. J., you are looking at me kind of funny; there isn't anything wrong, is there?"
    D. Stand up and say, "I can see that this interview is uncomfortable for you. We can continue it another time."

Correct Answer: A

Rationale: Silent attentiveness communicates that the person has time to think, to organize what he or she wishes to say without interruption from you. This "thinking silence" is the one health professionals interrupt most often.

Cognitive Level: Application

11. Ms. F. is discussing the problems she is having with her 2-year-old son. "He won't go to sleep at night and during the day he has several fits. I get so upset when that happens." Your best verbal response would be:
    A. "Yes, it can be upsetting when a child has a fit."
    B. "Fits? Tell me what you mean by this."
    C. "Don't be upset when he has a fit, every 2-year-old has fits."
    D. "Go on, I'm listening."

Correct Answer: B

Rationale: Clarification. Use this when the person's word choice is ambiguous or confusing, e.g., "Tell me what you mean by 'tired blood.'" Clarification is also used to summarize the person's words, simplify the words to make them clearer, then ask if you are on the right track.

Cognitive Level: Application

12. Ms. F. is describing how difficult it is to raise a 2-year-old by herself. During the course of the interview she states, "I can't believe he left me to do this by myself! What a terrible thing to do to me!" Which of the following responses utilizes empathy?
    A. "You can't believe he left you alone."
    B. "I would be angry too; raising a child alone is no picnic."
    C. "You feel alone?"
    D. "It must be so hard to face this all alone."

Correct Answer: D

Rationale: An empathetic response recognizes the feeling and puts it into words. It names the feeling and allows the expression of it. It strengthens rapport. Other empathetic responses are, "This must be very hard for you," "I understand," or just placing your hand on the person's arm.

Cognitive Level: Application

13. Mr. K. has been admitted to your unit for observation after being treated in the emergency room for a large cut on his forehead. As you work through the interview, one of the standard questions has to do with alcohol, tobacco, and drug use. When you ask him about tobacco use, he tells you, "I quit smoking after my wife died 7 years ago." As you observe him, however, you notice an open package of cigarettes in his shirt pocket. Utilizing confrontation, you could say:
    A. "Mr. K., I didn't realize your wife had died. Tell me more about that."
    B. "Mr. K., I know that you are lying."
    C. "Mr. K., you have said that you don't smoke, but I see that you have an open package of cigarettes in your pocket."
    D. "Mr. K., come on, tell me how much you smoke."

Correct Answer: C

Rationale: In the case of confrontation, you have observed a certain action, feeling, or statement and you now focus the person's attention on it. You give your honest feedback about what you see or feel. This may focus on a discrepancy. Or, you may confront the person when you notice parts of the story are inconsistent.

Cognitive Level: Application

14. You have used interpretation regarding a patient's statement or actions. After this, it would be best to:
    A. apologize, since this can be demeaning for the patient.
    B. allow the patient time to confirm or correct

your inference.

C. continue with your interview as though nothing had happened.

D. immediately restate your conclusion based on the patient's nonverbal response.

Correct Answer: B

Rationale: Interpretation. This statement is not based on direct observation as is confrontation, but it is based on your inference or conclusion. You do run a risk of making the wrong inference. If this is the case, the person will correct it. But even if the inference is corrected, interpretation helps to prompt further discussion of the topic.

Cognitive Level: Analysis

15. Mrs. P. says, "I have decided that I can no longer allow my children to live with their father's violence. I just can't seem to leave him, though." Using interpretation, your response would be:
    A. "It sounds as if you might be afraid of how your husband will respond."
    B. "It sounds as though you have made your decision. I think it is a good one."
    C. "If you're afraid for your children, why can't you leave?"
    D. "You're going to leave him?"

Correct Answer: A

Rationale: Interpretation. This statement is not based on your inference or conclusion. It links events, makes associations, or implies cause. Interpretation also ascribes feelings and helps the person understand his or her own feelings in relation to the verbal message.

Cognitive Level: Application

16. Mrs. A. states, "I just know labor will be so painful that I won't be able to stand it. I know it sounds awful, but I really dread going into labor." You respond by stating, "Oh, don't worry about labor so much. I have been through it and although it is painful there are many good medications to decrease the pain." Which statement is true regarding this response?
    A. It was a therapeutic response. By sharing something personal, the nurse gives hope to Mrs. A.
    B. It was a nontherapeutic response. By providing false reassurance, you have actually cut off further discussion of her fears.
    C. It was a therapeutic response. By providing information about the medications available, the nurse is giving information to Mrs. A.
    D. It was a nontherapeutic response. The nurse is essentially giving the message to Mrs. A. that labor cannot be tolerated without medication.

Correct Answer: B

Rationale: Providing false assurance or reassurance. This "courage builder" relieves your anxiety and give you the false sense of having provided comfort. But for the woman it actually closes off communication. It trivializes her anxiety and effectively denies any further talk of it.

Cognitive Level: Analysis

17. Mr. W. states, "The doctor just told me he thought I ought to stop smoking. He doesn't understand how hard I've tried. I just don't know the best way to do it. What should I do?" Your most appropriate response in this case would be:
    A. "Mr. W., would you like some information about the different ways a person can quit smoking?"
    B. "I'd quit. Dr. S. really knows what he is talking about."
    C. "Stopping your dependence on cigarettes can be very difficult. I understand how you feel."
    D. "Mr. W., why are you confused? Didn't Dr. S. give you the information about the smoking cessation program we offer?""

Correct Answer: A

Rationale: Clarification. Use this when the person's word choice is ambiguous or confusing. Clarification also is used to summarize the person's words, simplify the words to make them clearer, then ask if you are on the right track.

Cognitive Level: Application

18. As you enter a patient's room, you find her crying. She states that she has just found out that the lump in her breast is cancer and says, "I'm so afraid of, um, you know." As her nurse your most therapeutic response would be to gently say:
    A. "No, I'm not sure what you are talking about."
    B. "I can see that you are very upset, perhaps we should discuss this later."
    C. "I'll wait here until you get yourself under control and then we can talk."
    D. "You're afraid you might lose your breast?"

Correct Answer: D

Rationale: Reflection. This response echos the patient's words. Reflection is repeating part of what the person just said. Reflection also can help express feeling behind a person's words.

Cognitive Level: Application

19. You are assigned to take complete health histories on all the patients attending a wellness workshop. As a part of this history, you ask, "You don't smoke, drink, or take drugs do you?" This is an example of:
    A. using confrontation.
    B. using biased or leading questions.
    C. talking to much.
    D. using blunt language to deal with distasteful topics.

Correct Answer: B

Rationale: Using leading or biased questions. Asking, "You don't smoke, do you?" implies that one answer is "better" than another. If the person wants to please you, he or she is either forced to answer in a way corresponding to your values or is made to feel guilty when admitting the other answer.

Cognitive Level: Comprehension

20. When observing your patient's verbal and nonverbal communication, you notice a discrepancy. Which statement is true regarding this situation?
    A. You should focus on your patient's nonverbal behaviors since these are usually more reflective of a patient's true feelings.
    B. You should focus on your patient's verbal message and try to ignore the nonverbal behaviors.
    C. You should try to integrate the verbal and nonverbal messages and then interpret them as an "average."
    D. You should ask someone who knows the patient well to help you interpret this discrepancy.

Correct Answer: A

Rationale: When nonverbal and verbal messages are congruent, the verbal is reinforced. When they are incongruent, the nonverbal message tends to be the true one, because it is under less conscious control. Thus, it is important to study the nonverbal messages of patients and examiners and to understand their meanings.

Cognitive Level: Application

21. Mr. C. is sitting in an open position. As you begin to discuss his son's treatment, however, he suddenly crosses his arms against his chest and crosses his legs. This would suggest:
    A. Mr. C. is more comfortable in this position.
    B. Mr. C. is tires and needs a break in the interview.
    C. Mr. C. is uncomfortable talking about his son's treatment.
    D. Mr. C. is just changing positions.

Correct Answer: C

Rationale: Note the patient's position. An open position with extension of large muscle groups shows relaxation, physical comfort, and a willingness to share information. A closed position with arms and legs crossed tends to look defensive and anxious. Note any change in posture. If a person in a relaxed position suddenly tenses, it suggests possible discomfort with the new topic.

Cognitive Level: Analysis

22. Mrs. R. brings her 28-month-old daughter into your office for a well-child visit. At the beginning of the visit, you focus your attention away from the toddler but as the interview progresses, she begins to "warm up" and is smiling shyly at you. You will be most successful if you next:
    A. Tickle the toddler and get her to laugh.
    B. Stoop down to her level and ask her about the toy she is holding.
    C. Ask Mrs. R. to leave while you examine the toddler, since toddlers often fuss less if their parents aren't in view.
    D. Continue to ignore her until you are ready for the physical examination.

Correct Answer: B

Rationale: Although most of your communication is with the parent, do not ignore the child completely. You need to make contact to ease into the physical examination later. Begin by asking about the toys the child is playing with or about a special doll or teddy bear brought from home: "Does your doll have a name?" or "What can your truck do?" Stoop down to meet the child at his or her eye level.

Cognitive Level: Application

23. During your examination of a 3-year-old child, you will need to take her blood pressure. What might you do in order to try to gain her full cooperation?

A. Tell the child that the blood pressure cuff is asleep and cannot wake up.
B. Tell the child that the blood pressure cuff is going to give her arm a big hug.
C. Give the blood pressure cuff a name and refer to it by this name during your assessment.
D. Tell the child that by using the blood pressure cuff, you can see how strong her muscles are.

Correct Answer: D

Rationale: Use short, simple sentences with a concrete explanation. Take time to give a short, simple explanation for any unfamiliar equipment that will be used on the child. Preschoolers are animistic; they imagine inanimate objects can come alive and have human characteristics. Thus a blood pressure cuff can wake up and bite or pinch.

Cognitive Level: Application

24. T. H., 16, has just been admitted to your unit for overnight observation after being in an automobile accident. What is your best approach to communicating with him?
    A. Use slang language when you can since he'll think you're "cool" and will open up to you.
    B. Be totally honest with him, even if your information is unpleasant.
    C. Use periods of silence to communicate your respect for him.
    D. Tell him that you will keep everything that you talk about totally confidential.

Correct Answer: B

Rationale: Successful communication (with adolescents) is possible, and rewarding. The guidelines are simple. The first consideration is your attitude, which must be one of respect. Second, your communication must be totally honest. The adolescent's intuition is highly tuned and can detect phoniness or withholding of information. Always give them the truth.

Cognitive Level: Application

25. Mrs. B., 75, is at your clinic for a preoperative interview. This interview may take longer than interviews with younger persons. Why?
    A. As a person ages, they are unable to hear and thus interviewers usually need to repeat much of what is said.
    B. Aged persons lose much of their mental capacities and require greater time to complete an interview.
    C. An aged person has a longer story to tell.
    D. An aged person is usually lonely and likes to have someone to talk to.

Correct Answer: C

Rationale: The interview usually takes longer with older adults because they have a longer story to tell.

Cognitive Level: Comprehension

26. You are interviewing Mr. L., who has a hearing impairment. What techniques would be most beneficial in communicating with Mr. L.?
    A. Request a sign language interpreter before you meet with Mr. L. to help facilitate the communication.
    B. Speak loudly and with exaggerated facial movement when talking with Mr. L. since this helps with lip reading.
    C. Avoid using facial and hand gestures because most hearing-impaired people find this degrading.
    D. Assess the method of communication Mr. L. prefers.

Correct Answer: D

Rationale: Ask the deaf person the preferred way to communicate—by signing, lip reading, or writing. If the person prefers lip reading, be sure to face him or her squarely and have good lighting on your face. Do not exaggerate your lip movements because this distorts your words. Similarly, shouting distorts the reception of a hearing aid the person may wear. Speak slowly and supplement your voice with appropriate hand gestures or pantomime.

Cognitive Level: Comprehension

27. During a prenatal check, Mrs. P. begins to cry as you ask her about previous pregnancies. She states that she is remembering her last pregnancy, which ended in miscarriage. Your best response to her crying would be:
    A. "I can see that you are sad remembering this. It is all right to cry."
    B. "I can see that you feel sad about this; why don't we talk about something else?"
    C. "I'm so sorry for making you cry!"
    D. "Why don't I step out for a few minutes until you're feeling better?"

Correct Answer: A

Rationale: A beginning examiner usually feels horrified when the patient starts crying. When you say something that "makes the person cry," do not think you have hurt the person. You have just hit on a topic that is important. Do not go on to a new topic. Just let the person cry and express his or her feelings fully. You can offer a tissue and wait until the crying subsides to talk.

Cognitive Level: Application

28. You are interviewing Mr. A., who is a recent immigrant from Iran. During the course of the interview, Mr. A. leans forward and then finally moves his chair close enough that your knees are nearly touching. You begin to feel uncomfortable with his proximity. Which statement most closely reflects what you should do:
    A. Discreetly move your chair back until the distance suits you, then continue your interview.
    B. Laugh and tell Mr. A. that you are uncomfortable with his close proximity and ask him to move away from you.
    C. These behaviors are indicative of sexual aggression, and you should confront Mr. A. about them.
    D. Try to relax—these behaviors are culturally appropriate for Mr. A.

Correct Answer: D

Rationale: Both the patient's and your own sense of spatial distance are significant throughout the interview and physical examination, with culturally appropriate distance zones varying widely. For example, you may find yourself backing away from people of Hispanic, East Indian, or Middle Eastern origins who invade your personal space with regularity in an attempt to bring you closer into the space that is comfortable to them.

Cognitive Level: Analysis

29. Mrs. W., a Native American, has come to your clinic for diabetic follow-up teaching. During your interview, you notice that she never makes eye contact with you and speaks mostly to the floor. Which statement is true regarding this situation?
    A. Mrs. W. is showing that she is listening carefully to what you are saying.
    B. Mrs. W. has something to hide and is ashamed.
    C. Mrs. W. is nervous and embarrassed.
    D. Mrs. W. is showing inconsistent verbal and nonverbal behaviors.

Correct Answer: A

Rationale: Eye contact is perhaps among the most culturally variable nonverbal behaviors. Asian, Native American, Indochinese, Arab, and Appalachian people may consider direct eye contact impolite or aggressive, and they may avert their own eyes during the interview. Native Americans often stare at the floor during the interview, a culturally appropriate behavior indicating that the listener is paying close attention to the speaker.

Cognitive Level: Analysis

30. You have just begun your assessment of Mrs. L.'s newborn. Mrs. L. is Vietnamese. Which statement is true regarding this examination?
    A. Mrs. L. would prefer to have the results of the examination communicated directly to her husband.
    B. Mrs. L. will be offended if you touch the infant's diaper area during your examination.
    C. Mrs. L. will be offended if you examine the infant's fontanels.
    D. Mrs. L. would prefer to have you give her written material about growth and development rather than verbal explanation.

Correct Answer: C

Rationale: Touching children may also have associated meaning cross-culturally. Many Asians believe that one's strength resides in the head and touching the head is considered disrespectful. Thus, palpating the fontanel of an infant from Southeast Asian descent should be approached with sensitivity.

Cognitive Level: Analysis

31. You are performing a health interview on a patient who has a language barrier and no interpreter is available. Which of the following is the best example of an appropriate question to ask in this situation?
    A. "Do you have nausea and vomiting?"
    B. "He has been taking his medicine, hasn't he?"
    C. "Does Joe take medicine?"
    D. "Do you sterilize the bottles?"

Correct Answer: C

Rationale: In a situation where there is a language barrier and no interpreter available, use simple words avoiding medical jargon. Avoid using contractions and pronouns. Use nouns repeatedly and discuss one topic at a time.

Cognitive Level: Analysis

32. Mr. J. is at the clinic for an annual wellness physical. He is experiencing no acute health problems. Which of following statements is most appropriate when beginning the interview?
    A. "Why are you here today?"
    B. "How is your family?"
    C. "Tell me about your hypertension?"
    D. "How has your health been since your last visit?"

Correct Answer: D

Rationale: Open-ended questions are used for narrative information. Use this type of questioning to begin the interview, introduce a new section of questions, and whenever the person introduces a new topic.

Cognitive Level: Application

33. Critique the following statement made by the nurse. "I know it may be hard, but you should do what the doctor ordered, since he/she is the expert in this field."
    A. This statement is appropriate because members of the health care team are experts in the area of patient care.
    B. At times, it is necessary to utilize authority statements when dealing with patients, especially when they are undecided about an issue.
    C. This type of statement promotes dependency and inferiority on the part of the patient and is best avoided in an interview situation.
    D. This statement is inappropriate because it shows the nurse's bias.

Correct Answer: C

Rationale: Using authority responses promotes dependency and inferiority. It is best to avoid using authority. Even though the health care provider and patient do not have equal professional knowledge, both have equally worthy roles in the health process.

Cognitive Level: Analysis

Chapter 5

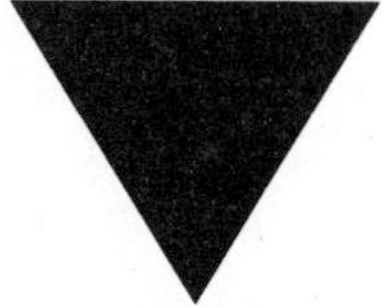

The Complete Health History

1. Which of the following statements best describes the purpose of a health history?
   A. To document the normal and abnormal findings of a physical assessment.
   B. To provide a database of subjective information about patient's past and present health.
   C. To provide a form for obtaining the patient's biographical information.
   D. To provide an opportunity for interaction between patient and nurse.

Correct Answer: B

Rationale: The purpose of the health history is to collect subjective data, what the person says about himself or herself.

Cognitive Level: Comprehension

2. In documenting the reliability of a patient's responses, which of the following would be appropriate?
   A. M.S. smiled throughout interview so is assumed reliable.
   B. M.S. has history of drug abuse so is not reliable.
   C. M.S. provided consistent information and is reliable.
   D. M.S. would not answer questions concerning stress so is not reliable.

Correct Answer: C

Rationale: A reliable person always gives the same answers, even when questions are rephrased, or are repeated later in the interview.

Cognitive Level: Application

3. J.M., a 59-year-old male, tells you he is here today to "check his ulcerative colitis." He has been having "black stools" for the last 24 hours. How would you document his reason for seeking care?
   A. J.M. is a 59-year-old male here for "black stools" for past 24 hours.
   B. J.M., a 59-year-old male, states he has ulcerative colitis and wants it checked.
   C. J.M. came into clinic complaining of black stools for past 24 hours.
   D. J.M. is a 59-year-old male here for "ulcerative colitis."

Correct Answer: A

Rationale: Reason for seeking care is a brief spontaneous statement in the person's own words that describes the reason for the visit. It states one (possibly two) signs or symptoms and their duration. It is enclosed in quotation marks to indicate the person's exact words.

Cognitive Level: Application

4. A patient tells you she has had abdominal pain for the past week. What would be your response?
   A. "We'll talk more about that later in the interview."
   B. "What have you had to eat in the last 24 hours?"
   C. "Have you ever had any surgeries on your abdomen?"
   D. "Can you point to where it hurts?"

Correct Answer: D

Rationale: Your final summary of any symptom the person has should include, among eight critical characteristics, "Location: specific"; ask the person to point to the location.

Cognitive Level: Application

5. P.M., a 29-year-old female, tells you she has "excruciating pain" in her back. Which of the following would be an appropriate response to her statement?
   A. "That must be terrible; you probably pinched a nerve."
   B. "How would you say the pain affects your ability to do your daily activities?"
   C. "How does your family react to your pain?"

D. "I've had back pain myself and it can be excruciating."

Correct Answer: B

Rationale: The symptom of pain is difficult to quantify because of individual interpretation. With pain, avoid adjectives and ask how it affects daily activities.

Cognitive Level: Application

6. In recording the childhood illnesses of a patient who denies having had any, which of the following would be most accurate?
   A. Patient denies usual childhood illnesses.
   B. Patient states sister had measles, but she didn't.
   C. Patient denies measles, mumps, rubella, chicken pox, pertussis or strep throat.
   D. Patient states she was a "very healthy" child.

Correct Answer: C

Rationale: Childhood illnesses include measles, mumps, rubella, chicken pox, pertussis, and strep throat. Avoid recording "usual childhood illnesses" because an illness common in the person's childhood may be unusual today, e.g., measles.

Cognitive Level: Knowledge

7. A female patient tells you she has had six pregnancies, four live births and two spontaneous abortions. How would you record this information?
   A. Patient has had four healthy babies.
   B. P-6, B-4, SAb-2
   C. Patient has been pregnant six times.
   D. G-6, P-4, SAb-2

Correct Answer: B

Rationale: Obstetric history should include number of pregnancies (gravidity), number of deliveries in which the fetus reached viability (parity), and number of incomplete pregnancies (abortions). This is recorded: G_P_Ab_. For each complete pregnancy, note the course of pregnancy; labor and deliver; sex, weight, and condition of each infant; and postpartum course. For any incomplete pregnancies, record the duration and whether the pregnancy resulted in spontaneous (S) or induced (I) abortion.

Cognitive Level: Comprehension

8. Your patient tells you he is allergic to penicillin. What would be your next response?
   A. "Are you allergic to any other drugs?"
   B. "I'll write your allergy on your chart so you won't receive any."
   C. "Would you describe what happens to you when you take penicillin?"
   D. "How often have you received penicillin?"

Correct Answer: C

Rationale: Note both the allergen (medication, food, or contact agent, such as fabric or environmental agent) and the reaction (rash, itching, runny nose, watery eyes, difficulty breathing). With a drug, this symptom should not be a side effect but a true allergic reaction.

Cognitive Level: Comprehension

9. When taking a family history, important diseases or problems to ask the patient about include:
   A. fractured bones.
   B. mental illness.
   C. head trauma.
   D. emphysema.

Correct Answer: B

Rationale: Specifically ask for any family history of: heart disease, high blood pressure, stroke, diabetes, blood disorders, cancer, sickle cell anemia, arthritis, allergies, obesity, alcoholism, mental illness, seizure disorder, kidney disease, and tuberculosis.

Cognitive Level: Knowledge

10. The review of systems provides the nurse with:
    A. physical findings related to each system.
    B. information regarding health promotion practices.
    C. an opportunity to teach the patient medical terms.
    D. information necessary for the nurse to diagnose the patient's medical problem.

Correct Answer: B

Rationale: "The purposes of this section are (1) to evaluate the past and present health state of each body system, (2) to double check in case any significant data were omitted in the present illness section, and (3) to evaluate health promotion practices."

Cognitive Level: Knowledge

11. Which of the following statements represents subjective data obtained from the patient regarding his skin?
    A. Skin appears dry.
    B. No obvious lesions.
    C. Denies color change.
    D. Lesion noted lateral aspect right arm.

Correct Answer: C

Rationale: Remember that the history should be limited to patient statements, or subjective data—factors that the person says were or were not present.

Cognitive Level: Comprehension

12. You are obtaining a history from a 30-year-old male and are concerned about health promotion activities. Which of the following questions would you ask?
    A. "Have you ever noticed any pain in your testicles?"
    B. "Do you perform testicular self exams?"
    C. "Do you have any history of sexually transmitted disease?"
    D. "Have you had any problems with passing your urine?"

Correct Answer: B

Rationale: Health promotion for a man would include performance of testicular self-examination.

Cognitive Level: Comprehension

13. Which of the following responses might you expect during a functional assessment of a patient whose leg is in a cast?
    A. "I'm able to transfer myself from the wheelchair to the bed without help."
    B. "The pain is getting less but I still need to take Tylenol."
    C. "I broke my right leg in a car accident 2 weeks ago."
    D. "I check the color of my toes every evening just like I was taught."

Correct Answer: A

Rationale: Functional assessment measures a person's self-care ability in the areas of general physical health, or absence of illness.

Cognitive Level: Application

14. In response to your question about stress, a 39-year-old female tells you that her husband and mother both died in the past year. Your response might include which of the following?
    A. "Having two family members die so close must have been hard."
    B. "I don't know how anyone could handle that much stress in 1 year!"
    C. "What did you do to cope with the loss of both your husband and mother?"
    D. "That is a lot of stress; now let's go on to the next section of your history."

Correct Answer: C

Rationale: Coping and stress management includes kinds of stresses in life, especially in the last year, any change in lifestyle or any current stress, methods tried to relieve stress, and whether these have been helpful.

Cognitive Level: Application

15. In response to your question regarding use of alcohol, a patient asks you why you need to know. What is your reason for needing this information?
    A. This is necessary to determine the patient's reliability.
    B. The nurse needs to be able to teach patient how bad alcohol is for him.
    C. Alcohol can interact with medications as well as make some diseases worse.
    D. It's not really necessary to have this information unless there is an obvious drinking problem.

Correct Answer: C

Rationale: Alcohol interacts adversely with all medications; is a factor in many social problems such as motor vehicle accidents, assaults, rapes, and child abuse; and is a major factor in the exacerbation of most medical illness (Meyer, et al., 1992).

Cognitive Level: Comprehension

16. The mother of a 16-month-old tells you her daughter has an earache. What would be an appropriate response?
    A. "I will check her ear for an ear infection."
    B. "Are you sure she is really having pain?"
    C. "Would you describe what she is doing to indicate she is having pain?"
    D. "Maybe she is just teething."

Correct Answer: C

Rationale: With a child, ask the parent, "How do you

know the child is in pain?" (E.g., pulling at ears alerts parent to ear pain.)

Cognitive Level: Application

17. In obtaining the history from the mother of a 2-year-old with pneumonia, you ask the mother if she smoked or used drugs during her pregnancy. Her response is, "What does that have to do with pneumonia?" How would you answer her question?
   A. "The use of tobacco during pregnancy could be the cause of your daughter's pneumonia."
   B. "It's not really that important, we just ask everyone the same questions."
   C. "You don't need to answer if it makes you uncomfortable."
   D. "Knowing about your pregnancy gives us a more complete picture of your daughter's health."

Correct Answer: D

Rationale: Record the mother's use of alcohol, street drugs, or cigarettes and any x-ray studies taken during pregnancy.

Cognitive Level: Application

18. A 5-year-old boy is being admitted to the hospital to have his tonsils removed. Information that would be helpful prior to procedure would include:
   A. the child's birth weight.
   B. reactions to previous hospitalizations.
   C. whether he has had the measles.
   D. age at which he crawled.

Correct Answer: B

Rationale: Assess how child reacted to hospitalization and any complications. (If child reacted poorly, he or she may be afraid now and will need special preparation for the examination that is to follow.)

Cognitive Level: Analysis

19. As part of the health history of a 12-year-old male here for a sports physical, you obtain his immunization record. His mother indicates he has had his OPV and DTP immunizations, tetanus was last year and MMR was at 15 months of age. What recommendation would you make?
   A. No further immunizations are needed.
   B. DTP needs to be repeated every 4 years until age 21.
   C. MMR needs to be repeated at age 12.
   D. You can't make a recommendation until you check with the physician.

Correct Answer: C

Rationale: Recommended schedule for immunization of healthy infants and children indicates MMR is needed at 15 months and again at 11-12 years of age.

Cognitive Level: Analysis

20. In obtaining a review of systems on a "healthy" 7-year-old girl, it would be important to include:
   A. frequency of breast self exam.
   B. limitations related to involvement in sports activities.
   C. last glaucoma exam.
   D. date of last electrocardiogram.

Correct Answer: B

Rationale: Cardiovascular system. You should ask whether there is any limitation of activity, or whether the child can keep up with peers.

Cognitive Level: Application

21. A description of whom a child lives with, method of discipline, and support system are all related to which part of the assessment?
   A. Review of systems
   B. Family history
   C. Functional assessment
   D. Reason for seeking care

Correct Answer: C

Rationale: Functional assessment includes interpersonal relationships and home environment.

Cognitive Level: Comprehension

22. When obtaining a health history on an 87-year-old female, which of the following questions would be most useful?
   A. Obstetric history
   B. Current health promotion activities
   C. General health for past 20 years
   D. Childhood illnesses

Correct Answer: B

Rationale: It is important for you to recognize positive health measures: what the person has been doing to help himself or herself stay well and to live to an older age.

Cognitive Level: Application

23. Which of the following statements regarding questions you would ask a 76-year-old patient during your review of systems is true?
    A. You start incorporating different questions at the age of 70 or older.
    B. Additional questions you would include are reflective of normal effects of aging.
    C. The questions you ask are identical for all ages.
    D. At this age, you don't do a review of systems, rather just focus on current problems.

Correct Answer: B

Rationale: The health history includes the same format as that described for the younger adult, as well as some additional questions. These questions address ways in which the ADLs may have been affected by normal aging processes or by the effects of chronic illness or disability.

Cognitive Level: Comprehension

24. A 90-year-old patient tells you he can't remember the names of the drugs he is taking or what they are for. An appropriate response would be:
    A. "Don't worry about it; you are only taking two."
    B. "Can you tell me what they look like?"
    C. "How long have you been taking each of the pills?"
    D. "Would you have your family bring in your medications?"

Correct Answer: D

Rationale: The person may not know drug name or purpose. When this occurs, ask the person to bring in the drug to be identified.

Cognitive Level: Application

25. In performing a functional assessment on an 82-year-old patient with a recent stroke, which of the following questions would be most important to ask?
    A. Do you wear glasses?
    B. Do you have any thyroid problems?
    C. How many times a day do you have a bowel movement?
    D. Are you able to dress yourself?

Correct Answer: D

Rationale: The impact of a disease on their daily activities and overall quality of life (called the disease burden) is more important to older people than the actual disease diagnosis or pathology (Bernstein, 1992).

Cognitive Level: Application

26. During your interview with a Native American patient you would:
    A. assume he is like most other Native Americans in his cultural beliefs.
    B. obtain a cultural assessment.
    C. know that since he is an American there is no reason to ask any cultural questions.
    D. not ask specific cultural questions at the risk of offending the patient.

Correct Answer: B

Rationale: One aspect of a comprehensive health history concerns the collection of data related to culturally based beliefs and practices about health and illness.

Cognitive Level: Application

27. Which of the following best describes the purpose of a functional assessment?
    A. It assesses how the individual is coping with life at home.
    B. It can identify any problems with memory the individual may be experiencing.
    C. It determines how children are meeting developmental milestones.
    D. It is very important, especially in the elderly, to determine how they are managing day-to-day activities.

Correct Answer: D

Rationale: The functional assessment, because it emphasizes function, is very important in assessing older people.

Cognitive Level: Knowledge

Chapter 6

Mental Status Assessment

1. When examining a patient, the nurse can assess mental status by:
   A. examining the patient's response to a specific set of questions.
   B. observing the patient and inferring health or dysfunction.
   C. examining the patient's EEG.
   D. observing the patient as he or she performs on IQ tests.

Correct Answer: B

Rationale: Mental status cannot be scrutinized directly like the characteristics of skin or heart sounds. Its functioning is inferred through assessment of an individual's behavior.

Cognitive Level: Comprehension

2. When assessing mental status in children, which of the following statements would be true?
   A. Children are highly labile and unstable until the age of 2.
   B. Children's mental status is impossible to assess until the child develops the ability to concentrate.
   C. All aspects of mental status in children are interrelated.
   D. Children's mental status is largely a function of their parent's level of functioning until the age of 7.

Correct Answer: C

Rationale: It is difficult to separate and trace the development of just one aspect of mental status. All aspects are interdependent. For example, consciousness is rudimentary at birth because the cerebral cortex is not yet developed; the infant cannot distinguish the self from the mother's body.

Cognitive Level: Comprehension

3. You are assessing Mr. P., a 75-year-old. As you begin the mental status portion of your assessment you would expect:
   A. Mr. P. will have had a decrease in his response time due to language loss and a decrease in general knowledge.
   B. Mr. P. will have no decrease in any of his abilities including response time.
   C. It may take Mr. P. a little longer to respond but his general knowledge and abilities should not have declined.
   D. Mr. P. will have difficulty on tests of remote memory since this typically decreases with age.

Correct Answer: C

Rationale: The aging process leaves the parameters of mental status mostly intact. There is no decrease in general knowledge and little or no loss in vocabulary. Response time is slower than in youth; it takes a bit longer for the brain to process information and react to it.

Cognitive Level: Analysis

4. In your assessment of aging adults, you know that one of the first things that you should assess prior to making judgments about their mental status is:
   A. sensory perceptive abilities.
   B. general intelligence.
   C. phobias.
   D. irrational thinking patterns.

Correct Answer: A

Rationale: Age-related changes in sensory perception can affect mental status. For example, vision loss (as detailed in Chapter 12) may result in apathy, social isolation, and depression. Hearing changes are common in older adults. This problem produces frustration, suspicion, and social isolation, and also makes the person look confused (Rossman, 1986).

Cognitive Level: Analysis

5. Which of the following statements is true with regard to mental status examination?
   A. It is usually necessary to perform a complete mental status examination in order to get a good idea of the patient's level of functioning.
   B. A patient's family is the best resource for information about the patient's coping skills.
   C. It is usually sufficient to gather mental status information during the health history interview.
   D. It would take an enormous amount of extra time to integrate mental status examination into the health history interview.

Correct Answer: C

Rationale: The full mental status examination is a systematic check of emotional and cognitive functioning. The steps described here, though, rarely need to be taken in their entirety. Usually, you can assess mental status through the context of the health history interview.

Cognitive Level: Application

6. Mrs. H. brings her husband to the clinic for an examination. She is particularly worried because after a recent fall, he seems to have lost a great deal of his memory for recent events. Which statement reflects your best course of action?
   A. You should plan to perform a complete mental status examination.
   B. You should plan to integrate the mental status examination into the history and physical examination.
   C. It would be most appropriate to refer Mr. H. to a psychometrician.
   D. You should reassure Mrs. H. that memory loss after a physical shock is normal and will subside soon.

Correct Answer: A

Rationale: It is necessary to perform a full mental status examination when you discover any abnormality in affect or behavior, and in the following situations: Family members are concerned about a person's behavioral changes, e.g., memory loss, inappropriate social interaction.

Cognitive Level: Application

7. In your interview with Mr. W. it will be important for you to ascertain some basic history information. Which of the following would you explore more fully with Mr. W.?
   A. Mr. W. states that he is currently not taking any medication.
   B. Mr. W. states that he "never did too good in school."
   C. Mr. W. states that he "sleeps like a baby."
   D. Mr. W. states that he has no health problems that he knows of.

Correct Answer: B

Rationale: In every mental status examination, note these factors from the health history that could affect your findings: any known illnesses or health problems, such as alcoholism, or chronic renal disease; current medications, whose side effects may cause confusion or depression; the usual educational and behavioral level—note that factor as the normal baseline, and do not expect performance on the mental status examination to exceed it; responses to personal history questions, indicating current stress, social interaction patterns, and sleep habits.

Cognitive Level: Analysis

8. Mrs. K. is admitted to your unit following an automobile accident. You begin her mental status examination and find that her speech is dysarthric and she is lethargic. Your best approach regarding this examination is:
   A. skip the language portion of the examination and go on to assess mood and affect.
   B. do an in-depth speech evaluation and defer the mental status examination to another time.
   C. go ahead and assess for suicidal thoughts since dysarthria is often accompanied by severe depression.
   D. plan to defer the rest of the mental status examination.

Correct Answer: D

Rationale: In the following examination the sequence of steps forms a hierarchy, in which the most basic functions (consciousness, language) are assessed first. The first steps must be accurately assessed to ensure validity for the steps to follow. That is, if consciousness is clouded, then the person cannot be expected to have full attention and to cooperate with new learning. Or if language is impaired, subsequent assessment of new learning or abstract reasoning (anything that requires language functioning) can give erroneous conclusions.

Cognitive Level: Analysis

9. Ms. J., 19, comes to your clinic at the insistence of her brother. She is wearing black combat boots and a black lace nightgown over the top of her other clothes. Her hair is dyed pink with black streaks throughout. She has several pierced holes in her nares and ears and is wearing an earring through her eyebrow as well as heavy black make up. You conclude:
   A. Ms. J. has manic syndrome due to her abnormal dress and grooming.
   B. Ms. J. probably doesn't have any problems at all.
   C. you will need to gather more information in order to decide whether her dress is appropriate or not.
   D. she is just trying to shock people and her dress should be ignored.

Correct Answer: C

Rationale: Grooming and hygiene should be noted. The person is clean and well groomed, hair is neat and clean, women have moderate or no make-up, men are shaved for beard or moustache are well groomed. Use care in interpreting clothing that is disheveled, bizarre, or in poor repair, because these sometimes reflect the person's economic status or a deliberate fashion trend.

Cognitive Level: Application

10. Mr. D. has been in the ICU for 10 days. He has just been moved to your floor and you are planning to perform a mental status examination on him. During the tests of cognitive function you would expect:
   A. Mr. D. will be oriented to place and person but may not be certain of the date.
   B. Mr. D. will state, "I am so relieved to be out of intensive care."
   C. Mr. D. may evidence some disruption in thought content.
   D. Mr. D. may evidence some clouding of his level of consciousness.

Correct Answer: A

Rationale: Cognitive Functions: Orientation. You can discern orientation through the course of the interview, or ask directly, using tact. "Some people have trouble keeping up with the dates while in the hospital. Do you know today's date?" Many hospitalized people normally have trouble with the exact date but are fully oriented on the remaining items.

Cognitive Level: Analysis

11. In order to assess affect, you should ask the patient:
   A. "Have these medications had any effect on your pain?"
   B. "How do you feel today?"
   C. "Has this pain affected your ability to perform activities of daily living, such as dressing?"
   D. "Would you please repeat the following words?"

Correct Answer: B

Rationale: Mood and affect. Judge this by body language and facial expression, and by asking directly, "how do you feel today," or "how do you usually feel?" The mood should be appropriate to the person's place and condition and change appropriately with topics.

Cognitive Level: Application

12. You are going to assess recent memory with Mr. F. The best way to do this would be to:
   A. ask Mr. F. to describe what TV show he was watching prior to coming to the clinic.
   B. ask Mr. F. to describe his first job to you.
   C. give Mr. F. the Four Unrelated Words Test.
   D. give Mr. F. the FACT Test.

Correct Answer: C

Rationale: Assess recent memory in the context of the interview by the 24-hour diet recall, or asking the time the person arrived at the agency. Ask questions you can corroborate. This screens for the occasional person who confabulates or makes up answers to fill in the gaps of memory loss. New learning – the Four Unrelated Words Test. This tests the person's ability to lay down new memories. It is a highly sensitive and valid memory test.

Cognitive Level: Application

13. Mrs. A., 45, is at your agency for a mental status assessment. In giving her the Four Unrelated Words Test, you would be concerned if:
   A. she could not invent four unrelated words within 5 minutes.
   B. she could not recall four unrelated words after 30-minute delay.
   C. she could not recall four unrelated words after a 60-minute delay.
   D. she could not invent four unrelated words within 30 seconds.

Correct Answer: B

Rationale: New Learning—the Four Unrelated Words Test. This tests the person's ability to lay down new memories. It is a highly sensitive and valid memory test. It requires more effort than does the recall of personal or historic events. To the person, say, "I am going to say four words. I want you to remember them. In a few minutes I will ask you to recall them." After 5 minutes, ask for the recall of the 4 words. The normal response for persons under 60 years is an accurate three- or four-word recall after a 5-, 10-, and 30-minute delay.

Cognitive Level: Analysis

14. Which of the following questions would best assess a person's judgment?
    A. "What would you do if you found a stamped, addressed envelope lying on the sidewalk?"
    B. "Tell me about what you plan to do once you are discharged from the hospital."
    C. "What does the statement, 'People in glass houses shouldn't throw stones' mean to you?"
    D. "Do you feel that you are being watched, followed, or controlled?"

Correct Answer: B

Rationale: A person exercises judgment when he or she can compare and evaluate the alternatives in a situation and reach an appropriate course of action. Rather than testing the person's response to a hypothetical situation, (e.g., "What would you do if you found a stamped, addressed envelope lying on the sidewalk?"), you should be more interested in the person's judgment about daily or long-term goals, the likelihood of acting in response to delusions or hallucinations, and the capacity for violent or suicidal behavior.

Cognitive Level: Application

15. Which of the following individuals would you consider to be at highest risk for a suicide attempt?
    A. An adolescent who has just broken up with her boyfriend and states that she would like to kill herself
    B. An elderly man who tells you that he is going to "join his wife in heaven" tomorrow and plans to use a gun
    C. A woman during an episode of major depression who has tried suicide in the past
    D. A man who jokes about death

Correct Answer: B

Rationale: When the person expresses feelings of sadness, hopelessness, despair or grief, it is important to assess any possible risk of physical harm to himself or herself. Begin with more general questions. If you hear affirmative answers, continue with more specific questions. A precise suicide plan to take place in the next 24 to 48 hours using a lethal method constitutes high risk.

Cognitive Level: Comprehension

16. You are performing a mental status assessment on R., a 5-year-old girl. Her parents are undergoing a bitter divorce and are worried about the effect it is having on R. Of the following information, which statement might lead you to worry about R.'s mental status?
    A. R. appears angry and will not make eye contact with you.
    B. R.'s mother states that she has begun to ride a tricycle.
    C. R.'s mother states that she has had to put R. in diapers again because she refuses to use the toilet.
    D. R. clings to her mother whenever you are in the room.

Correct Answer: C

Rationale: The mental status assessment of infants and children covers behavioral, cognitive, and psychosocial development, and examines how the child is coping with his or her environment. Essentially, you will follow the same A- B- C- T- guidelines as for the adult, with special consideration for developmental milestones. Your best examination "technique" arises from thorough knowledge of developmental milestones as described in Chapter 3. Abnormalities are often problems of omission; the child does not achieve a milestone you would expect.

Cognitive Level: Analysis

17. You would plan to use the Behavioral Checklist with a child who:
    A. is 8 years old.
    B. is having difficulty with gross motor skills.
    C. is 5 years old, just prior to kindergarten.
    D. is 18 years old.

Correct Answer: A

Rationale: For school-age children, ages 7 to 11, who

have grown beyond the age when developmental milestones are very useful, the "Behavioral Checklist" is an additional tool that can be given to the parent along with the history.

Cognitive Level: Knowledge

18. You are assessing orientation in Mr. J., 79. Which of the following responses would lead you to conclude that Mr. J. is oriented?
    A. "I know that my name is Mr. J., but to tell you the truth, I get kind of confused about the date."
    B. "I know that my name is Mr. J., I am at the hospital in Spokane. I couldn't tell you what date it is, but I know that it is February of a new year—2000."
    C. "I know that my name is Mr. J. I couldn't tell you where I am. I think it is 2000, though."
    D. "I know that my name is Mr. J.; I guess I'm at the hospital in Spokane. No, I don't know the date."

Correct Answer: B

Rationale: Many aging persons experience social isolation, loss of structure without a job, a change in residence, or some short-term memory loss. These factors affect orientation and this person may not provide the precise date or complete name of agency. You may consider aging persons oriented if they know generally where they are and the present period. That is, consider them oriented to time if the year and month are correctly stated. Orientation to place is accepted with the correct identification of the type of setting (e.g., the hospital) and the name of the town.

Cognitive Level: Application

19. You have decided to administer the Set Test to Mr. C., 70. To administer this test you should:
    A. ask him to name 10 fruits, animals, colors, and towns. Tell him that you will be available to help if he gets stuck.
    B. ask him to name 10 items based on the categories in the acronym FACT. Tell him this test is timed and he can only have 2 minutes to take it.
    C. ask him to name 10 items based on the categories in the acronym FACT. Tell him that there is no hurry to do this.
    D. ask him to name 10 items based on the categories in the acronym FACT. If he has difficulty, you may prompt his memory.

Correct Answer: C

Rationale: The Set Test was developed specifically for use with an aging population. The test is easy to administer and takes less than 5 minutes. Ask the person to name 10 items in each of four categories or sets: fruits, animals, colors, and towns (FACT). Do not coach, prompt, or hurry the person.

Cognitive Level: Application

20. Mrs. G. drifts off to sleep when she is not being stimulated. You can arouse her easily when you call her name but she remains looking drowsy during your conversation. The best description of Mrs. G.'s level of consciousness would be:
    A. semi-alert.
    B. lethargic.
    C. stuporous.
    D. obtunded.

Correct Answer: B

Rationale: Lethargic (or somnolent): Not fully alert, drifts off to sleep when not stimulated, can be aroused to name when called in normal voice but looks drowsy; responds appropriately to questions or commands but thinking seems slow and fuzzy, inattentive, loses train of thought; spontaneous movements are decreased.

Cognitive Level: Comprehension

21. Mr. S. has suffered a CVA (stroke). He is trying very hard to communicate with you. He seems driven to speak and says, "I buy obie get spirding and take my train." What is the best way to communicate with Mr. S.?
    A. Give him a pencil and paper since reading and writing abilities will not be impaired.
    B. Use speech, he will understand you even if you cannot understand him.
    C. Support his efforts to communicate and use pantomime and gestures to communicate when you can.
    D. Abandon all attempts to communicate with Mr. S.; his aphasia is irreversible.

Correct Answer: C

Rationale: The linguistic opposite of Broca's aphasia. Speech is fluent, effortless, and well articulated. Output has many paraphasias (word substitutions that are malformed or wrong) and neologisms (made-up words) and often lacks substantive words. Speech can be totally incomprehensible. Often there is a great urge to speak. Essentially, it is a defect of auditory comprehension. Repetition, reading, and writing also are impaired.

Cognitive Level: Analysis

22. As you talk with your patient, he seems to repeatedly have difficulty coming up with a word. He says, "I was on my way to work and when I got there, the thing that you step into that goes up in the air, was so full that I decided to take the stairs." You will note on his chart that he is using/experiencing:
    A. circumstantiality.
    B. blocking.
    C. neologism.
    D. circumlocution.

Correct Answer: D

Rationale: Circumlocution: Round-about expression, substituting a phrase when one cannot think of name of object.

Cognitive Level: Comprehension

23. Which of the following statements is an example of flight of ideas?
    A. "My stomach hurts. Hurts, spurts, burts."
    B. "Take this pill? The pill is red, I see red, red velvet is soft, soft as a baby's bottom."
    C. "I wash my hands, wash them, wash them. I usually go to the sink and wash my hands."
    D. "Kiss, wood, reading, ducks, onto, maybe."

Correct Answer: B

Rationale: Flight of ideas: Abrupt change, rapid skipping from topic to topic, practically continuous flow of accelerated speech. Topics usually have recognizable associations or are plays on words.

Cognitive Level: Comprehension

24. Your patient describes feeling an unreasonable, irrational fear of snakes. It is so persistent, that he can no longer comfortably even look at pictures of snakes and has made an effort to identify all the places he might encounter a snake and avoids these. You explain to him that:
    A. "You have what we call an obsession. In this case, it is with snakes."
    B. "You have a delusion that snakes are harmful. It must stem from an early traumatic incident involving snakes."
    C. "You are suffering from a snake-phobia."
    D. "You are a hypochondriac; snakes are usually harmless."

Correct Answer: C

Rationale: Phobia: Strong, persistent, irrational fear of an object or situation; person feels driven to avoid it.

Cognitive Level: Application

25. Your patient is schizophrenic. During a recent interview, he shows you a picture of a man holding a decapitated head. He describes this picture as horrifying and laughs loudly at the content. This behavior is a display of:
    A. depersonalization.
    B. irritability.
    C. inappropriate affect.
    D. ambivalence.

Correct Answer: C

Rationale: Inappropriate affect: Affect clearly discordant with the content of the person's speech.

Cognitive Level: Analysis

26. Which of the following examples would be a hallucination?
    A. A child sees a man standing in his closet. When the lights are turned on it is only a dry cleaning bag.
    B. A man believes that the dog has curled up on the bed but when he gets closer he sees that it is the blanket.
    C. A woman hears the doorbell ring and goes to answer it, but no one is there.
    D. A man believes that his dead wife is talking to him.

Correct Answer: D

Rationale: Hallucination: Sensory perceptions for which there are no external stimuli; may strike any sense: visual, auditory, tactile, olfactory, gustatory.

Cognitive Level: Knowledge

27. Mr. B., 20, has just been brought into the emergency department with heat stroke. He is experiencing delirium secondary to the fluid and electrolyte imbalance he has. You would assess Mr. B.'s:
    A. level of consciousness and cognitive abilities.

B. thought processes and memory.
C. affect and mood.
D. memory and affect.

Correct Answer: A

Rationale: Delirium: (A) Disturbance of consciousness (i.e., reduced clarity of awareness of the environment) with reduced ability to focus, sustain, or shift attention. (B) A change in cognition (such as memory deficit, disorientation, language disturbance) or the development of a perceptual disturbance. (C) The disturbance develops over a short period of time (usually hours to days) and tends to fluctuate during the course of the day.

Cognitive Level: Comprehension

28. Ms. L. has come to your agency to seek help with a substance abuse problem. She admits to using cocaine just prior to arrival. Which of the following describes what you would expect to find when you examine Ms. L.?
    A. Dilated pupils, unsteady gait, incoordination, aggressiveness
    B. Constricted pupils, euphoria, decreased temperature
    C. Dilated pupils, pacing and psychomotor agitation, hypervigilance
    D. Pupil constriction, lethargy, apathy, dysphoria

Correct Answer: C

Rationale: Cocaine: Appearance—Pupillary dilation, tachycardia or bradycardia, elevated or lowered blood pressure, sweating, chills, nausea, vomiting, weight loss. Behavior—Euphoria, talkativeness, hypervigilance, pacing, psychomotor agitation, impaired judgement, impaired social or occupational functioning, fighting, grandiosity, visual or tactile hallucinations.

Cognitive Level: Comprehension

29. Mr. H. states, "I feel so sad all of the time. I can't feel happy even doing things I used to like to do." He also states that he is tired, sleeps poorly, and has no energy. In order to differentiate between Dysthymic Disorder and a Major Depressive Disorder, what additional areas should you assess?
    A. "Are you having feelings of worthlessness?"
    B. "Are you having any thoughts of suicide?"
    C. "Have you had any weight changes?"
    D. "How long have you been feeling this way?"

Correct Answer: D

Rationale: Major Depressive Disorder is characterized by one or more Major Depressive Episodes (i.e., at least 2 weeks of depressed mood or loss of interest accompanied by at least four additional symptoms of depression). Dysthymic Disorder is characterized by at least 2 years of depressed mood for more days than not, accompanied by additional depressive symptoms.

Cognitive Level: Analysis

30. Ms. P., 26, was raped and beaten a month ago. She is returning to your clinic today for a follow-up assessment. You would want to be certain to ask Ms. P.:
    A. "Are you having any disturbing dreams about the rape?"
    B. "How are things going with your job?"
    C. "Tell me about your recent engagement!"
    D. "How are things going with the trial?"

Correct Answer: A

Rationale: Posttraumatic stress disorder: The person has been exposed to a traumatic event. The traumatic event is persistently reexperienced by: (1) recurrent and intrusive distressing recollections of the event, including images, thoughts, or perceptions; (2) recurrent distressing dreams of the event; (3) acting or feeling as if the traumatic event were recurring.

Cognitive Level: Application

31. Which of the following statements is true regarding the assessment of mental status?
    A. Mental status can be assessed directly, just like other systems of the body, e.g., cardiac and breath sounds.
    B. Mental disorders occur in response to everyday life stressors.
    C. Mental status functioning is inferred through assessment of an individual's behaviors.
    D. Mental status assessment diagnoses specific psychiatric disorders.

Correct Answer: C

Rationale: Mental status functioning is inferred through assessment of an individual's behaviors. It cannot be assessed directly like characteristics of the skin or heart sounds.

Cognitive Level: Comprehension

32. A 23-year-old patient in the clinic appears anxious. Her speech is rapid. She is fidgety and in constant motion. Which of the following questions or statements would be most appropriate to use in this situation to assess attention span?
    A. "I am going to say four words. In a few minutes, I will ask you to recall them."
    B. "Please describe the meaning of the phrase, "Looking through rose-colored glasses."
    C. "How do you usually feel? Is this normal behavior for you?"
    D. "Please pick up the pencil in your left hand, move it to your right hand, and place it on the table."

Correct Answer: D

Rationale: Attention span is evaluated by assessing the individual's ability to concentrate and complete a thought or task without wandering. Giving a series of directions to follow is one method used to assess attention span.

Cognitive Level: Application

33. You are planning health teaching for Mr. Smith, age 65, who has suffered a CVA and is aphasic. Which of the following questions is most important to utilize when assessing mental status in this situation?
    A. "Please point to articles in the room and parts of the body, as I name them."
    B. "Please count back from 100 by seven."
    C. "What would you do if you found a stamped, addressed envelope on the sidewalk?"
    D. "I will name three items and ask you to repeat them in a few minutes."

Correct Answer: A

Rationale: Additional tests for persons with aphasia include the following: word comprehension—asking the individual to point to articles in the room or parts of the body; reading—asking the person to read available print; and writing—asking the person to make up and write a sentence.

Cognitive Level: Application

34. A 30-year-old female patient is describing feelings of hopelessness and depression. She has attempted self-mutilation and has a history of prior suicide attempts. She describes difficulty sleeping at night and has lost 10 pounds in the past month. Which of the following is the nurse's best response in this situation?
    A. "How do other people treat you?"
    B. "Are you feeling so hopeless that you feel like hurting yourself now?"
    C. " Often times people feel hopeless, but the feelings resolve within a few weeks."
    D. "Do you have a weapon?"

Correct Answer: B

Rationale: When the person expresses feelings of hopelessness, despair, or grief, it is important to assess for risk of physical harm to himself or herself. Begin this process with more general questions. If the answers are affirmative, continue with more specific questions.

Cognitive Level: Application

35. Which of the following statements best describes the Mini-Mental State Examination?
    A. It is a good tool to evaluate mood and thought processes.
    B. It is useful for initial evaluation of mental status; additional tools are needed to evaluate cognition changes over time.
    C. It is a good tool to detect delirium and dementia and to differentiate these from psychiatric mental illness.
    D. Scores below 30 indicate cognitive impairment.

Correct Answer: C

Rationale: The Mini-Mental State is a quick, easy test of 11 questions. It is used for initial and serial evaluations and can demonstrate worsening or improvement of cognition over time and with treatment. It evaluates cognitive functioning and not mood or thought processes. It is a good screening tool to detect dementia, delirium, and to differentiate these from psychiatric mental illness.

Cognitive Level: Comprehension

Chapter 7

Nutritional Assessment

1. Of the following people, who is at greatest risk for undernutrition?
   A. A 30-year-old hospital administrator
   B. A 50-year-old female
   C. A 20-year-old college student
   D. A 5-month-old infant

Correct Answer: D

Rationale: Vulnerable groups are infants, children, pregnant women, recent immigrants, persons with low incomes, hospitalized people, and aging adults.

Cognitive Level: Knowledge

2. Optimal nutritional status is best defined as:
   A. sufficient nutrients to provide for the minimal body needs.
   B. sufficient nutrients to provide for daily body requirements as well as for increased metabolic demands.
   C. nutrients in excess of daily body requirements.
   D. sufficient nutrients for daily body requirements but not for increased metabolic demands.

Correct Answer: B

Rationale: Optimal nutritional status is achieved when sufficient nutrients are consumed to support day-do-day body needs and any increased metabolic demands due to growth, pregnancy, or illness.

Cognitive Level: Knowledge

3. You are providing nutrition information to a mother of a 1-year-old. Which of the following represents accurate information?
   A. The baby should be placed on skim milk so as to decrease risk of coronary artery disease when older.
   B. At this age the baby's growth is minimal so caloric requirements are decreased.
   C. The recommended dietary allowances for an infant are the same as for an adolescent.
   D. It is important to maintain adequate fat and caloric intake.

Correct Answer: D

Rationale: For this reason, infants and children younger than 2 should not drink skim or low-fat milk or be placed on low-fat diets—fat (calories and essential fatty acids) is required for proper growth and central nervous system development.

Cognitive Level: Application

4. Mrs. T. is pregnant and interested in breastfeeding her baby. She is interested in facts about breastfeeding. Which of the following is information you would want to share with her?
   A. It is safe for women who are HIV positive to breastfeed.
   B. Babies who are breast fed often require supplemental vitamins.
   C. Breastfeeding is recommended for infants for the first 2 years of life.
   D. Breast milk provides the nutrients necessary for growth as well as natural immunity.

Correct Answer: D

Rationale: Breastfeeding is recommended for full-term infants for the first year of life because breast milk is ideally formulated to promote normal infant growth and development and natural immunity. Women who are HIV positive should not breastfeed, since human immunodeficiency virus (HIV) can be transmitted through breast milk.

Cognitive Level: Application

5. A mother and her 13-year-old daughter express their concern related to the daughter's recent weight gain and increase in appetite. Which of the following represents information you would

want to discuss with them?

A. The importance of a low calorie diet to prevent the accumulation of fat
B. Suggestions for snacks high in protein, iron, and calcium
C. The necessity of exercise and dieting at this age
D. Teenagers who have a weight problem should not be allowed to snack

Correct Answer: B

Rationale: Following a period of slow growth in late childhood, adolescence is characterized by rapid physical growth and endocrine and hormonal changes. Caloric and protein requirements increase to meet this demand, and because of bone growth and increasing muscle mass (and, in girls, the onset of menarche), calcium and iron requirements also increase.

Cognitive Level: Application

6. You are assessing a 30-year-old unemployed immigrant from an underdeveloped country who has been in America for 1 month. Which of the following problems related to his nutritional status might you expect to find?
   A. Obesity
   B. Coronary artery disease
   C. Osteomalacia
   D. Hypotension

Correct Answer: C

Rationale: General undernutrition, hypertension, diarrhea, lactose intolerance, osteomalacia (soft bones), scurvy, and dental caries are among the more common nutrition-related problems of new immigrants from developing countries.

Cognitive Level: Application

7. During a nutritional assessment of a 22-year-old male refugee it is important to:
   A. obtain a 24-hour dietary recall.
   B. clarify what is meant by the term food.
   C. provide him with a standard dietary handbook.
   D. assume his diet is consistent with other refugees you have assessed.

Correct Answer: B

Rationale: Although you may assume that the term "food" is a universal concept, you should have the person clarify what is meant by the term.

Cognitive Level: Application

8. Which of the following statements is true concerning the nutritional assessment?
   A. It provides the nurse with physical findings related to all the systems.
   B. It identifies patients who are at risk for malnutrition.
   C. It is only useful in patients who are overweight.
   D. This assessment can only be thoroughly done by a dietician.

Correct Answer: B

Rationale: The purposes of nutritional assessment are to (1) identify individuals who are malnourished or are at risk of developing malnutrition; (2) provide data for designing a nutrition plan of care that will prevent or minimize the development of malnutrition; and (3) establish baseline data for evaluating the efficacy of nutritional care.

Cognitive Level: Knowledge

9. You are seeing a patient for the first time who has no history of nutrition-related problems. Your initial screening should include which of the following?
   A. Anthropometric measures
   B. Calorie count of nutrients
   C. Measurement of height and weight
   D. Complete physical examination

Correct Answer: C

Rationale: Minimal nutritional screening involves taking a health history regarding conditions that might interfere with adequate food intake, measurement of height and weight, and routine laboratory tests.

Cognitive Level: Application

10. A patient is asked to indicate on a form how many times he eats a specific food. This would describe which of the following methods for obtaining dietary information?
   A. Food diary
   B. Food frequency questionnaire
   C. 24-hour recall
   D. Calorie count

Correct Answer: B

Rationale: With this tool, information is collected on how many times per day, week, or month the individual eats particular foods.

Cognitive Level: Knowledge

11. You are providing care for a 68-year-old female who is complaining of constipation. Why would you be concerned about her nutritional status?
    A. The gastrointestinal problem will increase her caloric demand.
    B. The constipation may represent a food allergy.
    C. She may need emergency surgery for the problem.
    D. The absorption of nutrients may be impaired.

Correct Answer: D

Rationale: Gastrointestinal symptoms such as vomiting, diarrhea, or constipation may interfere with nutrient intake or absorption.

Cognitive Level: Application

12. Why is it important to ask a patient what medications they are taking when doing a nutritional assessment?
    A. Medications can affect their memory and ability to identify food eaten in the last 24 hours.
    B. Certain drugs can affect the metabolism of nutrients.
    C. You need to be able to assess the patient for allergic reactions.
    D. Medications need to be documented on the record so the physician can review.

Correct Answer: B

Rationale: Analgesics, antacids, anticonvulsants, antibiotics, diuretics, laxatives, antineoplastic drugs, and oral contraceptives are among the drugs that can interact with nutrients, impairing their digestion, absorption, metabolism, or utilization.

Cognitive Level: Comprehension

13. A patient tells you that his food just doesn't have any taste anymore. Your best response would be which of the following?
    A. "That must be really frustrating."
    B. "When did you first notice this change?"
    C. "My food doesn't always have a lot of taste either."
    D. "Sometimes that happens but your taste will come back."

Correct Answer: B

Rationale: With changes in appetite, taste, smell, or chewing or swallowing, examiner asks about type of change and when change occurred.

Cognitive Level: Comprehension

14. You are performing a nutrition assessment on a 15-year-old girl. As you are obtaining her weight, she tells you she is "so fat." She is 5'4" and weighs 110 pounds. Your appropriate response would be:
    A. "Don't worry about it, you're not that overweight."
    B. "The best thing for you would be to go on a diet."
    C. "How much do you think you should weigh?"
    D. "I used to always think I was fat when I was your age."

Correct Answer: C

Rationale: Because of adolescents' increased body awareness and self-consciousness, they are prone to develop eating disorders such as anorexia nervosa or bulimia, conditions in which the real or perceived body image does not compare favorably to an ideal image.

Cognitive Level: Application

15. When you and a child's mother are discussing appropriate foods for a 2-year-old, which of the following would you recommend?
    A. Foods easy to hold such as hot dogs, nuts, and grapes
    B. Foods that the child will eat no matter what they are
    C. Any foods as long as the rest of the family is eating them
    D. Finger foods that can't be aspirated and nutritious snacks

Correct Answer: D

Rationale: Use of small portions, finger foods, simple meals, and nutritious snacks are strategies to improve dietary intake. Foods likely to be aspirated should be avoided (e.g., hot dogs, nuts, grapes, round candies, popcorn).

Cognitive Level: Application

16. Which of the following factors is most likely to affect the nutritional status of an 82-year-old male?
    A. Change in cardiovascular status
    B. Increase in gastrointestinal motility and absorption
    C. Living alone on a fixed income

D. Increase in taste and smell

Correct Answer: C

Rationale: Socioeconomic conditions frequently have the greatest effect on the nutritional status of the aging adult; these factors should be closely evaluated. Physical limitations, income, and social isolation are frequent problems and can obviously interfere with the acquisition of a balanced diet.

Cognitive Level: Comprehension

17. The most common anthropometric measurements include:
   A. biceps skinfold thickness.
   B. height and weight.
   C. leg circumference.
   D. hip and waist measurement.

Correct Answer: B

Rationale: The most commonly used anthropometric measures are height, weight, triceps skinfold thickness, elbow breadth, and arm and head circumferences.

Cognitive Level: Knowledge

18. If a 29-year-old female weighs 146 pounds and you determine her ideal body weight to be 120 pounds, how would you classify her?
   A. Mildly overweight
   B. Obese
   C. Suffering from malnutrition
   D. Within appropriate range of ideal weight

Correct Answer: B

Rationale: Obesity is defined as greater than 120 percent ideal body weight.

Cognitive Level: Application

19. To perform a triceps skinfold assessment, you would do which of the following?
   A. Instruct patient to stand with back to you and arms folded across chest and pinch the skin on forearm.
   B. Gently pinch the skin and fat on anterior aspect of patient's arm; then apply calipers.
   C. After pinching the skin and fat, apply the calipers vertically to the fat fold.
   D. After applying the calipers, wait 3 seconds before taking a reading, then repeat procedure three times.

Correct Answer: D

Rationale: Release the lever of the calipers while holding the skinfold. Wait 3 seconds, then take a reading. Repeat three times and average the three skinfold measurements.

Cognitive Level: Comprehension

20. When assessing muscle mass and fat stores on a 40-year-old female, you would use:
   A. mid-upper arm circumference.
   B. triceps skinfold.
   C. mid-arm muscle area.
   D. percent ideal body weight.

Correct Answer: A

Rationale: Mid-upper arm circumference (MAC) estimates skeletal muscle mass and fat stores.

Cognitive Level: Comprehension

21. When interpreting mid-upper arm circumference and triceps skinfold on an 82-year-old male, it is important to remember that:
   A. measurements may be difficult to obtain if patient is unable to flex elbow to at least 90 degrees.
   B. derived weight measures may be difficult to interpret due to wide ranges of normal.
   C. these measurements are no longer necessary for the elderly.
   D. these measurements may not be accurate because of changes in skin and fat distribution.

Correct Answer: D

Rationale: Remember that accurate MAC and TCP measurements are difficult to obtain and interpret in older adults because of sagging skin, changes in fat distribution, and declining muscle mass.

Cognitive Level: Application

22. You are concerned about the skeletal protein reserves of a patient who has been hospitalized frequently for chronic lung disease. Which of the following measurements would be necessary to include in your assessment?
   A. Weight and height
   B. Mid-upper arm circumference and triceps skinfold
   C. Body mass index
   D. Ideal body weight and frame size

Correct Answer: B

Rationale: Mid-arm muscle area (MAMA) is a good indicator of lean body mass and skeletal protein reserves. These reserves are important in growing children and are especially valuable in evaluating persons who may be malnourished because of chronic illness, multiple surgeries, or inadequate dietary intake. The equation for calculating mid-arm muscle area includes mid-upper arm circumference and mid-upper arm muscle circumference.

Cognitive Level: Application

23. Which of the following best describes the technique for measuring frame size?
    A. With the patient's right arm extended forward and the elbow extended, measure distance from fingertips to condyle of the humerus.
    B. With the patient standing, measure the distance from the top of the head to the back of their heel.
    C. With the right arm extended forward and the elbow bent, use the calipers to measure the distance between the condyles of the humerus.
    D. With the patient in a sitting position, measure the distance from the condyle of the humerus to the clavicle.

Correct Answer: C

Rationale: Instruct person to extend right arm forward, perpendicular to body. Bend the elbow to a 90-degree angle, with the palm of the hand turned laterally. Facing the person, place the calipers on the condyles of the humerus. Read the distance between the condyles.

Cognitive Level: Knowledge

24. In teaching a female patient how to determine total body fat at home, you would tell her she needs measurements of her:
    A. frame size and weight.
    B. height and weight.
    C. waist and hip circumferences.
    D. mid-upper arm circumference and arm span.

Correct Answer: B

Rationale: Body mass index is a simple indicator of total body fat or obesity.

Body Mass Index = Weight ÷ Height^2

Cognitive Level: Comprehension

25. In evaluating patients for obesity-related diseases, which one of the following would be at increased risk?
    A. 29-year-old female whose percent ideal body weight is 125%, waist 33 inches and hips 36 inches
    B. 32-year-old male whose percent ideal body weight is 115%, waist 34 inches and hips 36 inches
    C. 46-year old whose percent ideal body weight is 130%, waist 30 inches and hips 38 inches
    D. 38-year-old male whose percent ideal body weight is 120%, waist 35 inches and hips 38 inches

Correct Answer: A

Rationale: The waist-to-hip ratio assesses body fat distribution as an indicator of health risk (Folstom et al., 1993). A waist-to-hip ratio of 1.0 or greater in men or 0.8 or greater in women is indicative of android (upper body obesity) and increasing risk for obesity-related disease and early mortality.

Cognitive Level: Analysis

26. The mother of an 8-year-old boy is concerned about the amount of weight her son has gained. To determine whether this is a problem, you will measure:
    A. mid-upper arm circumference.
    B. skinfold thickness.
    C. arm span.
    D. waist-to-hip ratio.

Correct Answer: B

Rationale: Determination of skinfold thickness and/or body mass index may be useful in evaluating childhood and teenage overnutrition.

Cognitive Level: Application

27. You need to determine the body index of an 80-year-old male confined to a wheelchair. Which of the following is true?
    A. Declining muscle mass will affect the triceps skinfold measure.
    B. Changes in fat distribution will affect the waist-to-hip ratio.
    C. Height measurements may not be accurate due to changes in bone.
    D. Mid-arm circumference is difficult to obtain because of loss of skin elasticity.

Correct Answer: C

Rationale: Height measures may not be accurate in individuals confined to a bed or wheelchair or those over 60 years of age (because of osteoporotic changes).

Cognitive Level: Application

28. After completing a diet assessment on a 30-year-old female, you suspect she may be deficient in iron. Lab studies you would want to obtain include:
    A. cholesterol and triglycerides.
    B. serum albumin and urinary urea nitrogen.
    C. creatinine and serum protein.
    D. hemoglobin and hematocrit.

Correct Answer: D

Rationale: The hemoglobin determination is used to detect iron deficiency anemia. Hematocrit, a measure of cell volume, is also an indicator of iron status.

Cognitive Level: Application

29. M.S. is a 50-year-old female with elevated cholesterol and triglyceride levels. What would be important to include in your patient teaching in relation to these tests?
    A. The fact that this is hereditary and there is nothing she can do to change the levels
    B. Information regarding a low-saturated fat diet
    C. Methods to reduce stress in her life
    D. The risks of undernutrition

Correct Answer: B

Rationale: Total cholesterol is measured to evaluate fat metabolism and to assess the risk of cardiovascular disease. Serum triglycerides are used to screen for hyperlipidemia and to determine the risk of coronary artery disease.

Cognitive Level: Application

30. J.G. is a 40-year-old male who has a recent weight loss of 20 pounds due to a quick loss diet and stress. He tells you that he keeps getting "colds and the flu." In addition to assessing his nutrition status you would also want to obtain:
    A. total lymphocyte count.
    B. serum-transferrin.
    C. serum albumin.
    D. cholesterol level.

Correct Answer: A

Rationale: Loss of immunocompetence is strongly correlated with malnutrition in stressed and starving patients. The most commonly used tests of immune function are total lymphocyte count (TLC) and skin testing, also called delayed cutaneous hypersensitivity.

Cognitive Level: Analysis

31. In order to obtain an accurate nitrogen balance and creatinine-height index, you must ensure that:
    A. the patient has not had anything by mouth for 8 hours prior to the test.
    B. an accurate 24-hour urine specimen has been collected.
    C. the patient's height and weight have been determined.
    D. the lab draws the blood specimen in the early morning.

Correct Answer: B

Rationale: The validities of CHI and nitrogen balance studies are dependent on the accuracy of the 24-hour urine collection.

Cognitive Level: Comprehension

32. When evaluating the results of lab tests, the following is true:
    A. Normal values do not vary according to age.
    B. Variations based on biocultural differences may exist.
    C. It is not necessary to repeat lab tests once malnutrition has been determined.
    D. Lab tests are more sensitive than other parts of your assessment, so they can be evaluated without consideration of other findings.

Correct Answer: B

Rationale: Biocultural variations occur with some laboratory tests, such as hemoglobin/hematocrit, serum cholesterol, and serum transferrin.

Cognitive Level: Comprehension

33. In performing an assessment on a 49-year-old female with altered nutrition secondary to dysphagia, which of the following signs and symptoms would you expect to find?
    A. Sore, inflamed buccal cavity
    B. Weight 10-20% over ideal
    C. Increase in hair growth
    D. Inadequate food intake

Correct Answer: D

Rationale: Altered nutrition less than body requirements would result from inadequate food intake.

Cognitive Level: Application

34. B.B. is a 21-year-old female who has been on a low-protein liquid diet for the past month. She has had adequate calories and appears well nourished. In further assessing her, what would you expect to find?
    A. Decreased serum albumin
    B. Poor skin turgor
    C. Increased lymphocyte count
    D. Triceps skinfold less than standard

Correct Answer: A

Rationale: Kwashiorkor (protein malnutrition) is due to diets that may be high in calories but that contain little or no protein, e.g., low protein liquid diets, fad diets, and long-term use of dextrose-containing intravenous fluids. Serum albumin <3.5 g/dl.

Cognitive Level: Analysis

35. You are performing a nutritional assessment on Mr. Jones, an 80-year-old male. You know that physiologic changes that directly affect the nutritional status of the elderly include:
    A. an increased sensitivity to spicy and aromatic foods.
    B. hyperstimulation of the salivary glands.
    C. decreased gastrointestinal absorption causing esophageal reflux.
    D. slowed gastrointestinal motility.

Correct Answer: D

Rationale: Normal physiologic changes in aging adults that affect nutritional status include: slowed gastrointestinal motility, decreased gastrointestinal absorption, diminished olfactory and taste sensitivity, decreased saliva production, decreased visual acuity, and poor dentition.

Cognitive Level: Knowledge

36. Which of the following interventions is most appropriate when planning nutritional interventions for Mrs. Adams, a healthy, active 74-year-old female?
    A. Increase the amount of soy and tofu in her diet to promote bone growth and reverse osteoporosis.
    B. Increase the amount of calories she is eating by approximately 200 kcal/day due to increased energy needs of the elderly.
    C. Continue with the same protein requirement that is recommended for younger adults.
    D. Decrease the amount of carbohydrates to prevent lean muscle catabolism.

Correct Answer: C

Rationale: Energy needs decrease by approximately 200 kcal/day between the ages of 51 and 75. The protein requirement of 0.8 g/kg/day for younger adults is appropriate for healthy older persons.

Cognitive Level: Application

37. Which of the following statements is true regarding routine laboratory testing in the following individuals?
    A. In infancy and childhood, laboratory tests should be performed at each well child check-up, regardless of whether the child is exhibiting signs of illness that affect nutritional status.
    B. During adolescence, unless disease is suspected, laboratory evaluation of hemoglobin and hematocrit levels and urinalysis for glucose and protein are adequate.
    C. In pregnancy, no laboratory testing is needed, unless problems with the pregnancy are suspected.
    D. In the elderly, laboratory values regarding cholesterol and triglycerides are the most important because of the risk of disease.

Correct Answer: B

Rationale: Unless disease is suspected, evaluation of hemoglobin and hematocrit levels and urinalysis for glucose and protein levels are adequate in adolescents. In infancy, laboratory tests are performed only if nutritional problems are suspected, or illnesses affect nutritional status. Many laboratory values are monitored during pregnancy and older adulthood.

Cognitive Level: Analysis

38. M.J. is a 16-year-old female being seen at the clinic for gastrointestinal complaints and weight loss. You determine that many of her complaints may be related to erratic eating patterns, eating predominantly fast foods, and high caffeine intake. In this situation, which of the following is most appropriate when collecting current dietary intake information?

A. Ask M.J. for a 24-hour diet recall and assume this is reflective of a typical day for her.
B. Utilize the food frequency questionnaire to identify the amount of intake of specific foods.
C. Schedule a time for direct observation of M.J. during meals.
D. Have M.J. complete a food diary for three days—two weekdays and one weekend day.

Correct Answer: D

Rationale: Food diaries require the individual to write down everything consumed for a certain time period. Due to the erratic eating patterns of this individual, assessing dietary intake over a few days would produce more accurate information regarding eating patterns. Direct observation is best utilized with young children or older adults.

Cognitive Level: Analysis

39. Which of the following individuals is most likely to have an anergic response when assessing skin test antigens?
    A. A healthy 80-year-old female
    B. An 8-year-old child
    C. An individual suffering from malnutrition
    D. An obese individual

Correct Answer: C

Rationale: Adequate immunity can be assessed by a positive reaction to multiple skin test antigens. Antigens are injected and the response is noted at 24 and 48 hours. Anergy occurs with malnutrition, hepatic failure, infection, and immunosuppressive drugs.

Cognitive Level: Comprehension

Chapter 8

Assessment Techniques and Approach to the Clinical Setting

1. When performing a physical assessment, the technique you will always use first is:
   A. palpation.
   B. percussion.
   C. auscultation.
   D. inspection.

Correct Answer: D

Rationale: The assessment of each body system begins with inspection.

Cognitive Level: Knowledge

2. The inspection phase of the physical assessment:
   A. requires a quick glance at the patient's body systems before proceeding on with palpation.
   B. yields little information.
   C. may be somewhat uncomfortable for the expert practitioner.
   D. takes time and reveals a surprising amount of information.

Correct Answer: D

Rationale: A focused inspection takes time and yields a surprising amount of data. Initially, the examiner may feel uncomfortable "staring" at the person without also "doing something."

Cognitive Level: Comprehension

3. You are assessing Mr. P.J.'s skin during an office visit. What technique should you use to best assess the temperature of his skin?
   A. Use your fingertips because they're more sensitive to small changes in temperature.
   B. Use the palmar surface of your hand because it is most sensitive to temperature variations due to increased nerve supply in this area.
   C. Use the dorsal surface of your hand because the skin is thinner here than on your palms.
   D. Use the ulnar portion of your hand, because there is increased blood supply that enhances temperature sensitivity.

Correct Answer: C

Rationale: The dorsa (backs) of hands and fingers are best for determining temperature because the skin here is thinner than on the palms.

Cognitive Level: Application

4. Which of the following techniques uses the sense of touch when assessing a patient?
   A. Auscultation
   B. Percussion
   C. Palpation
   D. Inspection

Correct Answer: C

Rationale: Palpation uses the sense of touch to assess the patient.

Cognitive Level: Knowledge

5. You are preparing to assess your patient's abdomen by palpation. How should you proceed?
   A. Begin the assessment with deep palpation, encouraging the patient to relax and take deep breaths.
   B. Quickly palpate the area to avoid any discomfort that the patient may experience.
   C. Start with light palpation to detect surface characteristics and to accustom the patient to being touched.
   D. Avoid palpation of reported "tender" areas as this may cause the patient pain.

Correct Answer: C

Rationale: Light palpation is done initially to detect any surface characteristics and to accustom the person to being touched.

Cognitive Level: Application

6. When would you use a bimanual palpation technique?
   A. When assessing pulsations and vibrations

B. To palpate the kidneys and uterus
C. To assess the presence of tenderness and pain
D. When palpating the thorax of an infant

Correct Answer: B

Rationale: Bimanual palpation requires the use of both hands to envelop or capture certain body parts or organs, such as the kidneys, uterus, or adnexa.

Cognitive Level: Application

7. The purpose of percussion is to:
   A. assess underlying tissue density.
   B. assess underlying tissue texture.
   C. assess underlying tissue consistency.
   D. assess underlying tissue turgor.

Correct Answer: A

Rationale: Percussion yields a sound that depicts the location, size, and density of the underlying organ.

Cognitive Level: Comprehension

8. How would you percuss the thorax of an adult?
   A. Use the direct percussion technique.
   B. Use the indirect percussion technique.
   C. Use the ulnar surface of your hand to percuss the thorax.
   D. Use the dorsal surface of your hand to percuss the thorax.

Correct Answer: B

Rationale: In direct percussion, the striking hand directly contacts the body wall. This procedure is used in percussing the infant's thorax or the adult's sinus areas. With indirect percussion, the striking hand contacts the stationary hand fixed on the person's skin. This technique is used most often.

Cognitive Level: Application

9. When percussing over the ribs of your patient you note a flat sound. You would:
   A. consider this an abnormal finding and refer the patient for additional treatment.
   B. reposition your hands and attempt to percuss in this area again.
   C. consider this a normal finding.
   D. palpate this area for an underlying mass.

Correct Answer: C

Rationale: Percussion over bones or large muscles will produce a flat sound.

Cognitive Level: Analysis

10. You are unable to identify any changes in sound when percussing over the abdomen of an obese patient. You would:
    A. decrease the amount of strength used when attempting to percuss over the abdomen.
    B. move to a new body location and attempt to percuss.
    C. consider this a normal finding and proceed with the abdominal assessment.
    D. ask the patient to take deep breaths to relax his or her abdominal musculature.

Correct Answer: C

Rationale: The thickness of the person's body wall will be a factor when attempting to percuss. You will need a stronger percussion stroke for persons with obese or very muscular body walls. Percussion vibrations penetrate about 5 cm deep. A relatively dense organ or adipose tissue will elicit a dull percussion note.

Cognitive Level: Analysis

11. You hear bilateral hyperresonant tones when percussing over the thorax of a 4-year-old child. You would:
    A. ask the child to take shallow breaths and percuss over the area again.
    B. palpate over the area for increased pain and tenderness.
    C. refer the child immediately, due to an increased amount of air in the lungs.
    D. consider this normal finding for a child this age and proceed with the examination.

Correct Answer: D

Rationale: Hyperresonant percussion notes are normally heard over the child's lung.

Cognitive Level: Analysis

12. Your patient has suddenly developed shortness of breath and appears to be in significant respiratory distress. You would:
    A. call for a chest x-ray and wait for the results before beginning your assessment.
    B. inspect the thorax for any new masses and bleeding associated with respirations.
    C. auscultate the thorax for increased pain with respirations.

D. percuss the thorax bilaterally noting any differences in percussion tones, which signal a change in density of the lung.

Correct Answer: D

Rationale: Percussion is always available, portable, and gives instant feedback regarding changes in underlying tissue density.

Cognitive Level: Analysis

13. Which of the following statements is true regarding the stethoscope and its use?
    A. The stethoscope does not amplify sound, but does block out extraneous room noise.
    B. The slope of the earpieces should point posteriorly (towards the occiput).
    C. The ideal tubing length should be 22 inches long in order to dampen distortion of sound.
    D. The fit and quality of the stethoscope are not as important as its ability to magnify sound.

Correct Answer: A

Rationale: The stethoscope does not magnify sound, but does block out extraneous room sounds. The slope of the earpieces should point forward toward the examiner's nose. Longer tubing will distort sound.

Cognitive Level: Comprehension

14. Which of the following statements is true regarding the diaphragm of the stethoscope?
    A. Use the diaphragm to listen for high-pitched sounds.
    B. Use the diaphragm to listen for low-pitched sounds.
    C. Hold the diaphragm lightly against the person's skin to listen for extra heart sounds and murmurs.
    D. Hold the diaphragm lightly against the person's skin to block out the low-pitched sounds.

Correct Answer: A

Rationale: The diaphragm of the stethoscope is best for listening to high-pitched sounds such as breath, bowel, and normal heart sounds. It should be held firmly against the person's skin, firmly enough to leave a ring.

Cognitive Level: Comprehension

15. Before auscultating the abdomen for the presence of bowel sounds on a patient, you would:
    A. warm the end piece of your stethoscope by placing it in warm water.
    B. check the temperature of the room and offer blankets to your patient if he or she feels cold.
    C. wet the hair of the abdomen to prevent distortion of sounds.
    D. make sure that the bell side of your stethoscope is turned on.

Correct Answer: B

Rationale: The examination room should be warm. If the patient shivers, the involuntary muscle contractions can make it difficult to hear the underlying sounds. The end of the stethoscope should be warmed between the examiner's hands. To avoid the friction from a male's hairy chest, wet the hair before auscultating the area. The diaphragm of the stethoscope would be used to auscultate for bowel sounds.

Cognitive Level: Application

16. Which technique of assessment is used to determine the presence of crepitus, swelling, and pulsations?
    A. Inspection
    B. Palpation
    C. Percussion
    D. Auscultation

Correct Answer: B

Rationale: Palpation applies the sense of touch to assess these factors: texture, temperature, moisture, organ location and size, as well as any swelling, vibration or pulsation, rigidity or spasticity, crepitation, presence of lumps or masses, and presence of tenderness or pain.

Cognitive Level: Comprehension

17. Which of the following statements is true regarding the otoscope?
    A. The otoscope directs light into the ear canal and onto the tympanic membrane.
    B. The otoscope is used to examine the structures of the internal ear.
    C. The otoscope uses a short broad speculum to visualize the ear.
    D. The otoscope is often used to direct light onto the sinuses.

Correct Answer: A

Rationale: The otoscope directs light into the ear canal and onto the tympanic membrane that divides the external and middle ear. A short, broad speculum is used to visualize the nares.

Cognitive Level: Knowledge

18. An examiner is using an ophthalmoscope to examine a patient's eyes. Her patient has an astigmatism and is nearsighted. Which of the following techniques would indicate the examination is being performed correctly?
    A. Rotating the lens selector dial to the black numbers to compensate for astigmatism
    B. Rotating the lens selector dial to the red numbers to compensate for nearsightedness
    C. Using the grid on the lens aperture dial to visualize the external structures of the eye
    D. Using the large full circle of light when assessing pupils that are undilated

Correct Answer: B

Rationale: The ophthalmoscope is used to examine the internal eye structures. It can compensate for nearsightedness or farsightedness, but will not correct for astigmatism. The red numbers indicate a negative lens and can compensate for myopia. The grid is used to assess size and location of lesions on the fundus. The large full spot of light is used to assess dilated pupils.

Cognitive Level: Analysis

19. You are unable to palpate the right radial pulse on a patient. You would:
    A. use a Doppler to check for pulsations over the area.
    B. use a goniometer to measure the pulsations.
    C. check for the presence of pulsations with a stethoscope.
    D. auscultate over the area with a fetoscope.

Correct Answer: A

Rationale: Dopplers are used to augment pulse or blood pressure measurements. Goniometers measure joint range of motion. A fetoscope is used to auscultate fetal heart tones. Stethoscopes are used to auscultate breath, bowel, and heart sounds.

Cognitive Level: Analysis

20. When performing the physical assessment the examiner should:
    A. examine tender or painful areas first to help relieve the patient's anxiety.
    B. follow the same examination sequence regardless of the patient's age or condition.
    C. organize the steps of the assessment so that the patient does not change positions too often.
    D. perform the examination from the left side of the bed.

Correct Answer: C

Rationale: The sequence of the steps of the assessment may differ depending on the age of the person and the examiner's preference. Tender or painful areas should be assessed last. The steps of the assessment should be organized so that the patient does not change positions too often.

Cognitive Level: Application

21. Mr. S. is at the clinic for a physical examination. He states that he is "very anxious" about the physical exam. What steps can the examiner take to make him more comfortable?
    A. Ask Mr. S. to change into an examining gown and take off his undergarments.
    B. Always stay in the room when Mr. S. undresses in case he needs assistance.
    C. Defer measuring vital signs until the end of the examination, which allows Mr. S. time to become comfortable.
    D. Appear unhurried and confident when examining Mr. S.

Correct Answer: D

Rationale: Anxiety can be reduced by an examiner who is confident and self assured, as well as considerate and unhurried. Familiar and relatively nonthreatening actions, such as measuring the person's vital signs, will gradually accustom the person to the examination.

Cognitive Level: Application

22. When performing a physical examination, safety must be considered to protect you and the patient against the spread of infection. Which of the following statements describes the most appropriate actions to be taken when performing a physical examination?
    A. Wash your hands at the beginning of the examination and any time that you leave and re-enter the room.
    B. Wash your hands between the examination of each body system to prevent the spread of bacteria from one part of the body to another.
    C. There is no need to wash your hands after

removing gloves, as long as the gloves are still intact.
D. Wear gloves throughout the entire examination to demonstrate to your patient your concern regarding the spread of infectious diseases.

Correct Answer: A

Rationale: The examiner should wash his or her hands at the beginning of the examination and each time he or she re-enters the room. Gloves should be worn when there is potential contact with any body fluids. Hands should be washed after gloves have been removed, even if the gloves appear to be intact.

Cognitive Level: Application

23. You are examining a patient's lower leg and note a draining ulceration. Which of the following actions is most appropriate in this situation?
    A. Continue to examine the ulceration, then wash your hands.
    B. Wash your hands, put on gloves, and continue with examination of the ulceration.
    C. Wash your hands and contact the physician.
    D. Wash your hands, proceed with rest of the physical examination, then continue with examination of the leg ulceration.

Correct Answer: B

Rationale: The examiner should wear gloves when there is potential contact with any body fluids. In this situation, you should wash your hands, put on gloves and continue examining the ulceration.

Cognitive Level: Analysis

24. During the examination, it is often appropriate to offer some brief teaching about the patient's body or your findings. Which of the following statements is most appropriate?
    A. "You have pitting edema and mild varicosities."
    B. "Your hypertension is under control."
    C. "I'm using my stethoscope to listen for any crackles, wheezes, or rubs."
    D. "Your pulse is 80 beats per minute; this is within the normal range."

Correct Answer: D

Rationale: Sharing of information builds rapport as long as the patient is able to understand the terminology. Use of medical jargon is exclusionary and paternalistic.

Cognitive Level: Analysis

25. The most important reason to share information and offer brief teaching while performing the physical examination is:
    A. to help the patient understand his disease process and treatment modalities.
    B. to build rapport and increase the patient's confidence in the examiner.
    C. to help the examiner feel more comfortable and gain control of the situation.
    D. to help the patient identify questions about his or her disease and potential areas of patient education.

Correct Answer: B

Rationale: Sharing of information builds rapport and increases the patient's confidence in you as an examiner. It also gives the patient a little more control in a situation in which it's easy to feel completely helpless.

Cognitive Level: Comprehension

26. In infants the Moro reflex should be elicited:
    A. at the end of the examination.
    B. approximately halfway through the examination.
    C. before auscultation of the thorax.
    D. when the infant is sleeping.

Correct Answer: A

Rationale: Elicit the Moro or "startle" reflex at the end of the examination because it may cause the baby to cry.

Cognitive Level: Comprehension

27. When preparing to perform a physical examination on an infant, you should:
    A. instruct the parent to feed the infant immediately before the exam.
    B. ask the parent to briefly leave the room when assessing the infant's vital signs.
    C. have the parent remove all clothing except the diaper on a boy.
    D. encourage the infant to suck on a pacifier during the abdominal exam.

Correct Answer: C

Rationale: The parent should always be present for the child's feeling of security and to understand normal growth and development. Timing of the examination should be 1 to 2 hours after feeding when the baby is not too drowsy nor too hungry. Infants do not object to being nude; clothing should be removed and a diaper left on a boy.

Cognitive Level: Application

28. P.Y., a 6-month old, has been brought to the Well-Child Clinic for a check-up. She is currently sleeping. What should you do first?
    A. Examine the infant's hips since this procedure is uncomfortable.
    B. Auscultate the lungs and heart while the infant is still sleeping.
    C. Wake the infant before beginning any portion of the examination to obtain the most accurate assessment of body systems.
    D. Begin with the assessment of the eye and continue with the remainder of the examination in a head-to-toe approach.

Correct Answer: B

Rationale: When the infant is quiet or sleeping is an ideal time to assess the cardiac, respiratory, and abdominal systems. Assessment of the eye, ear, nose, and throat are invasive procedures and should be performed at the end of the examination.

Cognitive Level: Application

29. B.B., a 2-year-old child is here for a Well-Child check-up. How should you proceed with the assessment?
    A. Allow the child to keep a security object such as a toy or blanket during the examination.
    B. Have the parent remove all of the child's clothing prior to the examination.
    C. Initially focus your interactions on the child, essentially "ignoring" the parent, until you have developed the child's trust.
    D. Ask the parent to place the child on the examining table.

Correct Answer: A

Rationale: Sitting on the parent's lap is the best place to examine the toddler. Toddlers understand symbols, so a security object is helpful. Initially, focus more on the parent. This allows the child to gradually adjust and become familiar with you. A 2-year-old does not like to take off his or her clothes; have the parent undress one body part at a time.

Cognitive Level: Application

30. Nurse N is examining a 2-year-old child and asks, "May I listen to your heart now?" Which critique of her technique is most accurate?
    A. This is an appropriate statement because children at this age like to have choices.
    B. Children at this age like to say "No." The examiner should not offer a choice when there is none.
    C. Asking the child for permission helps to develop a sense of trust.
    D. Asking questions enhances the child's autonomy.

Correct Answer: B

Rationale: Children at this age like to say "No." Do not offer a choice when there really is none. If the child says "No," and you go ahead and do it anyway, you lose trust. Autonomy is enhanced by offering a limited option, "Shall I listen to your heart next, or your tummy?"

Cognitive Level: Analysis

31. With which of the following patients would it be most appropriate to use games during the assessment, such as, having the patient "blow out" the light on the penlight?
    A. An infant
    B. An adolescent
    C. A preschool child
    D. A school-age child

Correct Answer: C

Rationale: When assessing preschool children, it is helpful to use games or allow them to play with the equipment to reduce their fears.

Cognitive Level: Comprehension

32. You are preparing to examine J.J., a 4-year-old child. You would:
    A. explain procedures in detail to alleviate the child's anxiety.
    B. not ask the child to remove his clothes, as children at this age are usually very private.
    C. perform examination of the ear, nose, and throat first; then examine the thorax and abdomen.
    D. give the child feedback and reassurance during the examination.

Correct Answer: D

Rationale: With preschool children use short, simple explanations. Children at this age are usually willing to undress. Examination of the head should be performed last. During the examination give the preschooler needed feedback and reassurance.

Cognitive Level: Comprehension

33. When examining a 16-year-old male you should:
    A. ask his parent to stay in room during the history and physical examination to answer any questions and alleviate his anxiety.
    B. discuss health teaching with the parent, since he is unlikely to be interested in promoting wellness.
    C. talk to him as you would a younger child. A teenager's level of understanding often does not match that of his or her speech.
    D. provide feedback that his body is developing normally and discuss the wide variation among teenagers on the rate of growth and development.

Correct Answer: D

Rationale: During the examination, the adolescent needs feedback that his or her body is healthy and developing normally. The adolescent has a keen awareness of body image, often comparing himself or herself to peers. Apprise the adolescent of the wide variation among teenagers on the rate of growth and development.

Cognitive Level: Application

34. When examining the aging adult you should:
    A. attempt to perform the entire physical during one visit.
    B. avoid touching the patient too much.
    C. arrange the sequence to allow as few position changes as possible.
    D. speak loud and slow, since most aging adults have hearing deficits.

Correct Answer: C

Rationale: When examining the aging adult it is best to arrange the sequence of the examination to allow as few position changes as possible. Physical touch is especially important with the aging person because other senses may be diminished.

Cognitive Level: Application

35. The most important step that you can take to prevent transmission of nosocomial infections in the hospital setting is to:
    A. wear gloves during any and all contacts with patients.
    B. wear protective eye wear at all times.
    C. wash your hands before and after contact with each patient.
    D. clean your stethoscope with an alcohol swab between patients.

Correct Answer: C

Rationale: The most important step to decrease the risk of microorganism transmission is to wash your hands promptly before and after physical contact with each patient. Stethoscopes should also be cleansed with an alcohol swab between patients, but the most important step in prevention of infection is hand washing.

Cognitive Level: Comprehension

36. Which of the following statements is true regarding the use of standard precautions in the health care setting?
    A. Standard precautions are intended for use with all patients regardless of their risk or presumed infection status.
    B. Standard precautions apply to all body fluids, including sweat.
    C. Airborne, droplet and contact transmission-based precautions are included in the use of standard precautions.
    D. Standard precautions are to be used only when there is non-intact skin, excretions contain visible blood, or contact with mucous membranes is expected.

Correct Answer: A

Rationale: Standard precautions are designed to reduce the risk of transmission of microorganisms from both recognized and unrecognized sources. They apply to blood; all body fluids, secretions and excretions, except sweat—whether or not they contain visible blood; non-intact skin; and mucous membranes.

Cognitive Level: Comprehension

37. You are preparing to assess a hospitalized patient who is experiencing significant shortness of breath. How should you proceed with the assessment?
    A. Perform a complete history and physical assessment now to obtain baseline information.
    B. Have the patient lie down to obtain an accurate cardiac, respiratory and abdominal

assessment.

C. Examine body areas appropriate to the problem. Complete the assessment after the shortness of breath has resolved.

D. Obtain a thorough history and physical assessment information from the patient's family member.

Correct Answer: C

Rationale: It may be necessary in this situation to alter the position of the patient during the examination and to collect a mini data base by examining the body areas appropriate to the problem. You may return later to complete the assessment after the distress is resolved.

Cognitive Level: Application

Chapter 9

General Survey, Measurement, Vital Signs

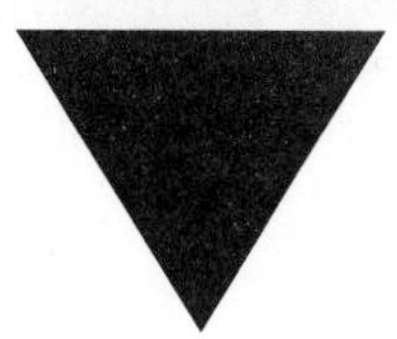

1. When performing a general survey the examiner is:
   A. observing the patient's body stature and nutritional status.
   B. measuring the patient's temperature, pulse, respirations, and blood pressure.
   C. observing specific body systems while performing the physical assessment.
   D. interpreting the subjective information the patient has reported.

Correct Answer: A

Rationale: The general survey is a study of the whole person that includes observation of physical appearance, body structure, mobility, and behavior.

Cognitive Level: Knowledge

2. When measuring a patient's weight:
   A. the patient may leave on his or her heavy coat and shoes as long as this is documented next to the weight.
   B. attempt to weigh the patient at approximately the same time of day, if a sequence of weights is necessary.
   C. always weigh the patient with only his or her undergarments on.
   D. it does not matter what type of scale is used, as long as the weights are similar from day to day.

Correct Answer: B

Rationale: A standardized balance scale is used to measure weight. The patient should remove his or her shoes and heavy outer clothing. If a sequence of repeated weights is necessary, aim for approximately the same time of day and type of clothing worn each time.

Cognitive Level: Comprehension

3. Gestational age is:
   A. the length (in weeks) of the pregnancy.
   B. the number of weeks from the first day of the mother's last menstrual period to the newborn's date of birth.
   C. the number of weeks from conception to birth.
   D. the projected delivery date minus the age of the child at birth.

Correct Answer: B

Rationale: Gestational age is the number of weeks from the first day of the mother's last menstrual period (LMP) to newborn's date of birth.

Cognitive Level: Knowledge

4. Physical growth is the best index of:
   A. a child's general health.
   B. a child's nutritional status.
   C. a child's genetic makeup.
   D. a child's activity and exercise patterns.

Correct Answer: A

Rationale: Physical growth is perhaps the best index of a child's general health.

Cognitive Level: Knowledge

5. J.J., a 1-month-old infant, has a head measurement of 34 cm and has a chest circumference of 32 cm. You would:
   A. consider this a normal finding for a 1-month-old infant.
   B. expect the chest circumference to be greater than the head circumference.
   C. refer the infant to a physician for further evaluation.
   D. ask the parent to return in 2 weeks to re-evaluate the head and chest circumferences.

Correct Answer: A

Rationale: The newborn's head measures about 32-38 cm and is about 2 cm larger than the chest circumference. Between 6 months and 2 years, both measurements are about the same, and after age 2, the chest circumference is greater than the head circumference.

Cognitive Level: Analysis

6. When assessing an 80-year-old male patient, which of the following findings would be considered normal?
   A. An increase in body weight from younger years
   B. Additional deposits of fat on the thighs and lower legs
   C. The presence of kyphosis and flexion in the knees and hips
   D. A change in overall body proportion; a longer trunk and shorter extremities

Correct Answer: C

Rationale: Changes that occur in the aging person include: more prominent bony landmarks, decreased body weight (especially in males), a decrease in subcutaneous fat from the face and periphery, and additional fat deposited on the abdomen and hips. Postural changes of kyphosis and slight flexion in the knees and hips also occur.

Cognitive Level: Application

7. You should avoid measuring rectal temperatures in which of the following patients?
   A. An unconscious patient
   B. A patient who is receiving oxygen by nasal cannula
   C. A patient with rectal bleeding
   D. An infant with a seizure disorder

Correct Answer: C

Rationale: Rectal temperatures should be taken when the other routes are not practical, e.g., for comatose or confused persons and for those who cannot close the mouth due to breathing or oxygen tubes. The rectal route is used with infants and children when the child is unable to cooperate, is agitated, unconscious, critically ill, or seizure prone.

Cognitive Level: Application

8. You are preparing to measure the length, weight, chest, and head circumference of a 6-month-old infant. You would:
   A. measure the infant's weight using an upright scale.
   B. measure the infant's length using a tape measure.
   C. measure the infant's head circumference, positioning the tape measure over the helices of the ears and around the frontal and occipital bones.
   D. measure the infant's chest circumference at the nipple line.

Correct Answer: D

Rationale: To measure chest circumference, encircle the tape around the chest at the nipple line. Length should be measured on a horizontal measuring board. Weight should be measured on a platform-type balance scale.

Cognitive Level: Application

9. The temperature of a toddler:
   A. is about the same as that of an adult.
   B. is usually lower than an adult's.
   C. is most accurate when taken with an oral mercury thermometer.
   D. is best taken with a tympanic membrane thermometer.

Correct Answer: D

Rationale: If this equipment is available, use it for any age child. Use an oral glass thermometer when the child is old enough to keep the mouth closed and does not bite on the thermometer.

Cognitive Level: Comprehension

10. Which of the following vital sign changes occur with aging?
    A. An increase in body temperature
    B. A widened pulse pressure
    C. A decrease in diastolic blood pressure
    D. An increase in pulse rate

Correct Answer: B

Rationale: With aging the systolic blood pressure increases, leading to widened pulse pressure. With many older people, both the systolic and diastolic pressures increase.

Cognitive Level: Knowledge

11. Cellular metabolism requires a stable core temperature. This requires a balance between heat production and heat loss. Which of the following is a mechanism of heat loss in the body?

A. Exercise
B. Food digestion
C. Radiation
D. Metabolism

Correct Answer: C

Rationale: The body maintains a steady temperature through a thermostat, or feedback mechanism, regulated in the hypothalamus of the brain. The hypothalamus regulates heat production (from metabolism, exercise, food digestion, external factors) with heat loss (through radiation, evaporation of sweat, convection, conduction).

Cognitive Level: Knowledge

12. Body temperature is influenced by:
    A. the diurnal cycle.
    B. constipation.
    C. emotional state.
    D. the nocturnal cycle.

Correct Answer: A

Rationale: Normal temperature is influenced by the diurnal cycle, exercise, and age.

Cognitive Level: Knowledge

13. The temperature of older adults:
    A. is about the same as that of a young child.
    B. varies widely owing to less effective heat control mechanisms.
    C. is lower than that of younger adults.
    D. depends on the type of thermometer used.

Correct Answer: C

Rationale: In older adults, temperature is usually lower than in other age groups, with a mean of 36.2° C.

Cognitive Level: Knowledge

14. M.J., a 60-year-old male, has been treated for pneumonia for the past 6 weeks. He is seen today in the clinic for an "unexplained" weight loss of 10 pounds over the last 6 weeks. You know that:
    A. unexplained weight loss often accompanies short-term illnesses.
    B. M.J.'s weight loss is probably due to a mental health dysfunction.
    C. chronic diseases such as hypertension cause weight loss.
    D. M.J.'s weight loss is probably due to unhealthy eating habits.

Correct Answer: A

Rationale: An unexplained weight loss may be a sign of a short-term illness, or a chronic illness such as endocrine disease, malignancy, or mental health dysfunction.

Cognitive Level: Analysis

15. When assessing L.H., a 15-year-old asthmatic patient, you note that he assumes a tripod position, leaning forward with arms braced on the chair. Based on this observation you would:
    A. assume that the patient is eager and interested in participating in the interview.
    B. recognize that a tripod position is often used when a patient is experiencing respiratory difficulties.
    C. assume that the patient is experiencing difficulty breathing and assist him to a supine position.
    D. evaluate the patient for abdominal pain, which may be exacerbated in sitting position.

Correct Answer: B

Rationale: Assuming a tripod position—leaning forward with arms braced on chair arms—occurs with chronic pulmonary disease.

Cognitive Level: Analysis

16. Which of the following describes the correct technique to use when assessing oral temperature with a mercury thermometer?
    A. Shake the mercury-in-glass thermometer down to 98° F before taking the temperature.
    B. Place the thermometer in front of the tongue and have the patient close his or her lips.
    C. Wait 30 minutes if the patient has ingested hot or iced liquids.
    D. Leave the thermometer in place 3-4 minutes if the patient is afebrile.

Correct Answer: D

Rationale: Leave the thermometer in place 3-4 minutes if the person if afebrile and up to 8 minutes if the person is febrile.

Cognitive Level: Application

17. Which of the following statements is true regarding use of the tympanic thermometer?
    A. There is a reduced risk of cross-contamination when compared to the rectal route.
    B. The tympanic membrane most accurately

reflects the temperature in the ophthalmic artery.
C. The tympanic method is more invasive and uncomfortable than the oral method.
D. A tympanic temperature is more time consuming than a rectal temperature.

Correct Answer: A

Rationale: The tympanic membrane thermometer is a noninvasive, nontraumatic device that is extremely quick and efficient. There is minimal chance of cross-contamination using the tympanic thermometer because the ear canal is lined with skin and not mucous membrane.

Cognitive Level: Comprehension

18. To accurately assess a rectal temperature on an adult you would:
   A. insert the thermometer 2-3 inches into the rectum.
   B. leave the thermometer in place up to 8 minutes if the patient is febrile.
   C. wait 2-3 minutes if the patient has recently smoked a cigarette.
   D. use a lubricated blunt tip thermometer.

Correct Answer: D

Rationale: Insert a lubricated rectal thermometer (with a short, blunt tip) only 2-3 cm (1 inch) into the adult rectum, and leave in place for $2\frac{1}{2}$ minutes.

Cognitive Level: Knowledge

19. In assessing the radial pulse of a patient, you would:
   A. count the pulse for 15 seconds and multiply by 4, if the rhythm is regular.
   B. count the pulse for 1 minute if the rhythm is irregular.
   C. count the initial pulse for a full 2 minutes to detect any variation in amplitude.
   D. count the pulse for 10 seconds and multiply by 6, if the patient has no history of cardiac abnormalities.

Correct Answer: B

Rationale: Recent research suggests that the 30-second interval multiplied by 2 is the most accurate and efficient when heart rates are normal or rapid, and when rhythms are regular.

Cognitive Level: Application

20. When assessing a patient's pulse you should note which of the following characteristics?
   A. Pallor
   B. Capillary refill time
   C. Timing in the cardiac cycle
   D. Force

Correct Answer: D

Rationale: The pulse is assessed for rate, rhythm, force, and elasticity.

Cognitive Level: Knowledge

21. When assessing the pulse of a 6-year-old boy, you note that his heart rate varies with his respiratory cycle, speeding up at the peak of inspiration and slowing to normal with expiration. You would:
   A. notify the physician.
   B. check the child's blood pressure and note any variation with respiration.
   C. consider this a normal finding in children and young adults.
   D. document that this child has bradycardia and continue with the assessment.

Correct Answer: C

Rationale: Sinus arrhythmia is commonly found in children and young adults. Here the heart rate varies with the respiratory cycle, speeding up at the peak of inspiration and slowing to normal with expiration.

Cognitive Level: Analysis

22. The force or strength of the pulse:
   A. is a reflection of the heart's stroke volume.
   B. reflects the blood volume in the arteries during diastole.
   C. demonstrates elasticity of the vessel wall.
   D. is usually recorded on a 0-2 scale.

Correct Answer: A

Rationale: The heart pumps an amount of blood (the stroke volume) into the aorta. The force flares the arterial walls and generates a pressure wave, which is felt in the periphery as the pulse.

Cognitive Level: Knowledge

23. You are assessing the vital signs of M.M., a 20-year-old runner. You document the following vital signs: temperature—97° F; pulse—48 BPM; respirations—14/minute; blood pressure—104/68. Which of the following statements is true?

A. These are normal vital signs for a healthy, athletic adult.
B. The patient is experiencing tachycardia.
C. The patient's pulse rate is not normal—his physician should be notified.
D. Based on today's readings, the patient should return to the clinic in 1 week.

Correct Answer: A

Rationale: In the adult, a heart rate less than 60 BPM is called bradycardia. This occurs normally in the well-trained athlete whose heart muscle develops along with the skeletal muscles.

Cognitive Level: Analysis

24. You are assessing the vital signs of a 3-year-old patient who appears to have an irregular respiratory pattern. How should you assess this child's respirations?
    A. Count the patient's respirations for 15 seconds and multiply by 4 to obtain the number of respirations per minute.
    B. Count the respirations for a full minute noting rate and rhythm.
    C. Check the child's pulse and respirations simultaneously for 30 seconds.
    D. Check the child's respirations for a minimum of 5 minutes in order to identify any variations in respiratory pattern.

Correct Answer: B

Rationale: Count respirations for 30 seconds or for 1 full minute if you suspect an abnormality.

Cognitive Level: Application

25. Mr. M.'s blood pressure is 118/82. He asks you to explain what the "numbers mean." You reply:
    A. "The numbers are within normal range and nothing to worry about."
    B. "The top number is the systolic blood pressure and reflects the pressure on the arteries when the heart contracts."
    C. "The bottom number is the diastolic pressure and reflects the stroke volume of the heart."
    D. "The concept of blood pressure is difficult to understand. The main thing to be concerned about is the top number, or systolic blood pressure."

Correct Answer: B

Rationale: The systolic pressure is the maximum pressure felt on the artery during left ventricular contraction, or systole. The diastolic pressure is the elastic recoil, or resting, pressure that the blood exerts constantly in between each contraction.

Cognitive Level: Analysis

26. Blood pressure is determined by:
    A. pulse pressure.
    B. pulse rate.
    C. peripheral vascular resistance.
    D. vascular output.

Correct Answer: C

Rationale: The level of blood pressure is determined by five factors: cardiac output, peripheral vascular resistance, volume of circulating blood, viscosity, and elasticity of vessel walls.

Cognitive Level: Knowledge

27. A school nurse is performing blood pressure screening for the senior students at a high school in a large metropolitan city. Which of the following does the nurse need to consider when assessing these students' blood pressures?
    A. After puberty, males usually show a lower blood pressure reading than females.
    B. A black adult's blood pressure is usually higher than that of whites of the same age.
    C. The blood pressure screening should be scheduled later in the afternoon when the students' blood pressures would be lower.
    D. Blood pressure measurements in the overweight students should be the same as those of normal weight students.

Correct Answer: B

Rationale: In the United States, a black adult's blood pressure is usually higher than that of whites of the same age. The incidence of hypertension is twice as high in blacks as in whites.

Cognitive Level: Application

28. You are preparing to check the blood pressure of an obese patient using a standard-sized blood pressure cuff. You would:
    A. expect the reading to be the same regardless of cuff size.
    B. expect the reading to yield a falsely high blood pressure due to increased pressure needed to compress the artery.
    C. check the blood pressure three times and average the numbers to obtain a more accurate reading.

D. expect the reading to yield a false low reading due to the difficulty in hearing the Korotkoff sounds.

Correct Answer: B

Rationale: Using a cuff that is too narrow yields a falsely high blood pressure because it takes extra pressure to compress the artery.

Cognitive Level: Comprehension

29. Mr. L. is late for his appointment and has rushed across campus to your clinic to have his vital signs assessed. Your first step should be to:
    A. check the blood pressure in both arms, expecting a difference in the readings due to his recent exercise.
    B. check his blood pressure in the supine position, since this will give you a more accurate reading and allow him to relax at the same time.
    C. allow Mr. L. time to relax and rest 5 minutes before checking his vital signs.
    D. monitor his vital signs immediately upon his arrival at the clinic, then 5 minutes later and note any differences.

Correct Answer: C

Rationale: A comfortable, relaxed person yields a valid blood pressure. Many people are anxious at the beginning of an examination; allow at least a 5-minute rest before measuring his blood pressure.

Cognitive Level: Analysis

30. The reason for performing a palpatory pressure prior to auscultating is to:
    A. avoid missing a falsely elevated blood pressure.
    B. hear the Korotkoff sounds more clearly.
    C. identify Phase IV of the Korotkoff sounds more readily.
    D. detect the presence of an auscultatory gap.

Correct Answer: D

Rationale: Inflation of the cuff 20-30 mm Hg beyond the point at which a palpated pulse disappears will avoid missing an auscultatory gap, which is a period when the Korotkoff sounds disappear during auscultation.

Cognitive Level: Comprehension

31. You are taking an initial blood pressure on a 72-year-old patient with documented hypertension. How should you proceed?
    A. Place the cuff on the patient's arm and inflate it 30 mm Hg above the patient's pulse rate.
    B. Inflate the cuff to 200 mm Hg in an attempt to obtain the most accurate systolic reading.
    C. Inflate the blood pressure cuff 30 mm Hg above the point at which the palpated pulse disappeared.
    D. Look at the patient's past blood pressure readings, and inflate the cuff 30 mm Hg above the highest systolic reading recorded.

Correct Answer: C

Rationale: An auscultatory gap occurs in about 5% of the people; most often in hypertension. To check for the presence of an auscultatory gap, inflate the cuff 20 to 30 mm Hg beyond the point at which the palpated pulse disappeared.

Cognitive Level: Analysis

32. You have collected the following information on Mrs. P.: palpated BP = 180; auscultated BP = 170/100; apical pulse = 60; radial pulse = 70. What is Mrs. P.'s pulse pressure?
    A. 10
    B. 70
    C. 80
    D. 100

Correct Answer: B

Rationale: Pulse pressure is the difference between systolic and diastolic blood pressure and reflects the stroke volume.

Cognitive Level: Application

33. When auscultating the blood pressure of a 25-year old, you hear the Phase I Korotkoff sounds begin at 200 mm Hg; at 100 mm Hg the Korotkoff sounds muffle; at 92 mm Hg the Korotkoff sounds disappear. How should you record this patient's blood pressure?
    A. 200/100/92
    B. 200/100
    C. 200/92
    D. 100/200/92

Correct Answer: C

Rationale: In adults, the last audible sound indicates diastolic pressure best. When a variance greater than 10-12 mm Hg exists between Phase IV and

V, record both phases along with the systolic reading, e.g., 142/98/80.

Cognitive Level: Analysis

34. Mr. A. is being seen in the clinic for complaints of "fainting episodes that started last week." How should you proceed with the examination?
    A. Assist Mr. A. to a lying position and begin taking his blood pressure.
    B. Take Mr. A.'s blood pressure in both arms and thighs.
    C. Record Mr. A.'s blood pressure in the lying, sitting, and standing positions.
    D. Record Mr. A.'s blood pressure in the lying and sitting positions and average these numbers to obtain a mean blood pressure.

Correct Answer: C

Rationale: If the person is known to have hypertension, is taking antihypertensive medications or reports a history of fainting or syncope, take the blood pressure reading in three positions—lying, sitting, and standing.

Cognitive Level: Application

35. Mr. T., a 65-year-old male, has a blood pressure of 150/90 in a lying position; 130/80 in a sitting position, and 100/60 in a standing position. Interpret these findings.
    A. This is a normal response due to changes in the patient's position.
    B. The change in blood pressure reading is considered within normal limits for the patient's age.
    C. The change in blood pressure readings is called orthostatic hypotension.
    D. The blood pressure reading in the lying position is within normal limits.

Correct Answer: C

Rationale: Orthostatic hypotension is a drop in systolic pressure of more than 20 mm Hg, which occurs with a quick change to a standing position. Aging people have the greatest risk of this problem.

Cognitive Level: Analysis

36. Which of the following statements is true regarding thigh pressure?
    A. If the blood pressure in the arm is high in an adolescent, compare it with the thigh pressure.
    B. The thigh pressure is lower than that in the arm due to distance away from the heart and the size of the popliteal vessels.
    C. The best position to measure thigh pressure is the supine position with the knee slightly bent.
    D. Auscultate over either the popliteal or femoral vessels to obtain a thigh pressure.

Correct Answer: A

Rationale: When blood pressure measured at the arm is excessively high, particularly in adolescents and young adults, compare it with thigh pressure to check for coarctation of the aorta.

Cognitive Level: Comprehension

37. You are preparing to measure the vital signs of L.M., a 6-month-old infant. You will:
    A. measure respirations, then pulse and temperature.
    B. measure vital signs more frequently than in an adult.
    C. allow the infant to become familiar with you by performing the physical examination first, then measure the vital signs.
    D. explain procedures and encourage the infant to handle the equipment.

Correct Answer: A

Rationale: Measure vital signs with the same purpose and frequency as you would in an adult. With an infant, reverse the order of vital sign measurement to respiration, pulse, and temperature.

Cognitive Level: Application

38. Q.W., a 4-month-old child, is at the clinic for a well-baby check-up and immunizations. Which of the following actions is most appropriate when assessing an infant's vital signs?
    A. Watch the infant's chest and count the respiratory rate for 1 minute because the respiratory pattern may vary significantly.
    B. Auscultate an apical rate for 1 minute and assess for any normal irregularities, such as sinus arrhythmia.
    C. Palpate the infant's radial pulse and note any fluctuations due to activity or exercise.
    D. Assess the infant's blood pressure using a stethoscope with a large diaphragm piece to hear the soft muffled Korotkoff sounds.

Correct Answer: B

Rationale: Palpate or auscultate an apical rate with

infants and toddlers. Count the pulse for 1 full minute to take into account normal irregularities, such as sinus arrhythmia.

Cognitive Level: Application

39. Which of the following statements is true regarding vital sign measurements in aging adults?
    A. Changes in the body's temperature regulatory mechanism leave the aging person more likely to develop a fever.
    B. The pulse is more difficult to palpate due to the stiffness of the blood vessels.
    C. An increased respiratory rate and a shallower inspiratory phase are expected findings.
    D. A decreased pulse pressure occurs due to changes in systolic and diastolic blood pressures.

Correct Answer: C

Rationale: Aging causes a decrease in vital capacity and decreased inspiratory reserve volume. You may note a shallower inspiratory phase and an increased respiratory rate.

Cognitive Level: Knowledge

40. In a patient with acromegaly, you will expect to observe:
    A. heavy, flattened facial features.
    B. growth retardation and delayed onset of puberty.
    C. increased height and weight and delayed sexual development.
    D. overgrowth of bone in the face, head, hands, and feet.

Correct Answer: D

Rationale: Table 9-6.

Cognitive Level: Knowledge

41. You have just finished measuring the blood pressure of Mr. Smith, age 60. His reading was 150/85. He has no personal or family history of hypertension, coronary artery disease, hypercholesterolemia, CVA, or diabetes. What should you tell Mr. Smith regarding his blood pressure follow-up?
    A. "You have Stage 1 hypertension and should be evaluated by your health care provider."
    B. "Your blood pressure is elevated today. You should have this re-checked within the next few weeks."
    C. "You must be anxious today. Let's re-check you blood pressure in 6 months."
    D. "Your blood pressure is within normal range for your age. We expect it to rise as you get older."

Correct Answer: B

Rationale: Diagnosis of hypertension should be based on the average of 2 or more readings taken at each of 2 or more visits. A systolic blood pressure of 140–159 should be evaluated within 2 months.

Cognitive Level: Analysis

42. Which of the following statements is true regarding measurement of blood pressure in children?
    A. The disappearance of phase V Korotkoff can be used for the diastolic reading in children and adults.
    B. The blood pressure guidelines for children are based on age.
    C. Use of the Doppler is recommended for accurate blood pressures until adolescence.
    D. Phase II Korotkoff sounds are the best indicator of systolic blood pressure in children.

Correct Answer: A

Rationale: JNC VI guidelines state that the disappearance of phase V Korotkoff sounds can be used for the diastolic reading in children as well as adults.

Cognitive Level: Knowledge

43. What type of blood pressure measurement error is most likely to occur if the examiner does not check for the presence of an auscultatory gap?
    A. The systolic blood pressure may be falsely high.
    B. The systolic blood pressure may be falsely low.
    C. The diastolic blood pressure may not be heard.
    D. The diastolic blood pressure may be falsely low.

Correct Answer: B

Rationale: If an auscultatory gap is undetected, a falsely low systolic or falsely high diastolic reading may result.

Cognitive Level: Comprehension

44. Which of the following best describes the concept of mean arterial pressure (MAP)?
    A. MAP is the pressure of the arterial pulse.
    B. It is an average of the systolic and diastolic blood pressures and reflects tissue perfusion.
    C. It is the pressure forcing blood into the tissues, averaged over the cardiac cycle.
    D. MAP reflects the stroke volume of the heart.

Correct Answer: C

Rationale: The MAP is the pressure forcing blood into the tissues, averaged over the cardiac cycle.

Cognitive Level: Knowledge

45. Mr. Jones, a 75-year-old male, has a history of hypertension and was recently changed to a new antihypertensive medication by his health care provider. He reports feeling dizzy at times. How should the nurse evaluate Mr. Jones' blood pressure?
    A. Take the blood pressure on the right arm, then 5 minutes later take the blood pressure on the left arm.
    B. Assess his blood pressure and pulse at the beginning and end of the examination.
    C. Assess blood pressure and pulse in the supine, sitting and standing positions.
    D. Have Mr. Jones walk around the room and assess his blood pressure after activity.

Correct Answer: C

Rationale: Orthostatic vital signs should be taken when the person is hypertensive or is taking antihypertensive medications, when the person reports fainting or syncope, or when volume depletion is suspected. The blood pressure and pulse is recorded in the supine, sitting, and standing positions.

Cognitive Level: Application

Chapter 10

Skin, Hair, and Nails

1. Because hair for humans is no longer needed for protection from cold or trauma, it is called:
   A. vestibule.
   B. vestigial.
   C. vellus.
   D. vagus.

Correct Answer: B

Rationale: Hair is vestigial for humans; it no longer is needed for protection from cold or trauma.

Cognitive Level: Knowledge

2. You are preparing an education module for your staff on the epidermal layer of skin. Which of the following would be included in your module?
   A. The epidermis is thick and tough.
   B. The epidermis is completely replaced every 4 weeks.
   C. The epidermis is very vascular.
   D. The epidermis is nonstratified.

Correct Answer: B

Rationale: The epidermis is thin, replaced every 4 weeks, avascular, and stratified into several zones.

Cognitive Level: Comprehension

3. You are preparing an education module for your staff on the dermis layer of skin. Which of the following would be included in your module?
   A. The dermis consists mostly of keratin.
   B. The dermis contains fat cells.
   C. The dermis contains nerves and sensory receptors.
   D. The dermis is completely replaced every 4 weeks.

Correct Answer: C

Rationale: The dermis consists mostly of collagen, has resilient elastic tissue that allows the skin to stretch, contains nerves, sensory receptors, blood vessels, and lymphatics.

Cognitive Level: Comprehension

4. You are discussing epidermal appendages with your patient. Which of the following would be included in your discussion?
   A. Skin
   B. Sweat glands
   C. Arms
   D. Parotid glands

Correct Answer: B

Rationale: Epidermal appendages include hair, sebaceous glands, sweat glands, and nails.

Cognitive Level: Comprehension

5. You are examining Mr. S. who tells you that, "I sure sweat a lot, especially on my face and feet but it doesn't have an odor." You know that this could be related to:
   A. the apocrine glands.
   B. a disorder of the stratum germinativum.
   C. the eccrine glands.
   D. a disorder of the stratum corneum.

Correct Answer: C

Rationale: The eccrine glands are coiled tubules that open directly onto the skin surface and produce a dilute saline solution called sweat. Apocrine glands are located mainly in the axillae, anogenital area, nipples, and naval and mix with bacterial flora to produce characteristic musky body odor.

Cognitive Level: Application

6. Mrs. R. brings in her newborn for a skin assessment. You are concerned about the possibility of fluid loss because you know:
   A. the newborn's skin is more permeable than that of the adult.
   B. sebaceous glands are overproductive in the newborn.

C. subcutaneous fat deposits are high in the newborn.
D. the amount of vernix caseosa rises dramatically in the newborn.

Correct Answer: A

Rationale: The newborn's skin is thin, smooth, and elastic and is relatively more permeable than that of the adult so the infant is at greater risk for fluid loss.

Cognitive Level: Application

7. You are bathing an 80-year-old man and you notice that his skin is wrinkled, thin, lax, and dry. This finding would:
   A. be related to an increase in elastin and a decrease in subcutaneous fat in the elderly.
   B. be related to an increased loss of elastin and a decrease in subcutaneous fat in the elderly.
   C. be related to increased numbers of sweat and sebaceous glands in the elderly.
   D. be related to increased vascularity of the skin in the elderly.

Correct Answer: B

Rationale: An accumulation of factors place the aging person at risk for skin disease and breakdown: the thinning of the skin, the decrease in vascularity and nutrients, the loss of protective cushioning of the subcutaneous layer, a lifetime of environmental trauma to skin, the social changes of aging, the increasingly sedentary lifestyle, and the chance of immobility.

Cognitive Level: Application

8. During the aging process, the hair can look gray or white and begin to feel thin and fine. This is because:
   A. the number of functioning phagocytes decreases.
   B. the number of functioning melanocytes decreases.
   C. the number of functioning fungacytes decreases.
   D. the number of functioning metrocytes decreases.

Correct Answer: B

Rationale: In the aging hair matrix, the number of functioning melanocytes decreases so the hair looks gray or white and feels thin and fine.

Cognitive Level: Comprehension

9. Mr. P., an Inuit visiting Nevada from Anchorage, has come to your clinic in July during the hottest part of the day and your air conditioning is broken. Which of the following is true about the Inuit culture?
   A. They don't sweat because their diet is so high in roughage that their apocrine glands are less efficient in hot climates.
   B. They will sweat profusely all over their bodies because they are not used to the hot temperatures.
   C. They will sweat more on their faces because this is an adaptation that has been made over time by their culture for survival in their environment.
   D. They have an overabundance of eccrine sweat glands and so you might expect them to have body odor because of the bacterial flora reacting with the apocrine sweat.

Correct Answer: C

Rationale: Inuits have made an interesting environmental adaptation whereby they sweat less than Caucasians on their trunks and extremities but more on their faces.

Cognitive Level: Application

10. You are caring for a black child who has been diagnosed with marasmus. You would expect:
    A. the lymph nodes in the groin to be enlarged and tender.
    B. the skin on the hands and feet to be scaly and tender.
    C. the hair to be less kinky and to be a copper-red color.
    D. the head to be larger than normal, with wide set eyes.

Correct Answer: C

Rationale: The hair of black children with severe malnutrition, e.g., marasmus, frequently changes not only in texture but in color—the child's hair becomes less kinky and assumes a copper-red color.

Cognitive Level: Application

11. A variety of terms are available to describe the moisture and texture of skin. The term that means excess dryness is:
    A. seborritus.
    B. xerosis.
    C. pruritus.
    D. scalosis.

Correct Answer: B

Rationale: Xerosis is the term used to describe skin that is excessively dry.

Cognitive Level: Knowledge

12. Mrs. A. comes to you complaining of severe sunburn and states that, "I was just out in the sun for a couple of minutes." You begin a medication review with Mrs. A. paying special attention to:
   A. the medication that she is taking for her hyperthyroidism.
   B. the medication that she is taking for her acne.
   C. the medication that she is taking for her menopause.
   D. the medication that she is taking for her pain.

Correct Answer: B

Rationale: Drugs that may increase sunlight sensitivity and give burn response include: sulfonamides, thiazide diuretics, oral hypoglycemic agents, and tetracycline.

Cognitive Level: Application

13. Mrs. P. is leaving on a trip to Hawaii and has come in for a checkup. During your examination you notice that she is diabetic and takes oral hypoglycemic agents. Your teaching would include:
   A. a discussion of the dangers of snorkeling on the island of Hilo.
   B. a video showing food preparation in the West Indies.
   C. a discussion of the importance of sunscreen and avoiding direct sunlight.
   D. a booklet discussing the native Hawaiian treatment for yeast infections.

Correct Answer: C

Rationale: Drugs that may increase sunlight sensitivity and give burn response include: sulfonamides, thiazide diuretics, oral hypoglycemic agents, and tetracycline.

Cognitive Level: Application

14. Ms. L., a 13-year old, is interested in obtaining information about the cause of her acne. You could provide her with the following information:
   A. Acne is caused by a poor diet.
   B. Acne has been found to be related to unsafe sexual practices.
   C. Acne is contagious.
   D. Acne is found in about 70% of all teens.

Correct Answer: D

Rationale: About 70% of teens will have acne, and while the cause is unknown, it is not caused by poor diet, oily complexion, contagion, nor is it related to sexual practices.

Cognitive Level: Comprehension

15. Mrs. Q., a 75-year old who has a history of diabetes and peripheral vascular disease, has been trying to remove a corn on the bottom of her foot with a scissors. You will encourage Mrs. Q. to stop trying to remove the corn with her scissors because:
   A. with her diabetes, she has increased circulation to her foot and it could cause severe bleeding.
   B. with her peripheral vascular disease, her range of motion is limited and she may not be able to reach the corn safely.
   C. she could be at increased risk for infection and lesions because of her chronic disease.
   D. because she is 75 years old, she is unable to see and so puts herself at greater risk for falling with the scissors.

Correct Answer: C

Rationale: A personal history of diabetes and peripheral vascular increases a person's risk for skin lesions in the feet or ankles.

Cognitive Level: Application

16. A thorough skin assessment is very important because the skin holds information about:
   A. socioeconomic status.
   B. psychological wellness.
   C. circulatory status.
   D. support systems.

Correct Answer: C

Rationale: The skin holds information about the body's circulation, nutritional status, and signs of systemic diseases as well as topical data on the integument itself.

Cognitive Level: Comprehension

17. Mrs. B. comes in for an assessment of her acne, and you notice that she is very flushed (red) in the face. You could attribute this to:

A. peripheral vasoconstriction.
B. peripheral vasodilation.
C. decreased arterial perfusion.
D. venous pooling.

Correct Answer: B

Rationale: Table 10-1.

Cognitive Level: Application

18. Mr. V. comes to your clinic and tells you that he has been confined to his recliner chair for about 3 days with his feet down and he wants you to evaluate his feet. During your evaluation, you might expect to find:
    A. increased capillary filling time.
    B. capillary pooling.
    C. distended arteries.
    D. distended veins.

Correct Answer: D

Rationale: Table 10-1.

Cognitive Level: Application

19. Your patient is especially worried about an area of skin on her feet that has turned white. You suspect that this is vitiligo and you explain to your patient that:
    A. vitiligo is caused by an excess of apocrine glands in her feet.
    B. vitiligo is related to impetigo, and that it can be treated with an ointment.
    C. vitiligo is caused by the complete absence of melanin pigment.
    D. vitiligo is caused by an excess of melanin pigment.

Correct Answer: C

Rationale: Vitiligo is the complete absence of melanin pigment in patchy areas of white or light skin on the face, neck, hands, feet, body folds, and around orifices—otherwise the depigmented skin is normal.

Cognitive Level: Application

20. Your patient tells you that he notices one of his nevi has started to burn and bleed. In your assessment of his skin, you would pay special attention to the danger signs for pigmented lesions, and you would expect to find:
    A. symmetry of lesions.
    B. border regularity.
    C. color variation.
    D. diameter less than 6 mm.

Correct Answer: C

Rationale: Abnormal characteristics of pigmented lesions are summarized in the mnemonic ABCD: asymmetry of pigmented lesion, border irregularity, color variation, and diameter greater than 6 mm.

Cognitive Level: Comprehension

21. Mr. A. comes to your clinic and states that he feels his skin is redder than normal. You understand this condition to be due to hyperemia, and know that it can be caused by:
    A. excess blood in the dilated superficial capillaries.
    B. excess blood in the underlying blood vessels.
    C. decreased perfusion to the surrounding tissues.
    D. decreased amounts of bilirubin in the blood.

Correct Answer: A

Rationale: Erythema is an intense redness of the skin due to excess blood (hyperemia) in the dilated superficial capillaries.

Cognitive Level: Analysis

22. During a skin assessment you notice that Mr. C., a Mexican-American patient, has skin that is yellowish-brown in color. However, the skin on the hard/soft pallet is a normal pink color. From this finding, you could probably rule out:
    A. pallor.
    B. cyanosis.
    C. jaundice.
    D. iron deficiency.

Correct Answer: C

Rationale: Jaundice is exhibited by a yellow color, indicating rising amounts of bilirubin in the blood and is first noticed in the junction of the hard and soft palate in the mouth, and in the sclera.

Cognitive Level: Analysis

23. Mrs. Z., an African American patient, is observed to have skin that is ashen/gray in color; she is oliguric and restless. You might suspect that Mrs. Z. may be experiencing:
    A. iron deficient anemia.
    B. pernicious anemia.
    C. impending shock.

D. renal failure.

Correct Answer: C

Rationale: Pallor in black-skinned people will appear ashen or gray. The pallor of impending shock is accompanied by other subtle manifestations, such as increasing pulse rate, oliguria, apprehension, and restlessness.

Cognitive Level: Analysis

24. Your patient has tingling sensations in her feet, and has noticed that her tongue has become very red and painful. You suspect that she is suffering from:
    A. pernicious anemia.
    B. iron deficiency anemia.
    C. polycythemia.
    D. micronicious anemia.

Correct Answer: A

Rationale: Pernicious anemia is indicated by neurologic deficits and a red, painful tongue along with a lemon yellow tint of the face and slightly yellow sclera.

Cognitive Level: Application

25. Ms. I. complains that she has noticed several small, punctuate, slightly raised, bright red dots on her chest. You would reassure her that they are probably:
    A. scleroderma.
    B. anascara.
    C. senile angioma.
    D. latent myeloma.

Correct Answer: C

Rationale: Cherry (senile) angiomas are small, punctate, slightly raised bright red dots that commonly appear on the trunk in all adults over 30.

Cognitive Level: Application

26. J.K., a 65-year-old male with emphysema and bronchitis, has come to your clinic for a skin assessment. You might expect to find the following:
    A. Scleroderma
    B. Clubbing of the nails
    C. Anasarca
    D. Erythema

Correct Answer: B

Rationale: Clubbing of the nails occurs with congenital chronic cyanotic heart disease and with emphysema and chronic bronchitis.

Cognitive Level: Analysis

27. Mrs. B.'s newborn has Down syndrome. During the skin assessment you notice a transient mottling in the trunk and extremities in response to the cooler examination room temperature. Mrs. B. notices the mottling and asks what it is. You tell her that it probably is:
    A. acrocyanosis.
    B. cutis marmorata.
    C. corotenemia.
    D. café au lait.

Correct Answer: B

Rationale: Persistent or pronounced cutis marmorata occurs with Down syndrome or prematurity and is a transient mottling in the trunk and extremities in response to cooler room temperatures.

Cognitive Level: Analysis

28. Ms. H., a 35-year-old pregnant woman, comes to you for a skin assessment. You notice that she has a brown patch of hyperpigmentation on her face, and you continue your skin assessment aware that you might also find:
    A. linea gravida.
    B. keratosis.
    C. linea nigra.
    D. mitoasma.

Correct Answer: C

Rationale: In pregnancy, skin changes can include striae, linea nigra, chloasma, and vascular spiders.

Cognitive Level: Analysis

29. Mr. P. has come in for a skin assessment because he is afraid he might have skin cancer. During Mr. P.'s skin assessment you notice several areas of pigmentation that look greasy, dark, and "stuck on" his skin. Which is the best prediction?
    A. He probably has acrochordons, precursors to squamous cell carcinoma.
    B. He probably has actinic keratoses, a precursor to basal cell carcinoma.
    C. He probably has seborrheic keratoses, which do not become cancerous.
    D. He probably has senile lentigines, which do not become cancerous.

Correct Answer: C

Rationale: Seborrheic keratoses look like dark, greasy, "stuck on" lesions that develop mostly on the trunk. These lesions do not become cancerous.

Cognitive Level: Analysis

30. Mr. Q.'s areas of patchy depigmentation are related to:
    A. destruction of melanocytes.
    B. absence of pigment melanin.
    C. decreased perfusion.
    D. decreased hematocrit.

Correct Answer: A

Rationale: Anemia is caused by decreased hematocrit, shock is caused by decreased perfusion and vasoconstriction. Albinism is the total absence of pigment melanin and vitiligo is a patchy depigmentation from destruction of melanocytes.

Cognitive Level: Comprehension

31. You notice that Mr. W. has a solid, elevated, circumscribed lesion that is less than 1 cm in diameter. In your charting, you would report this as a:
    A. nodule.
    B. wheal.
    C. papule.
    D. bulla.

Correct Answer: C

Rationale: A papule is something you can feel, is solid, elevated, circumscribed, less than 1 cm diameter, and is due to superficial thickening in the epidermis.

Cognitive Level: Comprehension

32. You have just read in Mrs. S.'s chart that she has a lesion that is confluent in nature. Upon examination, you would expect to find:
    A. lesions that are grouped or clustered together.
    B. annual lesions that have grown together.
    C. lesions arranged in a line along a nerve route.
    D. lesions that run together.

Correct Answer: D

Rationale: Grouped lesions are clustered together, polycyclic lesions are annular in nature, zosteriform lesions are arranged along a nerve route, and confluent lesions run together.

Cognitive Level: Comprehension

33. Mr. P. has had a "terrible itch" for several months that he has been scratching continuously. Upon examination, you might expect to find:
    A. a keloid.
    B. a fissure.
    C. a bulla.
    D. lichenification.

Correct Answer: D

Rationale: Lichenification results from prolonged intense scratching that eventually thickens the skin and produces tightly packed sets of papules.

Cognitive Level: Comprehension

34. Dr. K. has diagnosed Mrs. Q. with purpura. Dr. K. leaves the room and Mrs. Q. asks you what Dr. K saw that lead him to that diagnosis and you respond:
    A. "He is referring to that fiery red, star-shaped marking on your cheek that has a solid circular center."
    B. "He is referring to those tiny little areas of hemorrhage (<2 mm, round and discrete, dark red in color)."
    C. "He is referring to that confluent and extensive patch of petechiae and ecchymosis on your feet."
    D. "He is referring to that blue dilation of blood vessels in a star-shaped linear pattern on your legs."

Correct Answer: C

Rationale: Purpura is a confluent and extensive patch of petechiae and ecchymoses and a flat macular hemorrhage seen in generalized disorders such as thrombocytopenia and scurvy.

Cognitive Level: Comprehension

35. Your patient's mother has noticed that her son, who has been to a new babysitter, has some blisters and scabs on his face and buttocks. Upon examination, you notice moist, thin-roofed vesicles with a thin erythematous base and you suspect:
    A. diaper dermatitis.
    B. intertrigo.
    C. impetigo.
    D. eczema.

Correct Answer: C

Rationale: Impetigo is moist, thin-roofed vesicles with a thin erythematous base. This is a contagious bacterial infection of the skin; most common in infants and children.

Cognitive Level: Application

36. You notice that your patient has bluish white, red-based spots in her mouth, that are elevated about 1 to 3 mm. What other signs would you expect to find in this patient?
    A. Pink papular rash on the face and neck
    B. Pruritic vesicles
    C. Hyperpigmentation on chest, abdomen, and back of arms
    D. Red-purple maculopapular blotchy rash behind ears and on face

Correct Answer: D

Rationale: With measles (Rubeola), you would assess a red-purple blotchy rash on the third or fourth day of illness that appears first behind ears and spreads over face, then over neck, trunk, arms and legs; looks coppery and does not blanch. You would also find Kopliks spots in the mouth.

Cognitive Level: Analysis

37. Mr. Y. has AIDS, and you are assessing his skin. You notice a widely disseminated violet-colored tumor covering the skin and mucous membranes, and you would conclude that:
    A. he is in the first stage of AIDS.
    B. this person has been exposed to a viral infection.
    C. these lesions represent an advanced case of herpes zoster.
    D. he is in the advanced stage of AIDS.

Correct Answer: D

Rationale: In the advanced stage of AIDS, you may notice widely disseminated lesions involving skin and mucous membranes, and visceral organs.

Cognitive Level: Application

38. Mr. U., a farmer, comes in for a skin evaluation complaining of hair loss on his head. He has noticed that his hair seems to be breaking off in patches and that he has some scaling on his head. You would begin your examination suspecting:
    A. toxic alopecia.
    B. seborrheic dermatitis.
    C. tinea capitis.
    D. tinea corporis.

Correct Answer: C

Rationale: Tinea Capitis: rounded patchy hair loss on scale, leaving broken-off hairs, pustules, and scales on skin; due to fungal infection; lesions fluorescent under Wood's light. Usually seen in children and farmers; highly contagious.

Cognitive Level: Analysis

39. Ms. X. brings her child in to you for an examination of the scalp and hair. She states that this child has developed some places where there are irregularly-shaped patches with broken-off, stub-like hair and she is worried that this could be some form of premature baldness. She tells you that the child's hair is always kept very short. You reassure her by telling her that it is:
    A. folliculitis, and that it can be treated with an antibiotic.
    B. tinea capitis, and that it is highly contagious and needs immediate attention.
    C. trichotillomania, and that her child has probably developed a habit of twirling her hair absent-mindedly.
    D. traumatic alopecia that can be treated with antifungal medications.

Correct Answer: C

Rationale: Trichotillomania: self-induced hair loss usually due to habit. Forms irregularly-shaped patches, with broken-off, stublike hairs of varying lengths; person is never completely bald and occurs as child rubs or twirls area absently while falling asleep, reading, or watching television.

Cognitive Level: Application

40. Decreased skin turgor is an expected finding in which of the following conditions?
    A. During childhood growth spurts
    B. In cases of severe obesity
    C. With conditions of connective tissue disorders such as scleroderma
    D. In an individual who is severely dehydrated

Correct Answer: D

Rationale: Decreased skin turgor is associated with severe dehydration, aging, or extreme weight loss.

Cognitive Level: Comprehension

41. When performing an assessment of a 65-year-old male with a history of HTN, CVA, and CAD, you note the presence of pitting edema in the

lower legs bilaterally. The skin is puffy and tight, but of normal color. There is no increased redness or tenderness over his lower legs, and the peripheral pulses are equal and strong. In this situation, which of the following is the most likely cause of the edema?
A. A local inflammation
B. Blockage of lymphatic drainage
C. Heart failure
D. Venous thrombosis due to circulatory problems

Correct Answer: C

Rationale: Bilateral edema or edema that is generalized over the entire body is caused by a central problem such as heart failure or kidney failure. Unilateral edema usually has a local or peripheral cause.

Cognitive Level: Analysis

42. A 40-year-old female reports a change in mole size, accompanied by color changes, itching, burning and bleeding over the past month. She is dark complected and has no family history of skin cancer, but she has had many blistering sunburns in the past. You would:
A. tell the patient to watch the lesion over the next few months and report back if there are no changes.
B. refer the patient due to the suspicion of melanoma based on her symptoms.
C. suspect that this is a compound nevus, which is very common in young to middle-aged adults.
D. ask additional questions regarding environmental irritants that may have caused this condition.

Correct Answer: B

Rationale: The ABCD danger signs of melanoma are asymmetry, border irregularity, color variation, and diameter. In addition, individuals may report a change in size, development of itching, burning, bleeding, or a new pigmented lesion. Any of these signs raise suspicion of malignant melanoma and warrant referral.

Cognitive Level: Analysis

43. Which of the following assessment findings is most consistent with clubbing of the fingernails?
A. A nail base that is firm to palpation and slightly tender
B. A nail base that feels spongy with an angle of the nail base of 160 degrees
C. Curved nails with a convex profile and ridges across the nail
D. An angle of the nail base of 180 degrees or greater with a nail base that feels spongy

Correct Answer: D

Rationale: The normal nail is firm at its base and has an angle of 160 degrees. In clubbing, the angle straightens to 180 degrees or greater and the nail base feels spongy.

Cognitive Level: Comprehension

44. Jaundice is exhibited by a yellow skin color, indicating rising levels of bilirubin in the blood. Which of the following findings is indicative of true jaundice?
A. Yellow patches throughout the sclera
B. Skin which appears yellow when examined under low light
C. Yellow color of the sclera which extends up to the iris
D. Yellow deposits on the palms and soles of feet where jaundice first appears

Correct Answer: C

Rationale: The scleral yellow of jaundice extends up to the edge of the iris. Calluses on the palms and soles of feet often look yellow, but are not classified as jaundice.

Cognitive Level: Knowledge

45. When assessing inflammation in a dark-skinned person, it may be necessary to:
A. palpate the skin for edema and increased warmth.
B. assess the oral mucosa for generalized erythema.
C. assess the skin for cyanosis and swelling.
D. palpate for tenderness and local areas of ecchymosis.

Correct Answer: A

Rationale: Inflammation is not easily recognized, and it is often necessary to palpate the skin for increased warmth, taut surfaces that may be indicative of edema, and hardening of deep tissues or blood vessels.

Cognitive Level: Application

Chapter 11

Head and Neck, Including Regional Lymphatics

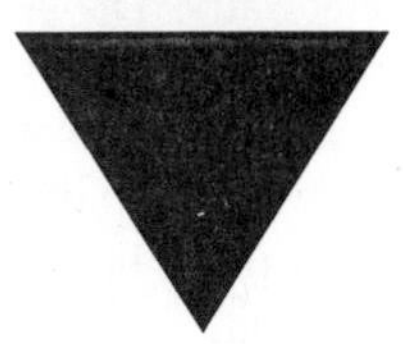

1. Dr. Jones, after examining his patient, tells you that the patient's vertebra prominens is tender, and asks that you re-evaluate the area in 1 hour. The area of the body you will assess is:
   A. the area just lateral to the knee cap.
   B. the area just above the diaphragm.
   C. the area at the level of the C7 vertebra.
   D. the area at the level of the T11 vertebra.

Correct Answer: C

Rationale: The C7 vertebra has a long spinous process that is palpable when the head is flexed, called the vertebra prominens.

Cognitive Level: Application

2. Mrs. Phillips brings in her 2-month-old daughter for an examination and says, "My daughter rolled over against the wall and now I have noticed that she has this spot that is soft on the top of her head. Is there something terribly wrong?" Your response would be:
   A. "That 'soft spot' is normal, and actually allows for growth of the brain during the first year of your baby's life."
   B. "That 'soft spot' you are referring to may be an indication of cretinism or congenital hypothyroidism."
   C. "Perhaps that could be a result of your dietary intake during pregnancy."
   D. "Your baby may have craniosynostosis, a disease of the sutures of the brain."

Correct Answer: A

Rationale: Membrane-covered "soft spots" allow for growth of the brain during the first year. They gradually ossify; the triangular-shaped posterior fontanel is closed by 1 to 2 months, and the diamond-shaped anterior fontanel closes between 9 months and 2 years.

Cognitive Level: Application

3. You notice that your patient's palpebral fissures are not symmetrical. Upon examination, you may find that there has been damage to:
   A. cranial nerve number five (V).
   B. cranial nerve number three (III).
   C. cranial nerve number seven (VII).
   D. cranial nerve number eight (VIII).

Correct Answer: C

Rationale: Facial muscles are mediated by cranial nerve VII (7).

Cognitive Level: Application

4. Your patient is unable to differentiate between sharp and dull stimulation to both sides of her face. You suspect:
   A. damage to the trigeminal nerve.
   B. frostbite with resultant paresthesia to cheeks.
   C. scleroderma with a pronounced proliferation of connective tissue in the face and cheeks.
   D. Bell's palsy.

Correct Answer: A

Rationale: Facial sensations of pain or touch are mediated by cranial nerve V, the trigeminal nerve.

Cognitive Level: Application

5. The two pairs of salivary glands that are accessible to examination on the face are:
   A. occipital and submental.
   B. parotid and jugulodigastric.
   C. submandibular and occipital.
   D. parotid and submandibular.

Correct Answer: D

Rationale: Two pairs of salivary glands accessible to examination on the face are the parotid glands in the cheeks over the mandible, anterior to and below the ear and the submandibular glands, beneath the mandible at the angle of the jaw.

Cognitive Level: Comprehension

6. Your patient comes to your clinic complaining of neck and shoulder pain, and is unable to turn her head. You suspect damage to the _____ cranial nerve, and proceed with your examination by:
   A. 12th; percussing the sternomastoid and submandibular neck muscles
   B. 11th; palpating the anterior and posterior triangles
   C. 12th; assessing for a positive Rhomberg
   D. 11th; asking the patient to shrug her shoulders against resistance

Correct Answer: D

Rationale: The major neck muscles are the sternomastoid and the trapezius; they are innervated by cranial nerve XI, the spinal accessory. The innervated muscles assist with head rotation and head flexion, movement of the shoulders and extension and turning of the head.

Cognitive Level: Analysis

7. The muscles in the neck that are innervated by cranial nerve XI are:
   A. spinal accessory and omohyoid.
   B. sternomastoid and trapezius.
   C. trapezius and sternomandibular.
   D. sternomandibular and spinal accessory.

Correct Answer: B

Rationale: The major neck muscles are the sternomastoid and the trapezius; they are innervated by cranial nerve XI, the spinal accessory.

Cognitive Level: Knowledge

8. Your patient's lab data reveal an elevated thyroxine level. You would proceed with an examination of:
   A. the thyroxine gland.
   B. the parotid gland.
   C. the thyroid gland.
   D. the adrenal gland.

Correct Answer: C

Rationale: The thyroid gland is a highly vascular endocrine gland that secretes thyroxine (T4) and triiodothyronine (T3).

Cognitive Level: Comprehension

9. Your patient says that she has recently noticed a lump in the front of her neck below her "Adam's apple" that seems to be getting bigger. During your assessment, the finding that reassures you that this may not be a cancerous thyroid nodule is that:
   A. the lump (nodule) is mobile and is not hard.
   B. the lump (nodule) is hard and is fixed to the surrounding structures.
   C. the lump (nodule) is tender.
   D. the lump (nodule) disappears when the patient smiles.

Correct Answer: A

Rationale: Suspect any painless, rapidly growing nodule, especially the appearance of a single nodule in a young person. Cancerous nodules tend to be hard and are fixed to surrounding structures.

Cognitive Level: Application

10. You notice that your patient's submental lymph nodes are enlarged. In an effort to identify the cause of the node enlargement, you would assess:
    A. the supraclavicular area.
    B. the infraclavicular area.
    C. the area proximal to the enlarged node.
    D. the area distal to the enlarged node.

Correct Answer: C

Rationale: When nodes are abnormal, check the area they drain for the source of the problem. Explore the area proximal (upstream) to the location of the abnormal node.

Cognitive Level: Analysis

11. The four areas in the body where lymph nodes are accessible are:
    A. head and neck, arms, breasts, axillae.
    B. arms, breasts, inguinal area, legs.
    C. head and neck, arms, inguinal area, axillae.
    D. head, breasts, groin, abdomen.

Correct Answer: C

Rationale: Nodes are located throughout the body, but are accessible to examination only in four areas: head and neck, arms, axillae, and inguinal region.

Cognitive Level: Knowledge

12. Ms. P. brings her newborn in for an assessment and asks, "Is there something wrong with my baby—his head seems so big." You know the following about relative proportions of the head and trunk of the newborn:
    A. head circumference should be greater than chest circumference at birth.
    B. at birth, the head is one-fifth the total length.

C. the head size reaches 90 percent of its final size when the child is 3.
D. when the anterior fontanel closes at 2 months, the size of the child's head will be reduced in size, and the head will be more proportioned to the body.

Correct Answer: A

Rationale: During the fetal period, head growth predominates. Head size is greater than chest circumference at birth and the head size grows during childhood, reaching 90 percent its final size when the child is age 6.

Cognitive Level: Comprehension

13. Your patient, an 85-year-old woman, is complaining about the fact that the bones in her face have become more noticeable. During your assessment, you attempt to reassure her by telling her what?
A. It is probably due to the fact that she doesn't use a dermatologically approved moisturizer.
B. Facial skin becomes more elastic with age and that this increased elasticity causes the skin to be more taught, drawing attention to the facial bones.
C. Diets low in protein and high in carbohydrates may cause enhanced facial bones.
D. It is probably due to a combination of factors such as decreased elasticity, subcutaneous fat, and moisture in her skin.

Correct Answer: D

Rationale: The facial bones and orbits appear more prominent in the aging adult, and the facial skin sags owing to decreased elasticity, decreased subcutaneous fat, and decreased moisture in the skin.

Cognitive Level: Comprehension

14. Your patient presents with excruciating headache pain on one side of his head especially around his eye, forehead, and cheek that lasts about ½ to 2 hours and occur once or twice each day. You suspect:
A. migraine headaches.
B. tension headaches.
C. cluster headaches.
D. hypertension.

Correct Answer: C

Rationale: Cluster headaches produce pain around the eye, temple, forehead and cheek, are unilateral and always on the same side of the head. They are excruciating and occur once or twice per day and last ½ to 2 hours each.

Cognitive Level: Application

15. You have been studying for an examination and you begin to notice that you have a severe headache in the frontotemporal area of your head that is throbbing and is somewhat relieved when you lie down. Your mother used to complain about these same symptoms. You suspect that you may be suffering from:
A. migraine headaches.
B. tension headaches.
C. cluster headaches.
D. hypertension.

Correct Answer: A

Rationale: Migraine headaches tend to be supraorbital, retro-orbital, or frontotemporal with a throbbing quality, are of a severe quantity, and are relieved by lying down.

Cognitive Level: Application

16. Mr. B. is complaining of a headache. He states that he just woke up from a nap and his headache is worse, his eyelids have started to droop, and the only thing that seems to help is walking around. Given those symptoms, you would suspect that Mr. B. has a:
A. migraine headache.
B. tension headache.
C. cluster headache.
D. head injury.

Correct Answer: C

Rationale: Cluster headaches produce pain around the eye, temple, forehead and cheek, are unilateral and always on the same side of the head. They are excruciating, occur once or twice per day, and are relieved by moving around.

Cognitive Level: Application

17. T.T.'s newborn baby's head is 1/3 of her total body length and even though her head. They are large, her face looks small. You tell T.T. that:
A. this is normal.
B. this could be craniosynostosis.
C. this could be hydrocephaly.
D. this could be microcephaly.

Correct Answer: C

Rationale: Obstruction of drainage of cerebrospinal fluid results in excessive accumulation, increasing intracranial pressure, and enlargement of the head. The face looks small compared with the enlarged cranium.

Cognitive Level: Application

18. The temporomandibular joint is just below the temporal artery and anterior to the:
    A. vagus.
    B. tragus.
    C. hyoid.
    D. mandible.

Correct Answer: B

Rationale: The temporomandibular joint is just below the temporal artery and anterior to the tragus.

Cognitive Level: Comprehension

19. Mr. T. has come in for an examination and states, "I have this spot in front of my ear lobe here on my cheek that seems to be getting bigger and is real tender—what do you think it is?" You reply:
    A. "It could be an inflammation of your submental lymph node."
    B. "It could be an inflammation of your thyroid gland."
    C. "It could be an inflammation of your occipital lymph node."
    D. "It could be an inflammation of your parotid gland."

Correct Answer: D

Rationale: Swelling with the parotid gland occurs below the angle of the jaw and is most visible when the head is extended. Painful inflammation occurs with mumps, and swelling also occurs with abscesses or tumors. Swelling occurs anterior to the lower ear lobe.

Cognitive Level: Application

20. Mr. A. has come in for an examination and he states, "I think that I have the mumps, and I am also HIV positive." You would begin by examining:
    A. the thyroid gland.
    B. the cervical lymph nodes.
    C. the mouth and skin for lesions.
    D. the parotid gland.

Correct Answer: D

Rationale: The parotid gland may become swollen with the onset of mumps, and parotid enlargement has been found with HIV.

Cognitive Level: Application

21. You suspect that your patient has hyperthyroidism and you know that thyroxine and triiodothyronine hormones are elevated. Which of the following findings would you most likely find?
    A. Constipation
    B. Tachycardia
    C. Atrophied nodular thyroid
    D. Rapid dyspnea

Correct Answer: B

Rationale: Thyroxine and triiodothyronine are thyroid hormones that stimulate the rate of cellular metabolism, and with an enlarged thyroid as in hyperthyroidism you might expect to find diffuse enlargement (goiter) or a nodular lump.

Cognitive Level: Analysis

22. Mr. F., a visitor from Poland who does not speak English and seems to be somewhat apprehensive about you examining his neck, would probably be most comfortable with you examining his thyroid:
    A. from behind, with your hands placed firmly around his neck.
    B. from the side, with your eyes averted towards the ceiling and your thumbs on his neck.
    C. from the front, with your thumbs placed on either side of his trachea and his head tilted backwards.
    D. from the front, with your thumbs placed on either side of his trachea and his head tilted forward.

Correct Answer: D

Rationale: Examining Mr. F's thyroid from the back may be unsettling for him, and so it will be best to examine his thyroid using the anterior approach, and asking him to tip his head forward and to the right and then the left.

Cognitive Level: Application

23. Mr. F.'s thyroid is enlarged, and you are going to auscultate the thyroid for the presence of a bruit. A bruit is:
    A. a loud, whooshing, blowing sound best heard

with the bell of the stethoscope.
B. a soft, whooshing, pulsatile sound best heard with the bell of the stethoscope.
C. a low gurgling sound best heard with the diaphragm of the stethoscope.
D. a high-pitched tinkling sound best heard with the diaphragm of the stethoscope.

Correct Answer: B

Rationale: If the thyroid gland is enlarged, auscultate it for the presence of a bruit, which is a soft, pulsatile, whooshing, blowing sound heard best with the bell of the stethoscope.

Cognitive Level: Knowledge

24. You notice that baby J. has a large soft lump on the side of his head and that the mother is very concerned. She tells you that she did notice this lump about 8 hours after baby J.'s birth, but that it seems to be getting bigger. One possible explanation for this is:
A. cephalhematoma.
B. caput succedaneum.
C. craniosynostosis.
D. hydrocephalus.

Correct Answer: A

Rationale: A cephalhematoma is a subperiosteal hemorrhage that is the result of birth trauma. It is soft, fluctuant, and well defined over one cranial bone. It appears several hours after birth and gradually increases in size.

Cognitive Level: Analysis

25. Mrs. T. brings in her newborn for an assessment and tells you that she has noticed that whenever her newborn's head is turned to the right side, she straightens out the arm and leg on the same side and flexes the opposite arm and leg. After finding this yourself upon examination, you would tell her that:
A. this is abnormal: the baby should be flexing the arm and leg on the right side of his body when the head is turned to the right.
B. this is normal and should disappear by the first year of life.
C. this is normal and should disappear between 3 and 4 months of age.
D. this is abnormal and is called the atonic neck reflex.

Correct Answer: C

Rationale: By 2 weeks the infant shows the tonic neck reflex when supine and the head is turned to one side (extension of same arm and leg, flexion of opposite arm and leg). The tonic neck reflex disappears between 3 and 4 months of age.

Cognitive Level: Analysis

26. Which of the following findings would indicate Paget's disease:
A. Positive Macewen's sign
B. Premature closure of the sagittal suture
C. Headache, vertigo, tinnitus and deafness
D. Elongated head with heavy eyebrow ridge

Correct Answer: C

Rationale: Paget's disease occurs more often in males and is characterized by bowed long bones, sudden fractures, and enlarging skull bones that press on cranial nerves causing symptoms of headache, vertigo, tinnitus, and progressive deafness.

Cognitive Level: Comprehension

27. Mr. J. approaches you to ask a question, and you notice that he seems to have an enlarged and rather thick skull. You wonder about acromegaly, and would continue to assess for:
A. bowed long bones.
B. an acorn-shaped cranium.
C. coarse facial features.
D. exophthalmos.

Correct Answer: C

Rationale: Acromegaly is excessive secretion of growth hormone that creates an enlarged skull and thickened cranial bones. Patients will have elongated heads, massive face, prominent nose and lower jaw, heavy eyebrow ridge, and coarse facial features.

Cognitive Level: Analysis

28. Children affected with chromosomal aberration (trisomy-21) Down syndrome may present with:
A. protruding thin tongue.
B. narrow and raised nasal bridge.
C. long, thin neck.
D. ear dysplasia.

Correct Answer: D

Rationale: With the chromosomal aberration (trisomy-21), head and face characteristics may include slanted eyes with inner epicanthal folds, flat nasal bridge, small broad flat nose, protruding thick tongue, ear dysplasia, and short broad neck with webbing.

Cognitive Level: Comprehension

29. Mr. S. has recently noticed that the left side of his mouth is paralyzed. He states that he cannot raise his eyebrow or whistle. You suspect that Mr. S. has:
    A. suffered a stroke (CVA).
    B. contracted Bell's palsy.
    C. Parkinson's syndrome.
    D. Cushing's syndrome.

Correct Answer: A

Rationale: With an upper motor neuron lesion (as with CVA) you will note paralysis of lower facial muscles, but upper half of face is not affected owing to the intact nerve from the unaffected hemisphere. The person is still able to wrinkle the forehead and to close the eyes.

Cognitive Level: Application

30. Ms. P. comes to your clinic and tells you that "her eyes have gotten so puffy, and that my eyebrows and hair have become coarse and dry." As you begin your examination, you suspect:
    A. scleroderma.
    B. cachecticia.
    C. myxedema.
    D. cretinism.

Correct Answer: C

Rationale: Myxedema (hypothyroidism) is a deficiency of thyroid hormone that when severe causes a nonpitting edema or myxedema. You will note puffy edematous face especially around eyes (periorbital edema), coarse facial features, dry skin, and dry, coarse hair and eyebrows.

Cognitive Level: Application

31. During your examination of Mrs. V. you note lymphadenopathy, and you suspect an acute infection. Acutely infected lymph nodes would be:
    A. hard and nontender.
    B. unilateral.
    C. firm but freely movable.
    D. clumped.

Correct Answer: C

Rationale: Acutely infected lymph nodes are bilateral, enlarged, warm, tender, and firm but freely movable.

Cognitive Level: Comprehension

32. With tracheal shift, the trachea is:
    A. pushed to the unaffected side with a tumor.
    B. pulled to the unaffected side with plural adhesions.
    C. pushed to the affected side with thyroid enlargement.
    D. pulled to the affected side with systole.

Correct Answer: A

Rationale: The trachea is pushed to the unaffected side with an aortic aneurysm, a tumor, unilateral thyroid lobe enlargement, and pneumothorax.

Cognitive Level: Comprehension

33. During your assessment of infant K., you note that the fontanels are depressed and sunken. You suspect:
    A. rickets.
    B. increased intracranial pressure.
    C. dehydration.
    D. mental retardation.

Correct Answer: C

Rationale: Depressed and sunken fontanels occur with dehydration or malnutrition.

Cognitive Level: Application

34. You are performing an assessment on a 7-year-old with symptoms of chronic watery eyes, sneezing, and clear nasal drainage. You note the presence of a transverse line across the bridge of the nose, dark blue shadows below the eyes, and a double crease on the lower eyelids. These findings are characteristic of:
    A. a sinus infection.
    B. an upper respiratory infection.
    C. nasal congestion.
    D. allergies.

Correct Answer: D

Rationale: Chronic allergies often develop chronic facial characteristics. These include: blue shadows below the eyes, a double or single crease on the lower eyelids, open-mouth breathing, and a transverse line on the nose.

Cognitive Level: Analysis

35. While performing a well child assessment on a 5-year-old, you note the presence of palpable bilateral cervical and inguinal lymph nodes. They are approximately 0.5 cm in size, round, mobile and non-tender. You suspect that:
    A. this is a normal finding for a well child of this age.
    B. this child may have an infection.
    C. this child has chronic allergies.
    D. this child should be referred for additional evaluation.

Correct Answer: A

Rationale: Palpable lymph nodes are normal in children until puberty when the lymphoid tissue begins to atrophy. Lymph nodes may be up to 1 cm in size in the cervical and inguinal areas, but are discrete, moveable, and nontender.

Cognitive Level: Analysis

36. You have just completed a lymph assessment on a 60-year-old healthy female patient. You expect to find that most lymph nodes in healthy adults are normally:
    A. rubbery, discrete, and mobile.
    B. shotty.
    C. not palpable.
    D. large, firm, fixed to the tissue.

Correct Answer: C

Rationale: Most lymph nodes are not palpable in adults. The palpability of lymph nodes decreases with age.

Cognitive Level: Application

Chapter 12

Eyes

1. The bulbar conjunctiva:
   A. is a thin mucous membrane that lines the lids.
   B. overlies the sclera.
   C. is visible at the inner canthus of the eye.
   D. covers the iris and pupil.

Correct Answer: B

Rationale: The bulbar conjunctiva overlies the eyeball, with the white sclera showing through.

Cognitive Level: Knowledge

2. Movement of the extraocular muscles:
   A. is stimulated by cranial nerves III (oculomotor), IV (trochlear) and VI (abducens).
   B. is impaired in a patient with cataracts.
   C. requires binocular vision.
   D. is decreased in the elderly.

Correct Answer: A

Rationale: Movement of the extraocular muscles is stimulated by three cranial nerves; cranial nerves III, IV, and VI.

Cognitive Level: Knowledge

3. Which of the following statements regarding the outer layer of the eye is true?
   A. The outer layer of the eye is darkly pigmented to prevent light from reflecting internally.
   B. The outer layer of the eye is very sensitive to touch.
   C. The trigeminal (CN V) and the trochlear (CN IV) are stimulated when the outer surface of the eye is stimulated.
   D. The visual receptive layer of the eye in which light waves are changed into nerve impulses is located in the outer layer of the eye.

Correct Answer: B

Rationale: The cornea and the sclera make up the outer layer of the eye. The cornea is very sensitive to touch.

Cognitive Level: Comprehension

4. Stimulation of the sympathetic branch of the autonomic nervous system:
   A. causes pupillary constriction.
   B. elevates the eyelid and dilates the pupil.
   C. causes contraction of the ciliary body.
   D. adjusts the eye for near vision.

Correct Answer: B

Rationale: Stimulation of the sympathetic branch dilates the pupil and elevates the eyelid.

Cognitive Level: Comprehension

5. Intraocular pressure is determined by the:
   A. contraction of the ciliary body.
   B. thickness or bulging of the lens.
   C. amount of aqueous produced and resistance to its outflow at the angle of the anterior chamber.
   D. posterior chamber as it accommodates for an increase in fluid.

Correct Answer: C

Rationale: Intraocular pressure is determined by a balance between the amount of aqueous produced and resistance to its outflow at the angle of the anterior chamber.

Cognitive Level: Knowledge

6. Which of the following statements regarding visual pathways and visual fields is true?
   A. The image formed on the retina is upside down and reversed from its actual appearance in the outside world.
   B. The light impulses are conducted through the optic nerve to the temporal lobes of the brain.

C. Light rays are refracted through the transparent media of the eye before striking the pupil.
D. The right side of the brain interprets vision for the right eye.

Correct Answer: A

Rationale: The image formed on the retina is upside down and reversed from its actual appearance in the outside world.

Cognitive Level: Knowledge

7. Accommodation refers to:
   A. pupillary dilation when looking at a far object.
   B. pupillary constriction when looking at a near object.
   C. involuntary blinking in the presence of bright light.
   D. changes in peripheral vision in response to light.

Correct Answer: B

Rationale: The muscle fibers of the iris contract the pupil in bright light and accommodate for near vision.

Cognitive Level: Knowledge

8. A patient has a normal pupillary light reflex. What does this mean?
   A. The eye focuses the image in the center of the pupil.
   B. The eyes converge to focus on the light.
   C. Constriction of both pupils occurs in response to bright light.
   D. Light is reflected at the same spot in both eyes.

Correct Answer: C

Rationale: The pupillary light reflex is the normal constriction of the pupils when bright light shines on the retina.

Cognitive Level: Comprehension

9. A mother asks when her newborn infant's eyesight will be developed. You reply:
   A. "Infants develop peripheral vision at about 8 months."
   B. "Most infants have uncoordinated eye movements for the first year of life."
   C. "By about 3 months infants develop more coordinated eye movements and can fixate on an object."
   D. "Vision is not totally developed until the age of 2 years."

Correct Answer: C

Rationale: By 3 to 4 months of age, the infant establishes binocularity and can fixate on a single image with both eyes simultaneously.

Cognitive Level: Application

10. Which of the following physiologic changes is responsible for presbyopia?
    A. Degeneration of the cornea
    B. Decreased distance vision abilities
    C. Loss of lens elasticity
    D. Decreased adaptation to darkness

Correct Answer: C

Rationale: The lens loses elasticity and decreases its ability to change shape in order to accommodate for near vision. This condition is called presbyopia.

Cognitive Level: Comprehension

11. Which of the following would you expect to find when examining the eyes of an African American patient?
    A. Narrowed palpebral fissures
    B. A dark retinal background
    C. Increased photosensitivity
    D. Increased night vision

Correct Answer: B

Rationale: There is a culturally based variability in the color of the iris and in retinal pigmentation, with darker irides having darker retinas behind them.

Cognitive Level: Comprehension

12. A 52-year-old patient describes the presence of occasional "floaters or spots" moving in front of his eyes. You:
    A. consider this an abnormal finding and refer him to an ophthalmologist.
    B. know that "floaters" are usually not significant and are caused by condensed vitreous fibers.
    C. presume the patient has glaucoma.
    D. examine the retina to determine the number of floaters.

Correct Answer: B

Rationale: Floaters are a common sensation with

myopia or after middle age owing to condensed vitreous fibers. Usually, they are not significant.

Cognitive Level: Analysis

13. You are preparing to assess the visual acuity of a 16-year-old patient. How would you proceed?
    A. Use the Snellen chart positioned 20 feet away from the patient.
    B. Ask the patient to read the print on a hand-held Jaeger card.
    C. Perform the confrontation test.
    D. Determine the patient's ability to read newsprint at a distance of 12-14 inches.

Correct Answer: A

Rationale: The Snellen alphabet chart is the most commonly used and accurate measure of visual acuity.

Cognitive Level: Analysis

14. A patient's vision is recorded as 20/30 using the Snellen eye chart. What does this mean?
    A. The patient can read from 30 feet what a person with normal vision can read from 20 feet.
    B. The patient can read the chart from 20 feet in the left eye and 30 feet in the right eye.
    C. At 30 feet the patient can read the entire chart.
    D. The patient can read at 20 feet what a person with normal vision can read at 30 feet.

Correct Answer: D

Rationale: The top number indicates the distance the person is standing from the chart, while the denominator gives the distance at which a normal eye can see.

Cognitive Level: Application

15. A patient is unable to read the 20/100 line on the Snellen chart. You would:
    A. shorten the distance between the patient and the chart and ask him or her to read the smallest line of print possible.
    B. assess whether the patient can count your fingers when they are placed in front of his or her eyes.
    C. refer the patient to an ophthalmologist.
    D. ask the patient to put on his or her reading glasses and attempt to read the Snellen chart again.

Correct Answer: C

Rationale: If vision is poorer than 20/30, refer the person to an ophthalmologist or optometrist.

Cognitive Level: Analysis

16. Interpret the findings of a vision examination recorded as 20/20 OU.
    A. The patient is presbyopic in the right eye.
    B. The patient is hyperopic in the left eye.
    C. The patient is myopic in both eyes.
    D. The patient is nearsighted in the right eye.

Correct Answer: C

Rationale: Normal visual acuity is 20/20 OU. The larger the denominator, the poorer the vision or myopic the person is.

Cognitive Level: Analysis

17. When performing the corneal light reflex assessment, you note that the light is reflected at 2 o'clock OU. You would:
    A. perform the confrontation test to validate your findings.
    B. document this as an asymmetrical light reflex.
    C. refer the individual for further evaluation.
    D. consider this a normal finding.

Correct Answer: D

Rationale: Reflection of the light on the corneas should be in exactly the same spot on each eye or symmetrical.

Cognitive Level: Analysis

18. Which of the following is an expected normal finding when performing the diagnostic positions test?
    A. Nystagmus in extreme superior gaze
    B. A slight amount of lid lag when moving the eyes from a superior to inferior position
    C. Parallel movement of both eyes
    D. Convergence and accommodation of the eyes

Correct Answer: C

Rationale: A normal response for the diagnostic positions test is parallel tracking of the object with both eyes.

Cognitive Level: Application

19. In assessing the sclera of a black patient, which of the following would be an expected finding?
    A. The presence of small brown macules on the sclera
    B. Yellow color of the sclera that extends up to the iris
    C. Pallor near the outer canthus of the lower lid
    D. Yellow fatty deposits over the cornea

Correct Answer: A

Rationale: In dark-skinned people, you normally may see small brown macules in the sclera.

Cognitive Level: Application

20. M.M., a 60-year-old Hispanic male, is at the clinic for an eye examination. You suspect that he has a ptosis of one eye. How would you check for this?
    A. Observe the distance between the palpebral fissures.
    B. Perform the corneal light test and look for symmetry of the light reflex.
    C. Assess the individual's near vision.
    D. Perform the confrontation test.

Correct Answer: A

Rationale: Ptosis is drooping of the upper eyelid that would be apparent by observing the distance between the upper and lower eyelids.

Cognitive Level: Analysis

21. What is the expected normal finding when assessing the lacrimal apparatus?
    A. The presence of tears along the inner canthus
    B. A slight swelling over the upper lid and along the bony orbit if the individual has a cold
    C. A blocked nasolacrimal duct in a newborn infant
    D. The absence of drainage from the puncta when pressing against the inner orbital rim

Correct Answer: D

Rationale: There should be no swelling, redness, or drainage from the puncta.

Cognitive Level: Application

22. Which technique is most correct to use when assessing the pupillary light reflex?
    A. Shine a penlight from directly in front of the patient and inspect for pupillary constriction.
    B. Shine a light across the pupil from the side and observe for direct and consensual pupillary constriction.
    C. Ask the patient to focus on a distant object; then ask the patient to follow your penlight to about 7 cm from the nose.
    D. Ask the patient to follow your penlight in eight directions and observe for bilateral pupil constriction.

Correct Answer: B

Rationale: To test the pupillary light reflex, advance a light in from the side and note the direct and consensual pupillary constriction.

Cognitive Level: Application

23. You are assessing a patient's eyes for the accommodation response. You would expect to see:
    A. a consensual light reflex.
    B. dilation of the pupils.
    C. conjugate movement of the eyes.
    D. convergence of the axes of the eyes.

Correct Answer: D

Rationale: The accommodation reaction includes (1) pupillary constriction and (2) convergence of the axes of the eyes.

Cognitive Level: Application

24. In using the ophthalmoscope to assess a patient's eyes, you note a red glow in the client's pupils. You would:
    A. check the light source of the ophthalmoscope to verify that it is functioning.
    B. consider this a normal reflection of the ophthalmoscope light off the inner retina.
    C. continue with the ophthalmoscopic examination and refer the patient for further evaluation.
    D. suspect that there is an opacity in the lens or cornea.

Correct Answer: B

Rationale: The red glow filling the person's pupil is the red reflex. This is caused by the reflection of the ophthalmoscope light off the inner retina.

Cognitive Level: Analysis

25. Which of the following is considered a normal finding in examination of the retina?
    A. Optic disc margins that are often difficult to visualize and blurred around the edges.
    B. The presence of pigmented crescents in the

macular area.
C. An optic disc that is a yellow-orange color.
D. The presence of the macula located on the nasal side of the retina.

Correct Answer: C

Rationale: The optic disc is located on the nasal side of the retina. It is a creamy yellow-orange to pink color.

Cognitive Level: Application

26. A 2-week-old infant can fixate on an object, but not follow a light or bright toy. You would:
    A. expect that a 2-week-old infant should be able to fixate and follow an object.
    B. consider this a normal finding.
    C. assess the pupillary light reflex for possible blindness.
    D. continue with the examination and assess visual fields.

Correct Answer: B

Rationale: By 2 to 4 weeks an infant can fixate on an object. By 1 month, the infant should fixate and follow a bright light or toy.

Cognitive Level: Analysis

27. To assess color vision on a male child, you would:
    A. begin color vision screening at the child's 2-year check-up.
    B. check color vision annually until the age of 18 years.
    C. test for color vision once between the ages of 4 and 8.
    D. ask the child to identify the color of his or her clothing.

Correct Answer: C

Rationale: Test only boys for color vision once between the ages of 4 and 8.

Cognitive Level: Application

28. You are performing an eye screening clinic at the day care center. You suspect that Y.T., a 2-year-old child, has a "lazy eye." You would:
    A. assess visual acuity using the Snellen E chart.
    B. assess the child's visual fields using the confrontation test.
    C. test for strabismus by performing the corneal light reflex test.
    D. examine the external structures of the eye.

Correct Answer: C

Rationale: Testing for strabismus is done by performing the corneal light reflex test. The light should be reflected at exactly the same spot in both eyes.

Cognitive Level: Application

29. You are performing an eye assessment on an 80-year-old patient. Which of the following findings is considered abnormal?
    A. Loss of the outer hair on the eyebrows due to a decrease in hair follicles
    B. The presence of arcus senilis seen around the cornea
    C. A decrease in tear production
    D. Unequal pupillary constriction in response to light

Correct Answer: D

Rationale: Pupils are small in old age, and the pupillary light reflex may be slowed, but pupillary constriction should be symmetrical.

Cognitive Level: Comprehension

30. You note the presence of periorbital edema when performing an eye assessment on a 70-year-old patient. You would:
    A. suspect that the patient has hyperthyroidism.
    B. check for the presence of exophthalmos.
    C. ask the patient if he or she has a history of congestive heart failure.
    D. assess for blepharitis as this is often associated with periorbital edema.

Correct Answer: C

Rationale: Periorbital edema occurs with local infections, crying, and systemic conditions such as congestive heart failure, renal failure, allergy, and hypothyroidism.

Cognitive Level: Analysis

31. When a light is directed across the iris of the eye from the temporal side, the examiner is assessing for:
    A. the presence of shadows, which may indicate glaucoma.
    B. a scattered light reflex, which may be indicative of cataracts.
    C. the presence of conjunctivitis over the iris.
    D. drainage from dacryocystitis.

Correct Answer: A

Rationale: The presence of shadows in the anterior chamber may be a sign of acute angle-closure glaucoma.

Cognitive Level: Application

32. In a patient who has anisocoria, you would expect to observe:
    A. excessive tearing.
    B. an uneven curvature of the lens.
    C. pupils of unequal size.
    D. dilated pupils.

Correct Answer: C

Rationale: Unequal pupil size is termed anisocoria. It exists normally in 5 percent of the population, but may also be indicative of central nervous system disease.

Cognitive Level: Comprehension

33. A 14-year-old junior high school student states that lately he has been having difficulty reading his school books because "the print is blurry." Your preliminary analysis, based on this history data, is that he may have:
    A. hyperopia.
    B. presbyopia.
    C. myopia.
    D. photophobia.

Correct Answer: A

Rationale: Hyperopia is difficulty with near vision, or reading distance of 12–14 inches away. Presbyopia is difficulty with near vision that occurs with aging as the lens loses elasticity and cannot accommodate for near vision. Myopia is difficulty with distance vision.

Cognitive Level: Analysis

34. What is happening physiologically to the image focus within the eye in the above (Question 33) situation?
    A. The image is focused in back of the retina.
    B. The image is focused in front of the retina.
    C. The image is focused on the retina.
    D. The image is focused on the pupil.

Correct Answer: A

Rationale: In hyperopia, the globe of the eye is shorter than normal. Light rays would focus behind the retina (if they could pass through).

Cognitive Level: Analysis

35. Johnny Jones, age 9, reports that he is having difficulty seeing the blackboard. He sits in the front row of the classroom, yet still reports that "the words are blurry." Your preliminary analysis based on this history data is that:
    A. Johnny has normal vision for a child of this age.
    B. Johnny has myopia.
    C. Johnny has hyperopia.
    D. Johnny has farsightedness.

Correct Answer: B

Rationale: Near vision is a distance of 14 inches away, any distance greater than 14 inches is distance vision. In myopia, or nearsightedness, the individual can see near, but has difficulty with distance vision.

Cognitive Level: Analysis

36. What is happening physiologically to image focus within the eye in the above (Question 35) situation?
    A. The image is scattered across the cornea.
    B. The image is focused on multiple points on the retina.
    C. The image is focused in front of the retina.
    D. The image is focused in back of the retina.

Correct Answer: C

Rationale: In myopia (nearsightedness), the individual has difficulty with distance vision. In this case, the globe is longer than normal and the light rays focus in front of the retina.

Cognitive Level: Analysis

37. When assessing the corneal light reflex of a 4-month-old infant, you note slight asymmetry with one light falling slightly off center of the pupil. The results of the cover test are normal. You would:
    A. consider this a normal finding for an infant of this age.
    B. have the infant return to the clinic in 1 month to be re-evaluated.
    C. refer the infant for further evaluation.
    D. ask additional history questions regarding family history of vision loss and visual problems.

Correct Answer: A

Rationale: Some asymmetry of the corneal light reflex (where one light falls off center) under age 6 months is normal.

Cognitive Level: Analysis

Chapter 13

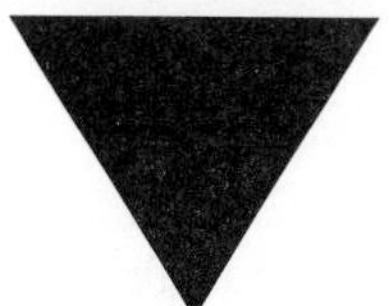

Ears

1. The portion of the ear that consists of movable cartilage and skin is called the:
   A. concha.
   B. outer meatus.
   C. auricle.
   D. mastoid process.

Correct Answer: C

Rationale: The external ear is called the auricle or pinna, and consists of movable cartilage and skin.

Cognitive Level: Knowledge

2. Which of the following statements about cerumen is correct?
   A. The purpose of cerumen is to protect and lubricate the ear.
   B. The presence of cerumen is indicative of poor hygiene.
   C. Sticky honey-colored cerumen in whites is a sign of infection.
   D. Cerumen is necessary for transmitting sound through the auditory canal.

Correct Answer: A

Rationale: It is lined with glands that secrete cerumen, a yellow waxy material that lubricates and protects the ear.

Cognitive Level: Knowledge

3. The tympanic membrane should appear:
   A. whitish with a small fleck of light in superior portion.
   B. pearly gray and slightly concave.
   C. pulled in at the base of the cone of light.
   D. light pink with a slight bulge.

Correct Answer: B

Rationale: It is a translucent membrane with a pearly gray color and a prominent cone of light in the anteroinferior quadrant, which is the reflection of the otoscope light. The drum is oval and slightly concave, pulled in at its center by one of the middle ear ossicles, the malleus.

Cognitive Level: Knowledge

4. Which of the following statements concerning the eustachian tube is true?
   A. It allows passage of air between the middle and outer ear.
   B. It remains open except when swallowing or yawning.
   C. It is responsible for the production of cerumen.
   D. It helps equalize air pressure on both sides of the tympanic membrane.

Correct Answer: D

Rationale: The eustachian tube allows equalization of air pressure on each side of the tympanic membrane so that the membrane does not rupture, e.g., during altitude changes in an airplane.

Cognitive Level: Knowledge

5. The middle ear functions to:
   A. increase amplitude of sound in order for the inner ear to function.
   B. conduct vibrations of sounds from the outer to the inner ear.
   C. interpret sounds as they enter the ear.
   D. maintain balance.

Correct Answer: B

Rationale: Among its other functions, the middle ear conducts sound vibrations from the outer ear to the central hearing apparatus in the inner ear.

Cognitive Level: Knowledge

6. Which of the following cranial nerves is responsible for conducting nerve impulses to your brain from the organ of Corti?
   A. cranial nerve I

B. cranial nerve III
C. cranial nerve VIII
D. cranial nerve X

Correct Answer: C

Rationale: The nerve impulses are conducted by the auditory portion of cranial nerve VIII to your brain.

Cognitive Level: Knowledge

7. Which of the following statements is true concerning air conduction?
   A. It is caused by the vibrations of bones in the skull.
   B. It is the most efficient pathway for hearing.
   C. A loss of air conduction is called a conductive hearing loss.
   D. The amplitude of sound determines the pitch that is heard.

Correct Answer: B

Rationale: The normal pathway of hearing is air conduction (AC) as described above; it is the most efficient.

Cognitive Level: Comprehension

8. Your patient has been shown to have a sensorineural hearing loss. During your assessment it would be important to:
   A. speak loudly so he can hear the questions.
   B. look for the source of the obstruction in the external ear.
   C. assess for middle ear infection as a possible cause.
   D. ask the patient what medications he is currently taking.

Correct Answer: D

Rationale: A simple increase in amplitude may not enable the person to understand words. Sensorineural hearing loss may be caused by presbycusis, a gradual nerve degeneration that occurs with aging and by ototoxic drugs, which affect the hair cells in the cochlea.

Cognitive Level: Application

9. During an interview, the patient states he has the sensation that "everything around him is spinning." The portion of the ear responsible for this sensation is:
   A. the organ of Corti.
   B. cranial nerve VIII.
   C. the bony labyrinth.
   D. the cochlea.

Correct Answer: C

Rationale: If the labyrinth ever becomes inflamed, it feeds the wrong information to the brain, creating a staggering gait and a strong, spinning, whirling sensation called vertigo.

Cognitive Level: Application

10. A patient in her first trimester of pregnancy is diagnosed with rubella. What is the significance of this in relation to the infant's hearing?
    A. Rubella may affect the mother's hearing but not the infant's.
    B. Rubella can damage the infant's organ of Corti, which will impair hearing.
    C. Rubella can impair the development of cranial nerve VIII and thus impact the hearing.
    D. Rubella is only dangerous to the infant in the second trimester of pregnancy.

Correct Answer: B

Rationale: If maternal rubella infection occurs during the first trimester, it can damage the organ of Corti and impair hearing.

Cognitive Level: Comprehension

11. The mother of a 2-year-old is concerned because her son has had three ear infections in the past year. What would be an appropriate response?
    A. "It is unusual for a small child to have frequent ear infections unless there is something else wrong."
    B. "Your son's eustachian tube is shorter and wider than yours because of his age, which allows for infections to develop more easily."
    C. "We need to check the immune system of your son to see why he is having so many ear infections."
    D. "Ear infections are not uncommon in infants and toddlers because they tend to have more cerumen in their external ear."

Correct Answer: B

Rationale: The infant's eustachian tube is relatively shorter and wider, and its position is more horizontal than the adult's, so it is easier for pathogens from the nasopharynx to migrate through to the middle ear.

Cognitive Level: Application

12. A 31-year-old patient tells you he has noticed a progressive loss in his hearing. It does seem to help when people speak louder or he turns up the volume. The most likely cause of his hearing loss is:
    A. otosclerosis.
    B. frequent ear infections.
    C. presbycusis.
    D. trauma to the bones.

Correct Answer: A

Rationale: Otosclerosis is a common cause of conductive hearing loss in young adults between the ages of 20 and 40.

Cognitive Level: Analysis

13. Your 70-year-old patient tells you he has noticed that he is having trouble hearing, especially in large groups. He can't "always tell where the sound is coming from" and the words often sound "mixed up." What might you suspect as the cause for this change?
    A. Scarring of the tympanic membrane
    B. Atrophy of the apocrine glands
    C. Cilia becoming coarse and stiff
    D. Nerve degeneration in the inner ear

Correct Answer: D

Rationale: Presbycusis is a type of hearing loss that occurs with aging, even in people living in a quiet environment. It is a gradual sensorineural loss caused by nerve degeneration in the inner ear or auditory nerve. This makes words sound garbled. The ability to localize sound is impaired also. This communication dysfunction is accentuated when background noise is present.

Cognitive Level: Analysis

14. During your assessment of a 20-year-old Asian patient you notice he has dry flaky cerumen in his canal. What is the significance of this finding?
    A. This represents poor hygiene and you need to do patient teaching.
    B. This is probably secondary to lesions from eczema in his ear.
    C. This is a normal finding and no further follow-up is necessary.
    D. this could be indicative of change in cilia so you should assess for conductive hearing loss.

Correct Answer: C

Rationale: Asians and Native Americans have an 84 percent frequency of dry cerumen, whereas blacks have a 99 percent and whites have a 97 percent frequency of wet cerumen (Overfield, 1985).

Cognitive Level: Application

15. In taking the history of a patient whom you suspect may have perforated an eardrum, what would be an important question?
    A. "Do you ever notice ringing or crackling in your ears?"
    B. "When was the last time you had your hearing checked?"
    C. "Was there any relation between the ear pain and the discharge you mentioned?"
    D. "Have you ever been told you have any type of hearing loss?"

Correct Answer: C

Rationale: Typically with perforation, ear pain occurs first, stops with a popping sensation, then drainage occurs.

Cognitive Level: Application

16. A 31-year-old patient tells you that he has noticed pain in his left ear when people speak loudly to him. What would be an appropriate response?
    A. "I would just cover my ear to help prevent the pain."
    B. "This is normal for people of your age."
    C. "Have you noticed any change in your ability to hear?"
    D. "I will check your ear for a middle ear infection."

Correct Answer: C

Rationale: Recruitment—a marked loss occurs when sound is at low intensity, but sound actually may become painful when repeated at a louder volume.

Cognitive Level: Analysis

17. While discussing the history of a 6-month-old infant, the mother tells you she took a great deal of aspirin while she was pregnant. What question would you want to include in your history?
    A. Has the child had any surgeries on the ears?
    B. How many ear infections has your baby had since birth?
    C. Have you noticed any drainage from her ears?

D. Does she seem to startle with loud noise?

Correct Answer: D

Rationale: Children at risk for hearing deficit include those exposed to maternal rubella, syphilis, cytomegalovirus, or toxoplasmosis or to maternal ototoxic drugs in utero; premature infants; low-birth-weight infants; trauma or hypoxia at birth; and infants with congenital liver or kidney disease.

Cognitive Level: Application

18. When performing an otoscopic examination on an adult, which of the following is true?
    A. You pull the pinna up and back before inserting speculum.
    B. Use the smallest speculum in order to decrease the amount of discomfort.
    C. Once the speculum is in the ear you may release the traction.
    D. Tilt the person's head forward as you do the exam.

Correct Answer: A

Rationale: Pull the pinna up and back on an adult or older child; this helps straighten the S-shape of the canal.

Cognitive Level: Knowledge

19. You are assessing a 16-year-old patient with head injuries from a recent motor vehicle accident. Which of the following statements indicates the most important reason for assessing for any drainage from the canal?
    A. His auditory canal many be occluded from increased cerumen.
    B. If the drum has ruptured, there will be purulent drainage.
    C. Bloody or clear watery drainage can indicate a basal skull fracture.
    D. There may be occlusion of the canal secondary to foreign bodies from the accident.

Correct Answer: C

Rationale: Frank blood or clear watery drainage (cerebrospinal leak) following trauma suggests basal skull fracture and warrants immediate referral.

Cognitive Level: Analysis

20. You are assessing an 80-year-old male with ear pain and are getting ready to ask him to hold his nose and swallow. You know that which of the following is true concerning this technique?
    A. This will cause the eardrum to bulge slightly and make landmarks more visible.
    B. This should not be used in an 80-year-old patient.
    C. This is especially useful in assessing a patient with an upper respiratory infection.
    D. This technique is helpful in assessing for otitis media.

Correct Answer: B

Rationale: The eardrum is flat, slightly pulled in at the center, and flutters when the person performs the Valsalva maneuver or holds the nose and swallows (insufflation). You may elicit these maneuvers to assess drum mobility. Avoid these with an aging person because they may disrupt equilibrium.

Cognitive Level: Application

21. In performing a voice test to assess hearing, which of the following would you do?
    A. Ask the patient to place his finger in his ear to occlude outside noise.
    B. Stand about 4 feet away to ensure the patient can really hear at this distance.
    C. Whisper two-syllable words and ask the patient to repeat them.
    D. Shield your lips so that the sound is muffled.

Correct Answer: C

Rationale: With your head 30 to 60 cm (1 to 2 ft) from the person's ear, exhale and whisper slowly some two-syllable words, such as Tuesday, armchair, baseball, and fourteen. Normally, the person repeats each word correctly after you say it.

Cognitive Level: Comprehension

22. In performing an examination of a 3-year-old with a suspected ear infection you would:
    A. pull the ear up and back before inserting the speculum.
    B. not do the otoscopic exam if the child has a fever.
    C. ask the mother to leave the room while you examine the child.
    D. perform the otoscopic examination at the end of the assessment.

Correct Answer: D

Rationale: In addition to its place in the complete examination, eardrum assessment is mandatory for any infant or child requiring care for illness or fever. For the infant or young child, the timing of the otoscopic examination is best toward the end of the complete examination.

Cognitive Level: Analysis

23. Which of the following would be true regarding the otoscopic exam of a newborn?
    A. An injected membrane would indicate infection.
    B. The normal membrane may appear thick and opaque.
    C. Immobility of the drum is a normal finding.
    D. The appearance of the membrane is identical to that of an adult.

Correct Answer: B

Rationale: During the first few days, the tympanic membrane often looks thickened and opaque. It may look "injected" and have a mild redness due to increased vascularity.

Cognitive Level: Comprehension

24. In assessing the hearing of a 7-month-old, what is the expected response when clapping your hands?
    A. Turns head to localize sound
    B. A startle and acoustic blink reflex
    C. Stops movement and appears to listen
    D. No obvious response to noise

Correct Answer: A

Rationale: With a loud sudden noise, you should note these responses: 6 to 8 months—infant turns head to localize sound, responds to own name.

Cognitive Level: Comprehension

25. Which of the following would be a normal finding in an 80-year-old patient?
    A. A shiny, pink tympanic membrane
    B. A high-tone frequency loss
    C. Increased elasticity of pinna
    D. A thin, translucent membrane

Correct Answer: B

Rationale: A high-tone frequency hearing loss is apparent for those affected with presbycusis, the hearing loss that occurs with aging.

Cognitive Level: Application

26. Your assessment of a 23-year-old patient reveals the following: an auricle that is tender and reddish-blue in color and has small vesicles. Information you would need to know includes which of the following?
    A. Any recent drainage from ear
    B. Recent history of trauma to the ear
    C. Any change in ability to hear
    D. Any prolonged exposure to extreme cold

Correct Answer: D

Rationale: Frostbite—Reddish-blue discoloration and swelling of auricle following exposure to extreme cold. Vesicles or bullae may develop, and the person feels pain and tenderness.

Cognitive Level: Analysis

27. While doing the otoscopic exam of a 3-year-old boy who has been pulling on his left ear, you find that his left tympanic membrane is bright red and the light reflex is not visible. The most likely cause is:
    A. fungal infection.
    B. rupture of the drum.
    C. acute otitis media.
    D. blood behind the drum.

Correct Answer: C

Rationale: Absent or distorted light reflex and a bright red color of the eardrum are indicative of acute otitis media.

Cognitive Level: Analysis

28. The mother of a 2-year-old is concerned about the upcoming placement of tympanostomy tubes in her son's ears. Your teaching would include which of the following?
    A. The tubes are permanently inserted during a surgical procedure.
    B. The purpose of the tubes is to decrease the pressure and allow for drainage.
    C. The tubes are placed into the inner ear.
    D. The tubes are used in children with sensorineural loss.

Correct Answer: B

Rationale: Polyethylene tubes are inserted surgically into the eardrum to relieve middle ear pressure and promote drainage of chronic or recurrent middle ear infections. Tubes extrude spontaneously in 6 months to 1 year.

Cognitive Level: Comprehension

29. During a hearing assessment you find that sound lateralizes to the patient's left ear with the Weber test. What can you conclude from this?
    A. He has conductive hearing loss in his right ear.
    B. Lateralization is a normal finding with the Weber test.
    C. He could have either a sensorineural or conductive loss.
    D. You must have made a mistake and so need to repeat the test.

Correct Answer: C

Rationale: It is necessary to perform the Weber and Rinne test to determine the type of loss. Conductive loss—sound lateralizes to "poorer" ear owing to background room noise. Sensorineural loss—sound lateralizes to "better" ear or unaffected ear.

Cognitive Level: Application

30. A patient states she is unable to hear well with her left ear. The Weber test shows lateralization to the right ear. Rinne has AC>BC with ratio of 2:1 in both ears, left-AC 10 sec and BC 5 sec, right-AC 30 sec and BC 15 sec. What would be your interpretation of these results?
    A. Patient may have sensorineural loss.
    B. Tests are reflective of normal hearing.
    C. Conduction of sound through bones is impaired.
    D. These results make no sense so further tests should be done.

Correct Answer: A

Rationale: With sensorineural loss sound lateralizes to "better" ear or unaffected ear. Normal ratio of AC>BC is intact but is reduced overall. That is, person hears poorly both ways.

Cognitive Level: Analysis

31. In an individual suffering from otitis externa, which of the following signs would you expect to find on assessment?
    A. Pain over the maxillary sinuses
    B. Rhinorrhea
    C. Enlargement of the superficial cervical nodes
    D. Periorbital edema

Correct Answer: C

Rationale: The lymphatic drainage of the external ear flows to the parotid, mastoid, and superficial cervical nodes. The signs are severe swelling of the canal, inflammation, and tenderness.

Cognitive Level: Comprehension

32. When performing an otoscopic examination of a 5-year-old child with a history of chronic ear infections, you note that his right tympanic membrane is amber-yellow in color and there are air bubbles behind the tympanic membrane. The child reports occasional hearing loss and a popping sound with swallowing. Your preliminary analysis based on this information is that:
    A. the child has an acute purulent otitis media.
    B. there is evidence of a resolving cholesteatoma.
    C. the child is experiencing the early stages of perforation.
    D. this is most likely a serous otitis media.

Correct Answer: D

Rationale: An amber-yellow color to the tympanic membrane suggests serum in the middle ear. Often an air/fluid level or bubbles behind the tympanic membrane are visible. The patient may experience feelings of fullness, transient hearing loss, and a popping sound with swallowing.

Cognitive Level: Analysis

33. You are performing an assessment on a 65-year-old male. He reports a crusty nodule behind the pinna. It bleeds intermittently and has not healed over the past 6 months. You note, on physical assessment, an ulcerated crusted nodule with an indurated base. Your preliminary analysis in this situation is that:
    A. this is most likely a benign sebaceous cyst.
    B. this could be a potential carcinoma and should be referred.
    C. this is a tophus, which is common in the elderly and is a sign of gout.
    D. this is most likely a Darwin's tubercle and is not significant.

Correct Answer: B

Rationale: An ulcerated crusted nodule with an indurated base that fails to heal is characteristic of a carcinoma. These lesions fail to heal and bleed intermittently. Individuals experiencing such symptoms should be referred for a biopsy.

Cognitive Level: Analysis

34. Early signs of otitis media include:
    A. a red, bulging TM.
    B. a retracted TM with landmarks clearly visible.
    C. a flat TM, slightly pulled in at the center that moves with insufflation.
    D. hypomobility of the TM.

Correct Answer: D

Rationale: An early sign of otitis media is hypomobility of the TM.

Cognitive Level: Knowledge

35. You are performing a middle ear assessment on a 15-year-old patient who has a history of chronic ear infections. When examining the right TM, you note the presence of dense white patches. The TM is otherwise unremarkable; it is pearly, with the light reflex at 5:00 and landmarks visible. You:
    A. refer the patient for the possibility of a fungal infection.
    B. consider that these findings may represent the presence of blood in the middle ear.
    C. know that these are scars caused from frequent ear infections.
    D. are concerned about the ability to hear because of this abnormality on the TM.

Correct Answer: C

Rationale: Dense white patches on the TM are sequelae of repeated ear infections. They do not necessarily affect hearing.

Cognitive Level: Analysis

Chapter 14

Nose, Mouth, and Throat

1. The primary purpose of the ciliated mucous membrane in the nose is to:
   A. filter coarse particles from inhaled air.
   B. facilitate movement of air through nares.
   C. filter out dust and bacteria.
   D. warm the inhaled air.

Correct Answer: C

Rationale: The nasal hairs filter the coarsest matter from inhaled air, whereas the mucous blanket filters out dust and bacteria.

Cognitive Level: Knowledge

2. The projections in the nasal cavity that increase the surface area are called the:
   A. Kiesselbach's plexus.
   B. turbinates.
   C. meatus.
   D. septum.

Correct Answer: B

Rationale: The lateral walls of each nasal cavity contain three parallel bony projections – the superior, middle, and inferior turbinates. They increase the surface area so that more blood vessels and mucous membrane are available to warm, humidify, and filter the inhaled air.

Cognitive Level: Knowledge

3. Which of the following is true in relation to a newborn?
   A. The maxillary and ethmoid sinuses are the only ones present at birth.
   B. The frontal sinuses are fairly well developed at birth.
   C. The sphenoid sinuses are full size at birth.
   D. The maxillary sinuses reach full size after puberty.

Correct Answer: A

Rationale: Only the maxillary and ethmoid sinuses are present at birth.

Cognitive Level: Knowledge

4. The tissue that connects the tongue to the floor of the mouth is the:
   A. uvula.
   B. palate.
   C. papillae.
   D. frenulum.

Correct Answer: D

Rationale: The frenulum is a midline fold of tissue that connects the tongue to the floor of the mouth.

Cognitive Level: Knowledge

5. The salivary gland that is located in the cheek in front of the ear is the:
   A. submandibular gland.
   B. parotid gland.
   C. Stenson's gland.
   D. sublingual gland.

Correct Answer: B

Rationale: The mouth contains three pairs of salivary glands. The largest, the parotid gland, lies within the cheeks in front of the ear extending from the zygomatic arch down to the angle of the jaw.

Cognitive Level: Knowledge

6. In assessing the tonsils of a 30-year-old, you note they are involuted, granular in appearance, and appear to have deep crypts. What would be your response to these findings?
   A. Nothing, this is the appearance of normal tonsils.
   B. Obtain a throat culture on the patient for possible strep infection.
   C. Refer patient to a throat specialist.
   D. Continue with assessment looking for any other abnormal findings.

Correct Answer: A

Rationale: The tonsils are the same color as the surrounding mucous membrane, although they look more granular and their surface shows deep crypts. Tonsillar tissue enlarges during childhood until puberty, then involutes.

Cognitive Level: Application

7. As you are obtaining a history on a 3-month-old infant, the mom states, "I think she is getting her first tooth because she has started drooling a lot." Your best response would be:
   A. "You're right, drooling is usually a sign of the first tooth."
   B. "She is just starting to salivate and hasn't learned to swallow the saliva."
   C. "It would be unusual for a 3-month-old to be getting her first tooth."
   D. "This could be the sign of a problem with the salivary glands."

Correct Answer: B

Rationale: In the infant, salivation starts at 3 months. The baby will drool periodically for a few months before learning to swallow the saliva. This drooling does not herald the eruption of the first tooth, although many parents think it does.

Cognitive Level: Comprehension

8. In your assessment of an 80-year-old male, you would expect to find:
   A. finer and less prominent nasal hair.
   B. increased production of saliva.
   C. decreased ability to identify odors.
   D. hypertrophy of the gums.

Correct Answer: C

Rationale: The sense of smell may diminish because of a decrease in the number of olfactory nerve fibers. The decrease in the sensation of smell occurs in the sixth and seventh decades, but especially during the eighth decade (Rossman, 1986).

Cognitive Level: Comprehension

9. You are doing an oral assessment on a 40-year-old black male. You note the presence of a 1 cm, nontender, grayish-white lesion on his left buccal mucosa. Which of the following is true concerning this lesion?
   A. This is the result of hyperpigmentation and is normal.
   B. This is torus palatinus and would normally only be found in smokers.
   C. This type of lesion is indicative of cancer and should be tested immediately.
   D. This is leukoedema and is common in blacks.

Correct Answer: D

Rationale: Leukoedema, a grayish-white benign lesion occurring on the buccal mucosa, is present in 68 to 90 percent of blacks but only 43 percent of whites (Martin and Crump, 1972).

Cognitive Level: Comprehension

10. During the history, your patient tells you he has frequent nosebleeds and asks the best way to get them to stop. What would be your response?
    A. "Lie on your back with your head tilted back and pinch your nose."
    B. "Sit up with your head tilted forward and pinch your nose."
    C. "While sitting up, place a cold compress over your nose."
    D. "Just let the bleeding stop on its own, but don't blow your nose."

Correct Answer: B

Rationale: With a nose bleed, person should sit up with head tilted forward, pinch nose between thumb and forefinger for 5 to 15 minutes.

Cognitive Level: Comprehension

11. A 92-year-old patient has suffered a stroke. The right side of his face is droopy. You might also suspect which of the following:
    A. Agenesis
    B. Epistaxis
    C. Dysphagia
    D. Xerostomia

Correct Answer: C

Rationale: Dysphagia is difficulty with swallowing.

Cognitive Level: Analysis

12. While obtaining a history from the mother of a 1-year-old, you notice that the baby has had a bottle in his mouth the entire time. The mother states, "it makes a great pacifier." Your response might be:
    A. "You're right, bottles make a very good pacifier."
    B. "Use of a bottle is better for the teeth than

thumb sucking."
C. "It's okay to do this as long as the bottle contains milk and not juice."
D. "Prolonged use of a bottle can increase the risk for tooth decay and ear infections."

Correct Answer: D

Rationale: Prolonged use of a bottle during day or when going to sleep places infant at risk for tooth decay and middle ear infections.

Cognitive Level: Application

13. Your patient is a 72-year-old female. She has a history of hypertension and chronic lung disease. An important question to include in her history would be:
    A. "At what age did you get your first tooth?"
    B. "Have you had tonsillitis in the last year?"
    C. "Have you noticed any dryness in your mouth?"
    D. "Do you use a fluoride supplement?"

Correct Answer: C

Rationale: Xerostomia (dry mouth) is a side effect of many drugs used by older people: antidepressants, anticholinergics, antispasmodics, antihypertensives, antipsychotics, bronchodilators.

Cognitive Level: Application

14. When using an otoscope to assess the nasal cavity, which of the following would you do?
    A. Keep the speculum tip medial to avoid touching the floor of the nares.
    B. Insert the speculum at least 3 cm into the vestibule.
    C. Gently displace the nose to the side you are examining.
    D. Avoid touching the nasal septum with the speculum.

Correct Answer: D

Rationale: Insert apparatus into the nasal vestibule, again avoiding pressure on the sensitive nasal septum.

Cognitive Level: Comprehension

15. You are doing an assessment on a 21-year-old male. You note that his nasal mucosa appears pale, gray, and swollen. What would be the most appropriate question to ask the patient?
    A. "Have you been having frequent nose bleeds?"
    B. "Do you have any allergies that you are aware of?"
    C. "Have you had any symptoms of a cold?"
    D. "Do you have an elevated temperature?"

Correct Answer: B

Rationale: With chronic allergy, mucosa looks swollen, boggy, pale, and gray.

Cognitive Level: Application

16. With palpation of the sinus areas, what would be a normal finding?
    A. Firm pressure
    B. Pain sensation behind eyes
    C. Pain during palpation
    D. No sensation

Correct Answer: A

Rationale: The person should feel firm pressure but no pain.

Cognitive Level: Knowledge

17. During your oral assessment of a healthy 30-year-old black male, you note bluish lips as well as a dark line along the gingival margin. What would you do in response to this finding?
    A. Check the patient's hemoglobin for anemia.
    B. Ask if he has been exposed to an excessive amount of carbon monoxide.
    C. Proceed with assessment, knowing this is a normal finding.
    D. Assess for other signs of insufficient oxygen supply.

Correct Answer: C

Rationale: Black persons normally may have bluish lips. Black people normally may have a dark melanotic line along the gingival margin.

Cognitive Level: Application

18. In your assessment of a 20-year-old patient with a 3-day history of nausea and vomiting you note the following: dry mucosa and deep fissures in the tongue. This is reflective of:
    A. a normal oral assessment.
    B. irritation of gastric juices.
    C. side effects from nausea medication.
    D. dehydration.

Correct Answer: D

Rationale: Dry mouth occurs with dehydration or fever; tongue has deep vertical fissures.

Cognitive Level: Application

19. A 32-year-old female is at the clinic for "little white bumps in my mouth." In her assessment you note she has a 0.5 cm white, nontender papule under her tongue and one on the mucosa of her right cheek. What would you tell the patient?
    A. "These could be indicative of a serious lesion so I will refer you to a specialist."
    B. "These bumps are fordyce's granules, which are sebaceous cysts and are not anything to be concerned about."
    C. "This is called leukoplakia and can be caused by chronic irritation such as smoking."
    D. "These spots are seen with infections such as strep throat."

Correct Answer: B

Rationale: Fordyce's granules are small, isolated white or yellow papules on the mucosa of cheek, tongue, and lips. These little sebaceous cysts are painless and not significant.

Cognitive Level: Application

20. Which of the following best describes the test performed to assess the function of cranial nerve X?
    A. Ask the patient to say "ahhh" and watch movement of soft palate and uvula.
    B. Have the patient stick out tongue and observe for tremors.
    C. Observe patient's ability to articulate specific words.
    D. Assess movement of the hard palate and uvula with the gag reflex.

Correct Answer: A

Rationale: Ask the person to say "ahhh" and note the soft palate and uvula rise in the midline. This tests one function of cranial nerve X, the vagus nerve.

Cognitive Level: Comprehension

21. A 10-year-old is at the clinic for "a sore throat lasting 6 days." Which of the following would be consistent with an acute infection?
    A. Tonsils 2+/1-4+ with small plugs of white debris
    B. Tonsils 3+/1-4+ with white coat covering
    C. Tonsils 3+/1-4+ with large white spots
    D. Tonsils 1+/1-4+ and pink

Correct Answer: C

Rationale: With an acute infection, tonsils are bright red, swollen, and may have exudate or large white spots. Tonsils are enlarged to 2+, 3+ or 4+ with an acute infection.

Cognitive Level: Comprehension

22. Immediately following birth, you are unable to suction the nares of a newborn. You attempt to pass a catheter through both nasal cavities with no success. What would be your best response?
    A. Wait a few minutes and try again once the newborn quits crying.
    B. Recognize this is a situation that requires immediate intervention.
    C. Contact the physician and request assistance when he gets a chance.
    D. Attempt to suction again using the bulb syringe.

Correct Answer: B

Rationale: It is essential to determine patency of the nares in the immediate newborn period because most newborns are obligate nose-breathers. Nares blocked with amniotic fluid are suctioned gently with a bulb syringe. If obstruction is suspected, a small lumen (5 to 10 Fr) catheter is passed down each naris to confirm patency. Inability to pass catheter through nasal cavity indicates choanal atresia, which needs immediate intervention.

Cognitive Level: Analysis

23. You notice that the mother of a 2-year-old boy brings him into the clinic quite frequently for various injuries. You suspect there may be some child abuse involved. In doing the inspection of his mouth, what would be important to assess for?
    A. Small, yellow papules along hard palate
    B. Swollen, red tonsils
    C. Ulcerations on the hard palate
    D. Bruising on the buccal mucosa or gums

Correct Answer: D

Rationale: Note any bruising or laceration on the buccal mucosa or gums of infant or young child. Trauma may indicate child abuse due to a forced feeding of bottle or spoon.

Cognitive Level: Application

24. You are assessing a 3-year-old who is here for "drainage from nose." You note that there is a purulent drainage from the left nares, which has a very foul odor to it. The child has no drainage from the right nares, is afebrile with no other symptoms. What would be your response?
    A. Perform otoscopic examination of the left nares.
    B. Refer to the physician for an antibiotic order.
    C. Have the mother bring the child back in 1 week.
    D. Tell mother that this is normal for children of this age.

Correct Answer: A

Rationale: Children are apt to put an object up the nose, producing unilateral purulent drainage and foul odor. Because some risk for aspiration exists, removal should be prompt.

Cognitive Level: Analysis

25. In your assessment of a 26-year-old at the clinic for "a spot on my lip I think is cancer" you note the following: a group of clear vesicles with an erythematous base around them located at the lip skin border. The patient tells you she just returned from Hawaii. What would be the most appropriate response?
    A. Tell the patient she will need to see a skin specialist.
    B. Discuss the benefits of having a biopsy done of any unusual lesion.
    C. Tell the patient this is herpes simplex I and will heal in 4 to 10 days.
    D. Tell the patient that this is most likely the result of a riboflavin deficiency and discuss nutrition.

Correct Answer: C

Rationale: The cold sores are groups of clear vesicles with a surrounding erythematous base. These evolve into pustules or crusts and heal in 4 to 10 days. The most likely site is the lip-skin junction; infection often recurs in same site. It may be precipitated by sunlight, fever, colds, allergy.

Cognitive Level: Analysis

26. While performing an assessment of the mouth, you notice the patient has a 1-cm ulceration that is crusted with an elevated border. It is located on the outer third of the lower lip. What other information would be most important to assess?
    A. Nutritional status
    B. When the patient first noticed the lesion
    C. Whether the patient has had a recent cold
    D. Whether the patient has had any recent exposure to sick animals

Correct Answer: B

Rationale: Carcinoma—The initial lesion is round and indurated, then it becomes crusted and ulcerated with an elevated border. The vast majority occur between the outer and middle thirds of lip. Any lesion that is still unhealed after 2 weeks should be referred.

Cognitive Level: Application

27. A pregnant female states she is concerned about her gums because she has noticed they are swollen and have started bleeding. What would be an appropriate response?
    A. "This is always indicative of a vitamin C deficiency."
    B. "This can be caused by the change in hormone balance in your system when you're pregnant."
    C. "You need to make an appointment with your dentist as soon as possible to have this checked."
    D. "I'm not sure what causes it but let me know if it's not better in a few weeks."

Correct Answer: B

Rationale: Gingivitis—Gum margins are red, swollen, and bleed easily. The condition may occur in pregnancy and puberty because of changing hormonal balance.

Cognitive Level: Application

28. A 40-year-old patient who has just finished chemotherapy for breast cancer tells you she is concerned about her mouth. In your assessment you find the following: areas of buccal mucosa that are raw and red with some bleeding as well as other areas that have a white, cheesy coating. You know that this abnormality is:
    A. leukoplakia.
    B. Koplik's spots.
    C. candidiasis.
    D. carcinoma.

Correct Answer: C

Rationale: Candidiasis—A white, cheesy, curdlike patch on the buccal mucosa and tongue. It scrapes off, leaving raw, red surface that bleeds easily. It also occurs after the use of antibiotics, corticosteroids, and in immunosuppressed persons.

Cognitive Level: Application

29. You are assessing a patient in the hospital who has received numerous antibiotics. You note that his tongue appears to be black and hairy. In response to his concern, what would you say?
   A. "This is an overgrowth of hair and will go away in a few days."
   B. "We need to get a biopsy and see what the cause is."
   C. "This is probably caused by the same bacteria you had in your lungs."
   D. "This is a fungal infection caused by all the antibiotics you've received."

Correct Answer: D

Rationale: Black Hairy Tongue—This is not really hair but the elongation of filiform papillae and painless overgrowth of mycelial threads of fungus infection on the tongue. It occurs following use of antibiotics, which inhibit normal bacteria and allow proliferation of fungus.

Cognitive Level: Analysis

30. You are assessing a patient with a history of intravenous drug abuse. In assessing his mouth you notice a dark red confluent macule on the hard palate. This could be an early sign of:
   A. measles.
   B. AIDS.
   C. leukemia.
   D. carcinoma.

Correct Answer: B

Rationale: Oral Kaposi's Sarcoma—Bruiselike, dark red or violet, confluent macule, usually on the hard palate, may be on soft palate or gingival margin. Oral lesions may be among the earliest lesions to develop with acquired immunodeficiency syndrome.

Cognitive Level: Comprehension

31. A mother brings her 4-month-old to the clinic with concerns regarding a small pad in the middle of the upper lip which has been there since 1 month of age. The infant has no health problems. On physical examination, you note a 0.5 cm fleshy, elevated area in the middle of the upper lip. There is no evidence of inflammation or drainage. What would you tell this mother?
   A. "This is an area of irritation caused from teething and is nothing to worry about."
   B. "This is a sucking tubercle caused from the friction of breast- or bottle-feeding and is very normal."
   C. "This is an abnormal finding and should be evaluated by another health care provider."
   D. "This is the result of chronic drooling and should resolve within the next month or two."

Correct Answer: B

Rationale: A normal finding in infants is the sucking tubercle, a small pad in the middle of the upper lip from friction of breast or bottle feeding.

Cognitive Level: Analysis

32. A mother is concerned that her 18-month-old has 12 teeth. She is wondering if this is normal for a child of this age. You reply:
   A. "Normally, by age 2½, 16 deciduous teeth are expected."
   B. "All 20 deciduous teeth are expected to erupt by age 4."
   C. " This is a normal number of teeth for an 18-month-old."
   D. "How many teeth did you have at this age?"

Correct Answer: C

Rationale: The guidelines for number of teeth for children under 2 years is as follows: the child's age in months minus the number 6 should be equal to the expected number of deciduous teeth. Normally, all 20 teeth are in by 2½ years old. In this instance, the child is 18 months old, minus 6, equals 12 deciduous teeth expected.

Cognitive Level: Application

33. Which of the following findings is due to the aging process?
   A. A small, painless lump on the dorsum of the tongue
   B. A tongue that looks smoother in appearance due to papillary atrophy
   C. Buccal mucosa that is beefy red in appearance
   D. Teeth that appear shorter, due to hypertrophy of the gingiva

Correct Answer: B

Rationale: In the aging adult, the tongue looks

smoother due to papillary atrophy. The teeth are slightly yellowed and appear longer due to receding of gingival margins.

Cognitive Level: Knowledge

34. When examining the nares of a 45-year-old female with complaints of rhinorrhea, itching of the nose and eyes, and sneezing, you note the following: pale turbinates, swelling of the turbinates, and clear rhinorrhea. Which of the following is most likely the cause?
    A. Acute sinusitis
    B. Nasal polyps
    C. Allergic rhinitis
    D. Nasal carcinoma

Correct Answer: C

Rationale: With allergic rhinitis, rhinorrhea, itching of the nose and eyes, and sneezing are present. On physical examination, there is serous edema, and the turbinates usually appear pale with a smooth, glistening surface.

Cognitive Level: Analysis

35. When assessing the tongue, which of the following is an abnormal finding?
    A. Raised papillae on the dorsal surface
    B. A smooth glossy dorsal surface
    C. A thin white coating
    D. Visible venous patterns on the ventral surface

Correct Answer: B

Rationale: The dorsal surface of the tongue is normally roughened from papillae. A thin white coating may be present.

Cognitive Level: Comprehension

36. Which of the following assessment findings would you be most concerned about?
    A. A painful vesicle inside the cheek x 2 days
    B. The presence of moist, non-tender Stenson's ducts
    C. Stippled gingival margins that adhere snugly to the teeth
    D. An ulceration under the tongue lasting longer than two weeks

Correct Answer: D

Rationale: An ulceration lasting longer than 2 weeks raises the suspicion of cancer and must be investigated.

Cognitive Level: Application

Chapter 15

Breasts and Regional Lymphatics

1. Which of the following statements is true regarding the internal structures of the breast?
   A. The breast is composed of fibrous, glandular, and adipose tissue.
   B. The breast is composed mostly of milk ducts, known as lactiferous ducts.
   C. The breast is mainly muscle, with very little fibrous tissue.
   D. The breast is composed of glandular tissue, which supports the breast by attaching to the chest wall.

Correct Answer: A

Rationale: The breast is composed of (1) glandular tissue, (2) fibrous tissue including the suspensory ligaments, and (3) adipose tissue.

Cognitive Level: Knowledge

2. In performing a breast examination on Mrs. J., you know that it is especially important to examine the upper outer quadrant of the breast. Why?
   A. The upper outer quadrant is more prone to injury and calcifications than other locations in the breast.
   B. The upper outer quadrant is where most of the suspensory ligaments attach.
   C. The upper outer quadrant is the location of most breast tumors.
   D. The upper outer quadrant is the largest quadrant of the breast.

Correct Answer: C

Rationale: In the upper outer quadrant, note the axillary tail of Spence, the cone-shaped breast tissue that projects up into the axilla, close to the pectoral group of axillary lymph nodes. The upper outer quadrant is the site of most breast tumors.

Cognitive Level: Application

3. In performing an assessment of Mrs. J.'s axillary lymph system, you will assess:
   A. central, axillary, and lateral nodes.
   B. central, lateral, pectoral, and subscapular nodes.
   C. lateral, pectoral, axillary, and suprascapular nodes.
   D. pectoral, lateral, anterior, and subscapular nodes.

Correct Answer: B

Rationale: The breast has extensive lymphatic drainage. Four groups of axillary nodes are present: (1) Central axillary nodes, (2) Pectoral (anterior), (3) Subscapular (posterior), and (4) Lateral. From the central axillary nodes, drainage flows up to the infraclavicular and supraclavicular nodes.

Cognitive Level: Application

4. If Mrs. R. reports a recent breast infection, you would expect:
   A. contralateral axillary node enlargement.
   B. inguinal and cervical node enlargement.
   C. nonspecific node enlargement.
   D. ipsilateral axillary node enlargement.

Correct Answer: D

Rationale: The breast has extensive lymphatic drainage. Most of the lymph, more than 75 percent, drains into the ipsilateral axillary nodes.

Cognitive Level: Application

5. T.R., 11, is in your clinic for a sports physical. After some initial shyness she finally asks, "Am I normal? I don't seem to need a bra yet and all my friends do. What if I never get breasts?" Your best response would be:
   A. "Don't worry, you still have plenty of time to develop."
   B. "I know just how you feel, I was a late bloomer myself."
   C. "I understand that it is hard to feel different

from your friends. Breasts usually develop between the ages of 8 and 13 years of age."

D. "You will probably get your periods before you notice any significant growth in your breasts."

Correct Answer: C

Rationale: Average breast development begins between 10 and 11 years of age, although the normal range is between 8 and 13 years.

Cognitive Level: Application

6. Mrs. B. contacts you and states that she is worried about her 10-year-old daughter having breast cancer. She describes a unilateral enlargement of the right breast with associated tenderness. She is worried because the left breast is not enlarged. What would be your best response?
   A. Tell Mrs. B. that she should bring her daughter in right away since breast cancer is fairly common in preadolescent girls.
   B. Tell Mrs. B. that it is unusual for breasts that are first developing to feel tender since they haven't developed much fibrous tissue.
   C. Tell Mrs. B. that breast development is usually fairly symmetric and she should be examined right away.
   D. Tell Mrs. B. that while you'd like to examine her daughter to rule out a problem, it is most likely normal breast development.

Correct Answer: D

Rationale: Occasionally, one breast may grow faster than the other, producing a temporary asymmetry. This may cause some distress; reassurance is necessary. Tenderness is common also.

Cognitive Level: Application

7. K.C., 14, is anxious about not having reached menarche. In your history you should ascertain which of the following?
   A. The age K.C. began to develop breasts
   B. The age K.C. began to develop axillary hair
   C. The age K.C. began to develop pubic hair
   D. The age K.C.'s mother developed breasts

Correct Answer: A

Rationale: Full development from stage 2 to stage 5 takes an average of 3 years, although the range is 1.5 to 6 years. The beginning of breast development precedes menarche by about 2 years. Menarche occurs in breast development stage 3 or 4, usually just after the peak of the adolescent growth spurt, which occurs around age 12.

Cognitive Level: Analysis

8. Ms. H., 23, nulliparous, is in the family planning clinic seeking birth control information. She states that her breasts "change all month long" and that she is worried that this is unusual. What is your best response?
   A. Tell her that it is unusual. The breasts of nonpregnant females usually stay pretty much the same all month long.
   B. Tell her that it is very common for breasts to change in response to stress and assess her life for stressful events.
   C. Tell her that breast changes normally occur only during pregnancy and that you would like to perform a pregnancy test on her.
   D. Tell her that due to the changing hormones during the monthly menstrual cycle, cyclic breast changes are common.

Correct Answer: D

Rationale: Breasts of the nonpregnant woman change with the ebb and flow of hormones during the monthly menstrual cycle.

Cognitive Level: Application

9. Mrs. W. has just learned that she is pregnant. What are some things you should teach her about her breasts?
   A. Breasts may begin secreting milk after the fourth month of pregnancy.
   B. During pregnancy, breast changes are fairly uncommon, most of the changes occur after the birth.
   C. Mrs. W. can expect her areolae to become larger and darker in color.
   D. Mrs. W. should inspect her breasts for visible veins and report this immediately.

Correct Answer: C

Rationale: The areolae become larger and grow a darker brown as pregnancy progresses and the tubercles become more prominent. (The brown color fades after lactation, but the areolae never return to the original color).

Cognitive Level: Comprehension

10. In teaching a pregnant woman about her breasts, which statement would be true?
   A. Colostrum, which is a thin, watery fluid, is

present day 4 and 5 postpartum (after the birth).

B. Colostrum is a fluid that contains antibodies and is usually present after the fourth month of pregnancy.

C. Breast milk is present immediately following delivery of the baby.

D. Breast milk is rich in protein and sugars (lactose) but has very little fat.

Correct Answer: B

Rationale: After the fourth month, colostrum may be expressed. This thick yellow fluid is the precursor of milk, containing the same amount of protein and lactose but practically no fat. The breasts produce colostrum for the first few days after delivery. It is rich with antibodies that protect the newborn against infection, so breastfeeding is important.

Cognitive Level: Application

11. Mrs. D., 65, remarks that she just can't believe that her breasts sag so much. She states it must be from lack of exercise. What explanation should you offer her?
    A. After menopause, the glandular and fat tissue atrophies and these changes diminish breast size and elasticity—so the breasts droop.
    B. After menopause, a diet that is high in fat will help maintain the fat envelope, which keeps the breasts from sagging.
    C. After menopause, sagging is usually due to decreased muscle mass within the breast.
    D. After menopause, only women with large breasts experience sagging.

Correct Answer: A

Rationale: After menopause, the glandular tissue atrophies and is replaced with connective tissue. The fat envelope atrophies also, beginning in the middle years and becoming marked in the eighth and ninth decades. These changes decrease breast size and elasticity so the breasts droop and sag, looking flattened and flabby.

Cognitive Level: Comprehension

12. In examining Mr. P., 70, you notice that he has bilateral gynecomastia. Which of the following describes your best course of action?
    A. Ignore it, it is not unusual for men to have benign breast enlargement.
    B. Recommend that Mr. P. see his doctor for a mammogram.
    C. Explain that this condition may be the result of hormonal changes and recommend that he see his physician.
    D. Tell Mr. P. that gynecomastia in the male is usually associated with prostate enlargement and recommend that he be screened thoroughly.

Correct Answer: C

Rationale: Gynecomastia may reappear in the aging male, and may be due to testosterone deficiency.

Cognitive Level: Analysis

13. When examining a 13-year-old black girl, which of the following would you expect to find based on Tanner's data on sexual maturity?
    A. She will be significantly slower in her development of secondary sex characteristics.
    B. Her secondary sex characteristics will appear to be in line with Tanner's data on sexual maturity.
    C. The development of secondary sex characteristics is inversely correlated with socioeconomic status.
    D. Her secondary sex characteristics will appear earlier than those of white girls her age.

Correct Answer: D

Rationale: One significant difference was that black girls were shown to develop secondary sex characteristics earlier than white girls of the same age.

Cognitive Level: Application

14. The incidence of breast cancer seems to vary among different countries. Researchers suspect that this is due to:
    A. dietary variations in different countries.
    B. self-care practices of women in different countries.
    C. breast health beliefs in different countries.
    D. genetic variations of women in different countries.

Correct Answer: A

Rationale: The incidence of breast cancer varies with different cultural groups. In the search for an environmental influence to account for this difference, researchers suspect a diet rich in fat. The high incidence of breast cancer rates in the United States, Britain, and the Netherlands correlates with a high amount of fat in the diet of those nations. In Japan, Peru, Singapore, and

Romania, where people eat a lean diet, the incidence of breast cancer is one-sixth to one-half that in the United States (American Cancer Society, 1994).

Cognitive Level: Comprehension

15. Which of the following statements is true with regard to breast cancer in black women?
    A. Breast cancer is not a threat to black women.
    B. Breast cancer is the leading cause of cancer death among black women.
    C. Breast cancer is the leading cause of death among black women.
    D. Breast cancer incidence in black women is much higher than that of white women.

Correct Answer: B

Rationale: Although breast cancer is the second leading cause of cancer death in women in the United States, it is the leading cause of cancer death among black women (Boring, et. al., 1992).

Cognitive Level: Comprehension

16. While performing a breast health interview with Mrs. J., she states that she has noticed pain in her left breast. Your most appropriate response to this would be:
    A. "Don't worry about the pain, breast cancer is not painful."
    B. "I would like some more information about the pain in your left breast."
    C. "Oh, I had pain like that after my son was born, it turned out to be a blocked milk duct."
    D. "Breast pain is almost always the result of fibrocystic breast tissue and so let's just ignore it."

Correct Answer: B

Rationale: Breast pain occurs with trauma, inflammation, or infection.

Cognitive Level: Analysis

17. When gathering history data on Mrs. L. she states that she has noticed a few drops of clear discharge from her right nipple. Which of the following actions would be most appropriate?
    A. Contact the physician immediately to report the discharge.
    B. Make a note of the discharge but ask no further questions since clear discharge is often found in healthy women.
    C. Ask Mrs. L. some additional questions about the medications she is taking.
    D. Discontinue the interview and refer her for a mammogram.

Correct Answer: C

Rationale: Note the use of medications that may cause clear nipple discharge, such as oral contraceptives, phenothiazines, diuretics, digitalis, and steroids. Also, tricyclic tranquilizers, reserpine, and methyldopa.

Cognitive Level: Application

18. Mrs. P., 45, states that she has had a crusty, itchy rash on her breast for about 2 weeks. In trying to determine the cause of the rash, which of the following would be important to determine?
    A. Is the rash raised and red?
    B. Does it appear to be cyclic?
    C. Where did it first appear—on the nipple, the areola, or on the surrounding skin?
    D. What was Mrs. P. doing when she first noticed the rash and do her actions make it worse?

Correct Answer: C

Rationale: Paget's disease starts with a small crust on the nipple apex, then spreads to areola. Eczema or other dermatitis rarely starts at nipple unless it is due to breastfeeding. It usually starts on the areola or surrounding skin and then spreads to the nipple.

Cognitive Level: Analysis

19. Ms. W. has been diagnosed with fibrocystic disease. You know this is significant. Why?
    A. Fibrocystic disease frequently turns into cancer in a woman's later years.
    B. Fibrocystic disease is usually diagnosed before a woman reaches childbearing age.
    C. Fibrocystic disease is easily reduced with hormone replacement therapy.
    D. Fibrocystic disease makes it more difficult to examine the breasts.

Correct Answer: D

Rationale: The presence of fibrocystic disease makes it more difficult to examine the breasts; the general lumpiness of the breast conceals a new lump.

Cognitive Level: Application

20. Mrs. S., 42, states that she doesn't perform monthly breast self-examinations. She tells you that she feels mammograms, "do a much better job than I ever could to find a lump." You should plan to explain to Mrs. S. that:
    A. she is correct, mammography is a good replacement for breast self-examination.
    B. mammography may not detect all palpable lumps.
    C. she doesn't need to perform breast self-examination as long as a physician checks her breasts yearly.
    D. breast self-examination is unnecessary until the age of 50.

Correct Answer: B

Rationale: The monthly practice of breast self-examination, and routine clinical breast examination and mammograms are complementary screening measures. Mammography can reveal cancers too small to be detected by the woman or by the most experienced examiner. However, mammography does not detect all palpable lumps, and interval lumps may become palpable between mammograms. (Foster, et. al., 1992).

Cognitive Level: Comprehension

21. Mrs. A. reveals that she is pregnant during your interview. She states that she is not sure if she will breast-feed her baby and asks for some information about this. Which of the following statements is accurate with regard to breast-feeding?
    A. Breast-fed babies tend to be more colicky.
    B. Breast-feeding is second nature and every woman can do it.
    C. Breast-feeding may actually reduce the risk of breast cancer in premenopausal women.
    D. Breast-fed babies eat more than infants on formula.

Correct Answer: C

Rationale: In addition to providing the perfect food and antibodies for the baby, promoting bonding, and providing relaxation, a recent study shows that lactation is also associated with a slight reduction in the risk of breast cancer among premenopausal women (Newcomb et. al., 1994).

Cognitive Level: Application

22. Which of the following women have risk factors that place them at a high risk for breast cancer?
    A. Mrs. J., 65, whose mother had breast cancer
    B. Mrs. W., 42, who has had ovarian cancer
    C. Mrs. R., 45, who has never been pregnant
    D. Mrs. T., 37, who is obese

Correct Answer: A

Rationale: High Risk: Mother and sister with history of breast cancer; Age over 60; Born in North America or northern Europe; Atypical hyperplasia detected on biopsy.

Cognitive Level: Application

23. During your examination of Mrs. S., you notice that her left breast is slightly larger than her right breast. Which of the following is true?
    A. This finding is not unusual but you should verify that this change is not new.
    B. This finding is very unusual and means Mrs. S. has an inflammation or growth.
    C. Breasts should always be symmetric.
    D. This is probably due to breast-feeding and is nothing to worry about.

Correct Answer: A

Rationale: Note symmetry of size and shape. It is common to have a slight asymmetry in size; often the left breast is slightly larger than the right. A sudden increase in the size of one breast signifies inflammation or new growth.

Cognitive Level: Analysis

24. Which of the following women reflect abnormal findings during the inspection phase of breast examination?
    A. A pregnant woman whose breasts have a fine blue network of veins visible under the skin.
    B. A nonpregnant woman whose skin is marked with linear striae.
    C. A woman whose nipples are in different planes (deviated).
    D. A woman whose left breast is slightly larger than her right.

Correct Answer: C

Rationale: The nipples should be symmetrically placed on the same plane on the two breasts. Deviation in pointing. An underlying cancer causes fibrosis in the mammary ducts, which pulls the nipple angle toward it.

Cognitive Level: Comprehension

25. During your physical examination, you note that Mrs. H. has an inverted left nipple. Which statement regarding this is most accurate?
    A. A unilateral inversion of a nipple is always a serious sign.
    B. It should be determined whether the inversion is a recent change.
    C. Nipple inversion is not significant unless accompanied by an underlying palpable mass.
    D. Normal nipple inversion is usually bilateral.

Correct Answer: B

Rationale: Nipples usually protrude, although some are flat and some are inverted. They tend to stay in their original condition. Distinguish a recently retracted nipple from one that has been inverted for many years or since puberty. Recent nipple retraction signifies acquired disease.

Cognitive Level: Analysis

26. Which of the following statements best describes the correct procedure to screen for nipple and/or skin retraction during a breast examination?
    A. Have the woman lie down on her left side and note any retraction.
    B. Have the woman shift from a supine position to a standing position, noting any lag or retraction.
    C. Have the woman slowly lift her arms above her head and note any retraction or lag in movement.
    D. Have the woman bend over and touch her toes.

Correct Answer: C

Rationale: Direct the woman to change position while you check the breasts for skin retraction signs. First ask her to lift the arms slowly over the head. Both breasts should move up symmetrically. Retraction signs are due to fibrosis in the breast tissue, usually caused by growing neoplasms. Note a lag in movement of one breast.

Cognitive Level: Application

27. Which of the following positions is most likely to make significant lumps more distinct during breast palpation?
    A. Supine with arms relaxed at the sides
    B. Sitting with arms relaxed at the sides
    C. Sitting with arms flexed and fingertips touching shoulders
    D. Supine with arms raised over head

Correct Answer: D

Rationale: Help the woman to a supine position. Tuck a small pad under the side to be palpated and raise her arm over her head. These maneuvers will flatten the breast tissue and displace it medially. Any significant lumps will then feel more distinct.

Cognitive Level: Application

28. Which of the following clinical situations would you consider to be outside of normal limits?
    A. Mrs. H. has never been pregnant. Her breast examination reveals large pendulous breasts that have a firm, transverse ridge along the lower quadrant in both breasts.
    B. Mrs. A. has never been pregnant. She reports that she should begin her period tomorrow. Her breast examination reveals breast tissue that is nodular and somewhat engorged. She states that the examination was slightly painful.
    C. Mrs. W. has had two pregnancies and she breastfed both of her children. Her youngest child is now 10 years old. Her breast examination reveals breast tissue that is somewhat soft and she has a small amount of thick yellow discharge from both nipples.
    D. Mrs. D. has had one pregnancy. She states that she feels she may be entering menopause. Her breast examination reveals breasts that are soft and sag slightly.

Correct Answer: C

Rationale: After palpating over the four breast quadrants, palpate the nipple. Note any induration or subareolar mass. Use your thumb and forefinger to apply gentle pressure or a stripping action to the nipple. If any discharge appears, note its color and consistency. Except in pregnancy and lactation, discharge is abnormal.

Cognitive Level: Analysis

29. Mrs. S. states in the interview that she noticed a new lump in the shower a few days ago. It was on her left breast near her axilla. You should plan to:
    A. palpate the unaffected breast first.
    B. palpate the lump first and try to get an idea of its size.
    C. avoid palpating the lump since it could be a cyst which might rupture.
    D. palpate the breast with the lump first but

plan to palpate the axilla last.

Correct Answer: A

Rationale: If the woman mentions a breast lump she has discovered herself, examine the unaffected breast first to learn a baseline of normal consistency for this individual.

Cognitive Level: Application

30. You have palpated a lump in Mrs. L.'s right breast. You document this as: A small, round, firm distinct, lump located at 2:00, 2 cm from the nipple. It is nontender and fixed. There is no associated retraction of skin or nipple, no erythema and no axillary lymphadenopathy. Which of the following statements reveals the information that is missing from the documentation?
    A. It is missing information about the shape of the lump.
    B. It is missing information about the exact size of the lump.
    C. It is missing information about whether the lump is solitary or multiple.
    D. It is missing information about the lump's consistency.

Correct Answer: B

Rationale: If you do feel a lump or mass, note these characteristics: (1) Location—Using the breast as a clock face, describe the distance in centimeters from the nipple, (2) Size—Judge in centimeters in three dimensions: width X length X thickness, (3) Shape—State if the lump is oval, round, lobulated, or indistinct, (4) Consistency—State if the lump is soft, firm or hard, (5) Moveable—Is the lump freely moveable, or is it fixed when you try to slide it over the chest wall? (6) Distinctness—Is the lump solitary or multiple? (7) Nipple—Is it displaced or retracted? (8) Note the skin over the lump—Is it erythematous, dimpled or retracted? (9) Tenderness—Is the lump tender to palpation? And (10) Lymphadenopathy—Are there any regional lymph nodes palpable?

Cognitive Level: Application

31. Which of the following statements indicates proper breast self-examination (BSE) instruction?
    A. Tell the woman that the best time to perform BSE is in the middle of her menstrual cycle.
    B. Tell the woman that the best time to perform BSE is 4-7 days after the first day of her menstrual period.
    C. Tell the woman that if she suspects that she is pregnant, she should not perform BSE until her baby is born.
    D. Tell the woman that she needs to do BSE only bi-monthly unless she has fibrocystic breast tissue.

Correct Answer: B

Rationale: Help each woman establish a regular schedule of self-care. The best time to conduct breast self-examination is right after the menstrual period, or the fourth through seventh day of the menstrual cycle, when the breasts are the smallest and least congested. Advise the pregnant or menopausal woman who is not having menstrual periods to select a familiar date to examine her breasts each month, for example her birthdate or the day the rent is due.

Cognitive Level: Application

32. Which of the following statements reflects the best approach to teaching a woman about breast self-examination (BSE)?
    A. "BSE is so important because 1 out of 9 women will develop breast cancer in her lifetime."
    B. "BSE will save your life since you are likely to find a cancerous lump between mammograms."
    C. "BSE on a monthly basis will help you feel familiar with your own breasts and their normal variations."
    D. "BSE is more important than ever for you since you have never had any children."

Correct Answer: C

Rationale: Stress that a regular monthly self-examination will familiarize her with her own breasts and their normal variation. This is a positive step that will reassure her of her healthy state. While teaching, focus on the positive aspects of breast self-examination. Avoid citing frightening mortality statistics about breast cancer. This may generate excessive fear and denial that actually obstructs a woman's self-care action.

Cognitive Level: Application

33. Mrs. J., a 55-year-old post-menopausal woman, is being seen in the clinic for a yearly examination. She is concerned about changes in her breasts that she has noticed over the past 5 years. She states that her breasts have decreased in size

and that the elasticity has changed so that her breasts seem "flat and flabby." You reply:

A. "This is a normal change that occurs as women get older. It is due to the absence of progesterone due to the aging process."
B. "This change occurs most often because of structural degeneration of the breast."
C. "Postural changes in the spine make it appear that your breasts have changed in shape. Exercises to strengthen the muscles of the upper back and chest wall will help to prevent the changes in elasticity and size."
D. "Decreases in progesterone and estrogen after menopause causes atrophy of the glandular tissue in the breast. This is a normal process of aging."

Correct Answer: D

Rationale: Ovarian secretion of estrogen and progesterone decreases after menopause. This causes the breast glandular tissue to atrophy.

Cognitive Level: Application

34. Which of the following statements regarding breast cancer is true?
    A. Breast cancer is the most common type of cancer in women.
    B. Breast cancer is the leading cause of death among black women in the United States.
    C. The leading cancer-caused death in women in the United States is breast cancer.
    D. There is little racial difference in mortality due to breast cancer.

Correct Answer: B

Rationale: Breast cancer is the leading cause of cancer death among black women in the United States. It is the second leading cause of cancer death in women in the United States.

Cognitive Level: Knowledge

35. M.J., a 43-year-old woman, is at the clinic for a routine examination. She reports that she has had a breast lump in her right breast for years. Recently, it has begun to change in consistency and is becoming harder. She reports that 5 years ago her physician evaluated the lump and determined that it "was nothing to worry about." Your examination validates the presence of a mass in the right upper outer quadrant at 1:00, approximately 5 cm from the nipple. It is firm, mobile, non-tender, with borders that are not well defined. Your recommendation to M.J. is:

    A. "This is probably nothing to worry about since it has been present for years and was determined to be non-cancerous at that time."
    B. "The changes you are experiencing could be related to your menstrual cycles. Keep track of changes in the mass related to your cycles."
    C. "Since you are experiencing no pain and the size has not changed, continue to monitor the lump and return to the clinic in 3 months."
    D. "Because of the change in consistency of the lump, it should be further evaluated by a physician."

Correct Answer: D

Rationale: A lump that has been present for years and is not exhibiting changes may not be serious but still should be explored. Any recent change or new lump should be evaluated.

Cognitive Level: Analysis

36. When discussing breast self examination with a 30-year-old woman, which of the following statements is most appropriate?

    A. "Examine your breasts every month on the same day of the month."
    B. "Examine your breasts shortly after your menstrual cycle each month."
    C. "The best time to examine your breasts is during ovulation."
    D. "The best time to examine your breasts is immediately prior to menstruation."

Correct Answer: B

Rationale: The best time to conduct breast self examination is shortly after the menstrual cycle when the breasts are the smallest and least congested.

Cognitive Level: Application

37. The best time for postmenopausal women to perform breast self examination is:
    A. daily, during the shower or bath.
    B. every year with annual gynecological examination.
    C. the same day every month.
    D. one week after her menstrual period.

Correct Answer: C

Rationale: Postmenopausal women are no longer experiencing regular menstrual cycles, but need to continue to perform breast self examination on a monthly basis. Choosing the same day of the month is a helpful reminder to perform breast self examination.

Cognitive Level: Comprehension

38. While inspecting Ms. R.'s breasts, you find that the left breast is slightly larger than the right, with the presence of Montgomery's glands bilaterally, and a fine venous pattern in both breasts. You would:

    A. consider these normal findings and proceed with the examination.
    B. continue with examination, then refer the patient for further evaluation of the Montgomery's glands.
    C. ask extensive history questions regarding the woman's breast asymmetry.
    D. palpate over the venous patterns, checking for drainage.

Correct Answer: A

Rationale: Normal findings of the breast include: one breast (most often the left) slightly larger than the other, the presence of Montgomery's glands across the areola, and a fine venous pattern visible, especially on fair-skinned individuals.

Cognitive Level: Analysis

Chapter 16

Thorax and Lungs

1. The vertebra prominens is:
   A. located next to the manubrium of the sternum.
   B. not palpable in most individuals.
   C. the spinous process of C7.
   D. opposite the interior border of the scapula.

Correct Answer: C

Rationale: The spinous process of C7 is the vertebra prominens. It is the most prominent bony spur protruding at the base of the neck. If two protrusions seem equally prominent, the upper one is C7 and the lower is T1. Counting ribs and intercostal spaces on the posterior thorax is difficult due to the muscles and soft tissue. The vertebra prominens is easier to identify and is used as a starting point in counting thoracic processes and identifying landmarks on the posterior chest.

Cognitive Level: Knowledge

2. When performing a respiratory assessment on your patient, you note a costal angle of approximately 90 degrees. This is:
   A. an expected finding in a patient with a barrel chest.
   B. a normal finding in a healthy adult.
   C. seen in patients with kyphosis.
   D. indicative of pectus excavatum.

Correct Answer: B

Rationale: The right and left costal margins form an angle where they meet at the xiphoid process. Usually, this angle is 90 degrees or less. The angle increases when the rib cage is chronically overinflated, as in emphysema.

Cognitive Level: Comprehension

3. The left lung:
   A. is shorter than the right lung because of the underlying stomach.
   B. consists of two lobes.
   C. consists primarily of an upper lobe on the posterior chest.
   D. is divided by the horizontal fissure.

Correct Answer: B

Rationale: The left lung consists of upper and lower lobes. It is narrower than the right lung because of the heart. The right lung is shorter than the left lung because of the presence of the liver. The right lung has three lobes: upper, middle, and lower lobes. The posterior chest is almost all lower lobe.

Cognitive Level: Comprehension

4. The apices of the lungs:
   A. rest on the diaphragm at the fifth intercostal space in the midclavicular line.
   B. are at the level of the second rib anteriorly.
   C. extend 3-4 cm above the inner third of the clavicles.
   D. are located at the sixth rib anteriorly and the eighth rib laterally.

Correct Answer: C

Rationale: The apex of the lung on the anterior chest is 3-4 cm Above the inner third of the clavicles. Posteriorly, the apices are at the level of C7.

Cognitive Level: Comprehension

5. The trachea bifurcates anteriorly at the:
   A. costal angle.
   B. xiphoid process.
   C. suprasternal notch.
   D. sternal angle.

Correct Answer: D

Rationale: The sternal angle marks the site of tracheal bifurcation into the right and left main bronchi; it corresponds with the upper border of the atria of the heart, and it lies above the fourth thoracic vertebra on the back.

Cognitive Level: Knowledge

6. Expected assessment findings in the normal adult lung include the presence of:
   A. increased tactile fremitus and dull percussion tones.
   B. adventitious sounds and limited chest expansion.
   C. muffled voice sounds and symmetrical tactile fremitus.
   D. absent voice sounds and hyperresonant percussion tones.

Correct Answer: C

Rationale: Normal lung findings include: symmetric chest expansion, resonant percussion tones, vesicular breath sounds over the peripheral lung fields, no adventitious sounds, and muffled voice sounds.

Cognitive Level: Comprehension

7. The primary muscles of respiration include the:
   A. diaphragm and intercostals.
   B. trapezius and rectus abdominus.
   C. sternomastoids and scaleni.
   D. external obliques and pectoralis major.

Correct Answer: A

Rationale: The major muscle of respiration is the diaphragm. The intercostal muscles lift the sternum and elevate the ribs during inspiration, increasing the anteroposterior diameter.

Cognitive Level: Knowledge

8. A 65-year-old patient with a history of heart failure comes to the clinic with complaints of "being awakened from sleep with shortness of breath." You:
   A. assure the patient that this is normal and will probably resolve within the next week.
   B. suspect that the patient is experiencing paroxysmal nocturnal dyspnea.
   C. obtain a detailed history of the patient's allergies and history of asthma.
   D. tell the patient to sleep on his/her right side to facilitate ease of respirations.

Correct Answer: B

Rationale: The patient is experiencing paroxysmal nocturnal dyspnea: Being awakened from sleep with shortness of breath and the need to be upright to achieve comfort. This is associated with congestive heart failure and not allergies or asthma.

Cognitive Level: Application

9. Over which of the following locations would it be normal to feel tactile fremitus most intensely?
   A. 2nd RICS @ SB
   B. 3rd RICS @ MAL
   C. 5th LICS @ MCL
   D. 7th RICS @ AAL

Correct Answer: A

Rationale: Normally, fremitus is most prominent between the scapulae and around the sternum. These are sites where the major bronchi are closest to the chest wall. Fremitus normally decreases as you progress down the chest because more tissue impedes sound transmission.

Cognitive Level: Comprehension

10. Tactile fremitus is produced by:
   A. sounds generated from the larynx.
   B. air in the subcutaneous tissues.
   C. moisture in the alveoli.
   D. blood flow through the pulmonary arteries.

Correct Answer: A

Rationale: Fremitus is a palpable vibration. Sounds generated from the larynx are transmitted through patent bronchi and the lung parenchyma to the chest wall where you feel them as vibrations.

Cognitive Level: Knowledge

11. A dull percussion note elicited in the left lower lobe of the lung is most likely due to:
   A. increased density of lung tissue.
   B. shallow breathing.
   C. normal lung tissue.
   D. decreased adipose tissue.

Correct Answer: A

Rationale: A dull percussion note indicates an abnormal density in the lungs, as with pneumonia, pleural effusion, atelectasis, or tumor. Resonance is the expected finding in normal lung tissue.

Cognitive Level: Comprehension

12. The most important technique when progressing from one auscultatory site on the thorax to another is:
   A. top to bottom comparison.
   B. side to side comparison.
   C. posterior to anterior comparison.
   D. interspace by interspace comparison.

Correct Answer: B

Rationale: Side to side comparison is most important when auscultating the chest. Listen to at least one full respiration in each location.

Cognitive Level: Comprehension

13. When auscultating the lungs of an adult patient, you note that over the posterior lower lobes you hear low pitched, soft breath sounds with inspiration being longer than expiration. You know that these are:
    A. bronchial breath sounds and are normal in that location.
    B. bronchovesicular breath sounds and are normal in that location.
    C. vesicular breath sounds and are normal in that location.
    D. sounds normally auscultated over the trachea.

Correct Answer: C

Rationale: Vesicular breath sounds are low pitched, soft sounds with inspiration being longer than expiration. These breath sounds are expected over peripheral lung fields where air flows through smaller bronchioles and alveoli.

Cognitive Level: Application

14. When auscultating the chest in an adult you would:
    A. use the bell of the stethoscope held lightly against the chest to avoid friction.
    B. use the diaphragm of the stethoscope held firmly against the chest.
    C. instruct the patient to breathe in and out through his/her nose.
    D. instruct the patient to take deep, rapid breaths.

Correct Answer: B

Rationale: The diaphragm of the stethoscope held firmly on the chest is the correct way to auscultate breath sounds. The patient should be instructed to breathe through his/her mouth, a little deeper than usual, but not to hyperventilate.

Cognitive Level: Knowledge

15. Percussion of an atelectatic lung would reveal:
    A. resonance.
    B. hyperresonance.
    C. dullness.
    D. tympany.

Correct Answer: C

Rationale: A dull percussion note signals an abnormal density in the lungs, as with pneumonia, pleural effusion, atelectasis, or tumor.

Cognitive Level: Comprehension

16. Decreased breath sounds would most likely be heard:
    A. when the bronchial tree is obstructed.
    B. when adventitious sounds are present.
    C. in conditions of consolidation (e.g., pneumonia).
    D. in conjunction with whispered pectoriloquy.

Correct Answer: A

Rationale: Decreased or absent breath sounds occur when the bronchial tree is obstructed; in emphysema; and when sound transmission is obstructed as in pleurisy, pneumothorax, or pleural effusion.

Cognitive Level: Comprehension

17. You note hyperresonant percussion tones when percussing the thorax of an infant. You would:
    A. notify the physician.
    B. monitor the infant's respiratory rate and rhythm.
    C. suspect a pneumothorax.
    D. consider this a normal finding.

Correct Answer: D

Rationale: The percussion note of hyperresonance occurs normally in the infant and young child owing to the relatively thin chest wall. Anything less than hyperresonance would have the same clinical significance as would dullness in the adult.

Cognitive Level: Application

18. A normal finding when assessing the respiratory system of an elderly adult is:
    A. a decreased anteroposterior diameter.
    B. bronchovesicular breath sounds throughout the lungs.
    C. increased thoracic expansion.
    D. decreased mobility of the thorax.

Correct Answer: D

Rationale: The costal cartilages become calcified with aging, resulting in a less mobile thorax.

Cognitive Level: Comprehension

19. A mother brings her 3-month-old infant to your clinic for evaluation of a "cold and runny nose for 1 week." When performing the physical assessment you note that the child has nasal flaring and sternal and intercostal retractions. You:
    A. assure the mother that these are normal symptoms of a cold.
    B. recognize that these are serious signs and refer the child immediately.
    C. perform a complete cardiac assessment as these are probably signs of early congestive heart failure.
    D. recognize that these are symptoms of rachitic rosary and refer the infant within the week.

Correct Answer: B

Rationale: The infant is an obligatory nose breather until the age of 3 months. Normally there is no flaring of the nostrils and no sternal or intercostal retractions. Marked retractions of the sternum and intercostal muscles, and nasal flaring indicate increased inspiratory effort, as in pneumonia, acute airway obstruction, asthma, and atelectasis.

Cognitive Level: Analysis

20. When assessing the respiratory system of a 4-year-old, which of the following findings would be expected?
    A. An irregular respiratory pattern and a respiratory rate of 40 breaths per minute at rest
    B. The presence of bronchovesicular breath sounds in the peripheral lung fields
    C. No diaphragmatic excursion due to a child's decreased inspiratory volume
    D. Crepitus palpated at the costochondral junctions

Correct Answer: B

Rationale: Bronchovesicular breath sounds in the peripheral lung fields of the infant and young child up to age 5 or 6 is a normal finding. Their thin chest walls with underdeveloped musculature do not dampen the sound as do the thicker chest walls of adults, so breath sounds are louder and harsher.

Cognitive Level: Application

21. When inspecting the anterior chest you should assess for:
    A. diaphragmatic excursion.
    B. symmetrical chest expansion.
    C. the shape and configuration of the chest wall.
    D. the presence of breath sounds.

Correct Answer: C

Rationale: The anterior chest is inspected for: the shape and configuration of the chest wall, level of consciousness, skin color and condition, quality of respirations, retraction and bulging of the intercostal spaces, and use of accessory muscles. The other techniques listed are percussion, palpation, and auscultation techniques.

Cognitive Level: Comprehension

22. You would most likely auscultate fine crackles:
    A. in a healthy 5-year-old.
    B. in the immediate newborn period.
    C. in the pregnant patient.
    D. in association with a pneumothorax.

Correct Answer: B

Rationale: Fine crackles are commonly heard in the immediate newborn period due to the opening of the airways and clearing of fluid.

Cognitive Level: Application

23. Unequal chest expansion occurs when:
    A. part of the lung is obstructed or collapsed.
    B. the patient is obese.
    C. accessory muscles are used to augment respiratory effort.
    D. bulging of the intercostal spaces is present.

Correct Answer: A

Rationale: Unequal chest expansion occurs when part of the lung is obstructed or collapsed, as with pneumonia, or guarding to avoid postoperative incisional pain or atelectasis.

Cognitive Level: Comprehension

24. Bronchophony heard upon auscultation is associated with:
    A. pulmonary consolidation.
    B. decreased breath sounds.
    C. hyperresonance.
    D. pneumothorax.

Correct Answer: A

Rationale: Pathology that increases lung density will enhance transmission of voice sounds.

Cognitive Level: Comprehension

25. Bronchovesicular breath sounds are:
    A. similar to bronchial sounds except they are shorter in duration.
    B. usually pathologic.
    C. expected near the major airways.
    D. musical in quality.

Correct Answer: C

Rationale: Bronchovesicular sounds are heard over major bronchi where fewer alveoli are located: posteriorly, between the scapulae especially on the right; anteriorly, around the upper sternum in the first and second intercostal spaces.

Cognitive Level: Comprehension

26. Air passing through narrowed bronchioles would produce which of the following adventitious sounds?
    A. Whispered pectoriloquy
    B. Wheezes
    C. Bronchophony
    D. Bronchial

Correct Answer: B

Rationale: Wheezes are caused by air squeezed or compressed through passageways narrowed almost to closure by collapsing, swelling, secretions, or tumors.

Cognitive Level: Comprehension

27. Your patient has a long history of chronic obstructive pulmonary disease. You are most likely to observe:
    A. an anteroposterior:transverse diameter ratio of 1:1.
    B. atrophied neck and trapezius muscles.
    C. unequal chest expansion.
    D. increased tactile fremitus.

Correct Answer: A

Rationale: An anteroposterior:transverse diameter of 1:1 or "barrel chest" is seen in individuals with chronic obstructive pulmonary disease due to hyperinflation of the lungs. The ribs are more horizontal and the chest appears as if held in continuous inspiration. Neck muscles are hypertrophied from aiding in forced respiration. Chest expansion is decreased, but is symmetrical. Decreased tactile fremitus occurs due to decreased transmission of vibrations.

Cognitive Level: Application

28. A teenage patient comes to the emergency room with complaints of an "inability to breathe and a sharp pain in my left chest." Your assessment findings include the following: Cyanosis, tachypnea, tracheal deviation to the right, decreased tactile fremitus on the left, hyperresonance on the left, and decreased breath sounds on the left. This description is consistent with:
    A. acute pneumonia.
    B. an asthmatic attack.
    C. bronchitis.
    D. a pneumothorax.

Correct Answer: D

Rationale: With a pneumothorax, free air in the pleural space causes partial or complete lung collapse. If the pneumothorax is large, tachypnea and cyanosis are seen. Unequal chest expansion, decreased or absent tactile fremitus, tracheal deviation to the unaffected side, decreased chest expansion, hyperresonant percussion tones, and decreased or absent breath sounds are assessed.

Cognitive Level: Analysis

29. An adult patient with a history of allergies comes to the clinic complaining of wheezing and difficulty breathing when working in his yard. Your assessment findings include the following: tachypnea, use of accessory neck muscles, prolonged expiration, intercostal retractions, decreased breath sounds, and expiratory wheezes. This description is consistent with:
    A. lobar pneumonia.
    B. atelectasis.
    C. congestive heart failure.
    D. asthma.

Correct Answer: A

Rationale: Asthma is allergic hypersensitivity to certain inhaled particles that produces inflammation and a reaction of bronchospasm, which increases airway resistance, especially during expiration. Increased respiratory rate, use of accessory muscles, retraction of intercostal muscles, prolonged expiration, decreased breath sounds, and expiratory wheezing are all characteristic of asthma.

Cognitive Level: Analysis

30. Which of the following describes normal changes in the respiratory system of the older adult?
    A. Respiratory muscle strength increases to compensate for a decreased vital capacity.

B. The lungs are less elastic and distensible, decreasing their ability to collapse and recoil.
C. There is a decrease in small airway closure, leading to problems with atelectasis.
D. Severe dyspnea is experienced on exertion, due to changes in the lungs.

Correct Answer: B

Rationale: In the aging adult the lungs are less elastic and distensible, decreasing their ability to collapse and recoil. There is a decreased vital capacity and a loss of intraalveolar septa, causing less surface area for gas exchange. The lung bases become less ventilated, and the older person is at risk of developing dyspnea with exertion, but this should not be severe (which would suggest the possibility of pathology).

Cognitive Level: Comprehension

31. A 26-week pregnant woman states that she is "not really short of breath," but feels that she is aware of her breathing and the need to breathe. What is your best reply?
A. "The increase in estrogren levels during pregnancy often causes a decrease in the diameter of the rib cage and makes it difficult to breathe."
B. "This is normal as the fetus grows because of the increased oxygen demand on the mother's body and results in an increased respiratory rate."
C. "The diaphragm becomes fixed during pregnancy, making it difficult to take in a deep breath."
D. "It is normal to experience an increased awareness of the need to breathe. Some women may interpret this as shortness of breath, but it is a normal finding and nothing is wrong structurally."

Correct Answer: D

Rationale: During pregnancy, the woman may develop an increased awareness of the need to breathe. Some women may interpret this as dyspnea, even though structurally nothing is wrong. Estrogen increases relax the chest cage ligaments, causing an increase in transverse diameter. The diaphragm is elevated, but not fixed. It moves with breathing even more during pregnancy.

Cognitive Level: Application

32. Which of the following statements is true with regard to cultural differences in the respiratory system?
A. The largest chest volumes are found in blacks.
B. Lung maturity in the fetus is reached 1 week earlier in blacks than in whites.
C. Asian infants have a much lower risk of respiratory distress syndrome than blacks.
D. Racial differences are of no significance when determining lung maturity of a fetus.

Correct Answer: B

Rationale: Lung maturity is reached 1 week earlier in blacks than in whites. The largest chest volumes are whites, then blacks, Asians, and Native Americans. Racial differences should be considered when determining lung maturity of a fetus.

Cognitive Level: Comprehension

33. Mr. H., a 35-year-old Asian immigrant, is being seen in the clinic for complaints of a cough that is associated with rust-colored sputum, low-grade afternoon fevers, and night sweats for the past 2 months. Your preliminary analysis based on this history is that Mr. H. may be suffering from:
A. pulmonary edema.
B. pneumonia.
C. bronchitis.
D. tuberculosis.

Correct Answer: D

Rationale: Sputum is not diagnostic alone, but some conditions have characteristic sputum production. Tuberculosis often produces rust-colored sputum in addition to other symptoms of night sweats and low-grade afternoon fevers. Asian immigrants have a high incidence of tuberculosis. Their tuberculosis usually peaks in the first 2 months of entry into the U.S.

Cognitive Level: Analysis

34. A 70-year-old male is being seen in the clinic for severe exacerbation of his congestive heart failure. Which of the following findings are you most likely to observe in this situation?
A. SOB, orthopnea, PND, ankle edema
B. Productive cough, dyspnea, weight loss, anorexia
C. Fever, dry non-productive cough, bronchial breath sounds

D. Rasping cough, thick mucoid sputum, wheezing

Correct Answer: A

Rationale: Heart failure often presents with increased respiratory rate, SOB on exertion, orthopnea, PND, nocturia, ankle edema and pallor in light-skinned individuals.

Cognitive Level: Application

Chapter 17

Heart and Neck Vessels

1. The sac that surrounds and protects the heart is called the:
   A. endocardium.
   B. myocardium.
   C. pericardium.
   D. pleural space.

Correct Answer: C

Rationale: The pericardium is a tough fibrous double-walled sac that surrounds and protects the heart. It has two layers that contain a few milliliters of serous pericardial fluid.

Cognitive Level: Knowledge

2. The direction of blood flow through the heart is best described by which of the following?
   A. right atrium—right ventricle—pulmonary vein—lungs—pulmonary artery—left atrium—left ventricle
   B. right atrium—right ventricle—pulmonary artery—lungs—pulmonary vein—left atrium—left ventricle
   C. vena cava—right atrium—right ventricle—lungs—pulmonary artery—left atrium—left ventricle
   D. aorta—right atrium—right ventricle—lungs—pulmonary vein—left atrium—left ventricle—vena cava

Correct Answer: B

Rationale: Returning blood from the body empties into the right atrium and flows into the right ventricle and then goes to the lungs via the pulmonary artery. The lungs oxygenate the blood and it is then returned to the left atrium via the pulmonary vein. It goes from there to the left ventricle and then out to the body through the aorta.

Cognitive Level: Knowledge

3. Which of the following best describes what is meant by atrial kick?
   A. The atria contract during systole and attempt to push against closed valves.
   B. The contraction of the atria at the beginning of diastole can be felt as a palpitation.
   C. The atria contract toward the end of diastole and push the remaining blood into the ventricles.
   D. This is the pressure exerted against the atria as the ventricles contract during systole.

Correct Answer: C

Rationale: Toward the end of diastole, the atria contract and push the last amount of blood (about 25 percent of stroke volume) into the ventricles. This active filling phase is called presystole, or atrial systole, or sometimes the "atrial kick".

Cognitive Level: Knowledge

4. The valve closures that can BEST be heard at the base of the heart are:
   A. mitral, tricuspid.
   B. mitral, pulmonic.
   C. tricuspid, aortic.
   D. aortic, pulmonic.

Correct Answer: D

Rationale: The second heart sound (S2) occurs with closure of the semilunar valves and signals the end of systole. Although it is heard over all the precordium, S2 is loudest at the base.

Cognitive Level: Knowledge

5. Which of the following describes the closure of the valves in a normal cardiac cycle?
   A. Both the tricuspid and the pulmonic valve close at the same time.
   B. The tricuspid valve closes slightly later than the mitral valve.

C. The aortic valve closes slightly before the tricuspid valve.
D. The pulmonic valve closes slightly before the aortic valve.

Correct Answer: B

Rationale: Also, events occur just slightly later in the right side of the heart due to the route of myocardial depolarization. As a result, two distinct components to each of the heart sounds exist, and sometimes you can hear them separately. In the first heart sound, the mitral component (M1) closes just before the tricuspid component (T1).

Cognitive Level: Comprehension

6. The component of the conduction system referred to as the pacemaker of the heart is the:
   A. SA node.
   B. AV node.
   C. bundle of His.
   D. bundle branches.

Correct Answer: A

Rationale: Specialized cells in the sinoatrial (SA) node near the superior vena cava initiate an electrical impulse. (Because the SA node has an intrinsic rhythm, it is the "pacemaker.")

Cognitive Level: Knowledge

7. The electrical stimulus of the cardiac cycle follows which sequence?
   A. AV node—SA node—bundle of His
   B. bundle of His—AV node—SA node
   C. SA node—AV node—bundle of His—bundle branches
   D. AV node—SA node—bundle of His—bundle branches

Correct Answer: C

Rationale: Specialized cells in the sinoatrial (SA) node near the superior vena cava initiate an electrical impulse. The current flows in an orderly sequence, first across the atria to the AV node low in the atrial septum. There, it is delayed slightly so that the atria have time to contract before the ventricles are stimulated. Then the impulse travels to the bundle of His, the right and left bundle branches, and then through the ventricles.

Cognitive Level: Comprehension

8. The findings from your assessment of a 70-year-old male with swelling in his ankles include jugular venous pulsations 5 cm above the sternal angle when elevated 45 degrees. This would indicate:
   A. increased pressure in right side of heart.
   B. decreased fluid volume.
   C. narrowing of jugular veins.
   D. increased cardiac output.

Correct Answer: A

Rationale: Since no cardiac valve exists to separate the superior vena cava from the right atrium, the jugular veins give information about activity on the right side of the heart. They reflect filling pressures and volume changes. Normal jugular venous pulsation is 2 cm or less above the sternal angle. Elevated pressure is more than 3 cm above the sternal angle while at 45 degrees, and occurs with right-sided congestive heart failure.

Cognitive Level: Analysis

9. Which of the following would be true concerning the circulation of a newborn who is just 5 minutes old?
   A. The foramen ovale closes just minutes before birth and the ductus arteriosus closes immediately after.
   B. The circulation of a newborn is identical to that of an adult.
   C. There is an opening in the atrial septum where blood can flow into the left side of the heart.
   D. The left ventricle is larger and weighs more than the right.

Correct Answer: C

Rationale: First, about two-thirds of it is shunted through an opening in the atrial septum, the foramen ovale into the left side of the heart, where it is pumped out through the aorta. The foramen ovale closes within the first hour because of the new lower pressure in the right side of the heart than in the left side.

Cognitive Level: Application

10. A pregnant 25-year-old in her fifth month has a blood pressure of 100/70. In reviewing her previous exam, you note that her blood pressure in her second month was 124/80. In evaluating this change what do you know to be true?

A. This is not an expected finding as it would mean a decreased cardiac output.
B. This would mean a decrease in circulating blood volume, which is dangerous for fetus.
C. This is the result of peripheral vasodilatation and is an expected change.
D. Because of increased cardiac output, the blood pressure should be higher this time.

Correct Answer: C

Rationale: Despite the increased cardiac output, arterial blood pressure decreases in pregnancy, due to peripheral vasodilatation. The blood pressure drops to its lowest point during the second trimester, then rises after that.

Cognitive Level: Analysis

11. In assessing a 70-year-old male you find the following: BP 140/100; HR 104 and slightly irregular; split S2; increased cardiac output. Which of these findings can be explained by expected hemodynamic changes related to age?
    A. Increase in resting heart rate
    B. Increase in cardiac output
    C. Increase in diastolic blood pressure
    D. Increase in systolic blood pressure

Correct Answer: D

Rationale: From age 20 to 80, systolic blood pressure tends to increase within the normal range by 25 to 30 percent. No significant change in diastolic pressure occurs with age. No change in resting heart rate occurs with aging. Cardiac output at rest is not changed with aging.

Cognitive Level: Analysis

12. A 45-year-old male is here for "a routine physical." During the history the patient states he's been having difficulty sleeping. "I'll be sleeping great and then I wake up and feel like I can't get my breath." Your best response to this would be:
    A. "It's probably because it's been so hot at night."
    B. "Have you had a recent sinus infection or upper respiratory infection?"
    C. "Do you have any history of problems with your heart?"
    D. "When was your last electrocardiogram?"

Correct Answer: C

Rationale: Paroxysmal nocturnal dyspnea (PND) occurs with congestive heart failure. Lying down increases volume of intrathoracic blood, and the weakened heart cannot accommodate the increased load. Classically, the person awakens after 2 hours of sleep, arises, and flings open a window with the perception of needing fresh air.

Cognitive Level: Application

13. In assessing a patient's MAJOR risk factors for heart disease, which would you want to include in your history?
    A. Alcohol consumption, obesity, diabetes, stress, high cholesterol
    B. Family history, hypertension, stress, age
    C. Smoking, hypertension, obesity, diabetes, high cholesterol
    D. Personality type, high cholesterol, diabetes, smoking

Correct Answer: C

Rationale: Risk factors for coronary artery disease—collect data regarding elevated serum cholesterol, elevated blood pressure, blood sugar levels above 130 or known diabetes mellitus, obesity, cigarette smoking, low activity level.

Cognitive Level: Application

14. The mother of a 3-month-old states her daughter has not been gaining weight. With further questioning you find that the infant falls asleep after nursing and wakes up after a short amount of time hungry. What other information would you want to have?
    A. Presence of dyspnea or diaphoresis when sucking
    B. Sibling history of eating disorders
    C. Amount of background noise when eating
    D. Position that baby sleeps in

Correct Answer: A

Rationale: To screen for heart disease in an infant, focus on feeding. Note fatigue during feeding. Infant with congestive heart failure takes fewer ounces each feeding; becomes dyspneic with sucking; may be diaphoretic, then falls into exhausted sleep; awakens after a short time hungry again.

Cognitive Level: Analysis

15. In assessing the carotid arteries of a patient with cardiovascular disease, you would:
    A. palpate both arteries simultaneously to compare amplitude.

B. listen with the bell of stethoscope to assess for bruits.
C. instruct patient to take slow deep breaths during auscultation.
D. palpate artery in the upper one third of the neck.

Correct Answer: B

Rationale: For persons middle aged or older or who show symptoms or signs of cardiovascular disease, auscultate each carotid artery for the presence of a bruit.

Cognitive Level: Application

16. In your assessment of a 68-year-old male with recent onset of right-sided weakness, you hear a blowing, swishing sound with the bell of the stethoscope over the left carotid artery. This would indicate:
    A. a valvular disorder.
    B. blood flow turbulence due to narrowing.
    C. ventricular hypertrophy.
    D. volume overload.

Correct Answer: B

Rationale: A bruit is a blowing, swishing sound indicating blood flow turbulence, normally none is present.

Cognitive Level: Analysis

17. During inspection of the precordium of an adult patient, you notice the chest moving in a forceful manner along the 4th-5th left intercostal space at the midclavicular line. This most likely suggests:
    A. an enlarged left ventricle.
    B. a normal heart.
    C. a systolic murmur.
    D. enlargement of the right ventricle.

Correct Answer: D

Rationale: A heave or lift is a sustained forceful thrusting of the ventricle during systole. It occurs with ventricular hypertrophy due to increased workload. A right ventricular heave is seen at the sternal border; a left ventricular heave is seen at the apex.

Cognitive Level: Application

18. In your assessment of a normal adult, where would you expect to palpate the apical impulse?
    A. Third left intercostal space at the midclavicular line
    B. Fifth left intercostal space at the midclavicular line
    C. Fourth left intercostal space at the sternal border
    D. Fourth left intercostal space at the anterior axillary line

Correct Answer: B

Rationale: Location—the apical impulse should occupy only one interspace, the fourth or fifth, and be at or medial to the midclavicular line.

Cognitive Level: Knowledge

19. In percussing the left cardiac border, you would expect to hear dullness at the:
    A. third left intercostal space midclavicular line and fifth left intercostal space left sternal border.
    B. fourth left intercostal space medial to midclavicular line and second left intercostal space midclavicular line.
    C. fifth left intercostal space midclavicular line and second left intercostal space sternal border.
    D. fifth left intercostal space sternal border and second right intercostal space midclavicular line.

Correct Answer: C

Rationale: Normally, the left border of cardiac dullness is at the midclavicular line in the fifth interspace and slopes in toward the sternum as you progress upward so that by the second interspace the border of dullness coincides with the left sternal border.

Cognitive Level: Comprehension

20. In performing auscultation of heart sounds, which sequence would you use?
    A. aortic area—pulmonic area—erbs point—tricuspid area—mitral area
    B. pulmonic area—erbs point—tricuspid area—pulmonic area—mitral area
    C. aortic area—tricuspid area—erbs point—mitral area—pulmonic area
    D. pulmonic area—aortic area—erbs point—tricuspid area—mitral area

Correct Answer: A

Rationale: Sounds produced by the valves may be heard all over the precordium. Thus, learn to inch your stethoscope in a Z pattern, from the base of the heart across and down, then over to the apex.

Or start at the apex and work your way up.

Cognitive Level: Comprehension

21. While counting the apical pulse on a 16-year-old patient, you note an irregular rhythm. His rate speeds up on inspiration and slows on expiration. What would be your response?
    A. Refer the patient to a cardiologist for further testing.
    B. No further response needed as this is a normal finding.
    C. Talk with patient about his intake of caffeine.
    D. Do an electrocardiogram following the exam.

Correct Answer: B

Rationale: The rhythm should be regular, although sinus arrhythmia occurs normally in young adults and children. With sinus arrhythmia, the rhythm varies with the person's breathing, increasing at the peak of inspiration, and slowing with expiration.

Cognitive Level: Analysis

22. Which of the following statements concerning S1 is true?
    A. S1 is caused by closure of the semilunar valves.
    B. S1 is louder than S2 at the base.
    C. S1 indicates the beginning of diastole.
    D. S1 coincides with the carotid artery pulse.

Correct Answer: D

Rationale: S1 is louder than S2 at the apex; S2 is louder than S1 at the base. S1 coincides with carotid artery pulse. Feel the carotid gently as you auscultate at the apex; the sound you hear as you feel each pulse is S1.

Cognitive Level: Comprehension

23. During the cardiac auscultation you hear a sound occurring immediately after S2 at the second left intercostal space. To further assess this sound what would you do?
    A. Ask patient to hold his breath while you listen again.
    B. Watch patient's respirations while listening for effect on the sound.
    C. No further assessment needed as you know it is an S3.
    D. Have patient turn to left side and listen with the bell.

Correct Answer: B

Rationale: A split S2 is a normal phenomenon that occurs toward the end of inspiration in some people. A split S2 is heard only in the pulmonic valve area, the second left interspace. When you first hear the split S2, do not be tempted to ask the person to hold his or her breath so that you can concentrate on the sounds. Breath holding will only equalize ejection times in the right and left sides of the heart and cause the split to go away. Instead, concentrate on the split as you watch the person's chest rise up and down with breathing.

Cognitive Level: Analysis

24. Which of the following could be an expected finding in a cardiac assessment on a 4-year-old?
    A. Palpable apical impulse in fifth left intercostal space lateral to midclavicular line
    B. Murmur at second left intercostal space when supine
    C. S3 when sitting up
    D. Persistent tachycardia>150

Correct Answer: B

Rationale: Some murmurs are common in healthy children or adolescents and are termed innocent or functional. The contractile force of the heart is greater in children. This increases blood flow velocity. The increased velocity plus a smaller chest measurement makes an audible murmur. The innocent murmur is heard at the second or third left intercostal space and disappears with sitting, and the young person has no associated signs of cardiac dysfunction.

Cognitive Level: Application

25. While auscultating heart sounds on a 7-year-old here for "routine physical" you hear the following: an S3, a soft murmur at left midsternal border and a venous hum when standing. Which of the following would be true regarding the findings?
    A. S3 is indicative of heart disease in children.
    B. These can all be normal findings in a child.
    C. These are indicative of congenital problems.
    D. The venous hum most likely indicates an aneurysm.

Correct Answer: B

Rationale: Physiologic S3 is common in children. A venous hum, due to turbulence of blood flow in the jugular venous system, is common in normal children and has no pathologic significance. Heart murmurs that are innocent (or functional) in origin are very common through childhood.

Cognitive Level: Analysis

26. During the precordial assessment on an 8-month pregnant patient, you palpate the apical impulse at the fourth left intercostal space lateral to the midclavicular line. This would indicate:
    A. displacement of heart due to elevation of the diaphragm.
    B. right ventricular hypertrophy.
    C. increased volume and size of heart due to pregnancy.
    D. increased blood flow through the internal mammary artery.

Correct Answer: A

Rationale: Palpation of the apical impulse is higher and lateral compared with the normal position, as the enlarging uterus elevates the diaphragm and displaces the heart up and to the left and rotates it on its long axis.

Cognitive Level: Analysis

27. In assessing for an S4, you would:
    A. listen with bell of stethoscope at apex with patient in left lateral position.
    B. listen with bell of stethoscope in pulmonic area with patient supine.
    C. listen with diaphragm in aortic area with patient sitting.
    D. listen with bell of stethoscope at base with patient leaning forward.

Correct Answer: A

Rationale: The S4 is a ventricular filling sound. It occurs when atria contract late in diastole. It is heard immediately before S1. This is a very soft sound, of very low pitch. You need a good bell, and you must listen for it. It is heard best at the apex, with the person in left lateral position.

Cognitive Level: Comprehension

28. The vital signs of a 70-year-old patient with a history of hypertension are: BP 180/100 and HR 90. You hear an extra heart sound at the apex immediately before S1. You can only hear it with the bell while patient is in left lateral position. With these findings and the patient's history, this extra heart sound is most likely:
    A. summation sound.
    B. atrial gallop.
    C. split S1.
    D. diastolic murmur.

Correct Answer: B

Rationale: A pathologic S4 is termed an atrial gallop or an S4 gallop. It occurs with decreased compliance of the ventricle, and with systolic overload (afterload), including outflow obstruction to the ventricle (aortic stenosis) and systemic hypertension. A left-sided S4 occurs with these conditions. It is heard best at the apex, in the left lateral position.

Cognitive Level: Analysis

29. You are performing a cardiac assessment on a 65-year-old patient 3 days after her myocardial infarction. Heart sounds are normal when supine but with the patient sitting and leaning forward, you hear a high-pitched, scratchy sound at the apex with the diaphragm. It disappears on inspiration. You suspect:
    A. another myocardial infarction.
    B. ventricular hypertrophy due to muscle damage.
    C. inflammation of the precordium.
    D. increased cardiac output.

Correct Answer: C

Rationale: Inflammation of the precordium gives rise to a friction rub. The sound is high-pitched and scratchy, like sandpaper being rubbed: It is best heard with the diaphragm, with the person sitting up and leaning forward, and with the breath held in expiration. A friction rub can be heard any place on the precordium but usually is best heard at the apex and left lower sternal border, places where the pericardium comes in close contact with the chest wall.

Cognitive Level: Analysis

30. The mother of a 10-month-old tells you that she has noticed that her son becomes blue when he is crying and that the frequency of this is increasing. He is also not crawling yet. In your exam you palpate a thrill at the left lower sternal border and auscultate a loud systolic murmur in the same area. What would be the most likely cause of these findings?
    A. Patent ductus arteriosus

B. Ventricular septal defect
C. Tetralogy of fallot
D. Atrial septal defect

Correct Answer: C

Rationale: Tetralogy of fallot subjective findings include: Severe cyanosis, not in first months of life but develops as infant grows and RV outflow (i.e., pulmonic) stenosis gets worse. Cyanosis with crying and exertion at first, then at rest. Development slowed. Objective: thrill palpable at left lower sternal border. S1 normal, S2 has A2 loud and P2 diminished or absent. Murmur is systolic, loud, crescendo-decrescendo.

Cognitive Level: Analysis

31. A 30-year-old female with a history of mitral valve problems states that she has been "very tired." She has started waking up at night and feels like her "heart is pounding." During her assessment, you palpate a thrill and lift at the fifth left intercostal space midclavicular line. In the same area you also auscultate a blowing, swishing sound right after S1. These findings would be most consistent with:
    A. congestive heart failure.
    B. mitral regurgitation.
    C. aortic stenosis.
    D. pulmonary edema.

Correct Answer: B

Rationale: Mitral regurgitation subjective: Fatigue, palpitation, orthopnea, PND. Objective: Thrill in systole at apex. Lift at apex. Apical impulse displaced down and to left. S1 diminished, S2 accentuated, S3 at apex often present. Murmur: asystolic, often loud, blowing, best heard at apex, radiates well to left axilla.

Cognitive Level: Analysis

32. During a cardiac assessment on an adult male in the hospital for "chest pain," you find the following: jugular vein pulsations 4 cm above sternal angle when elevated at 45 degrees, BP 98/60, HR 130; pale gray, cool, moist skin; difficulty breathing when supine; and an S3 on auscultation. Which of the following best explains the cause of these findings?
    A. Myocardial infarction
    B. Fluid overload
    C. Decreased cardiac output
    D. Atrial septal defect

Correct Answer: C

Rationale: Decreased cardiac output occurs when the heart fails as a pump, and the circulation becomes backed up and congested. Signs and symptoms include pale, gray or cyanotic skin; dyspnea, orthopnea, decreased blood pressure, cough; wheezes, crackles; nausea and vomiting; ascites; dependent, pitting edema; anxiety; confusion; jugular vein distention; fatigue, S3 gallop, tachycardia; enlarged spleen and liver, decreased urine output; weak pulse; cool, moist skin.

Cognitive Level: Analysis

33. Normal splitting of the second heart sound is associated with:
    A. inspiration.
    B. expiration.
    C. exercise state.
    D. low resting heart rate.

Correct Answer: A

Rationale: Normal or physiologic splitting of the second heart sound is associated with inspiration, due to the increased blood return to the right side of the heart, delaying closure of the pulmonic valve.

Cognitive Level: Comprehension

34. In cardiovascular assessment a "thrill" is:
    A. a murmur that is palpable.
    B. a murmur auscultated at the third intercostal space.
    C. associated with ventricular hypertrophy.
    D. palpated in the right epigatric area.

Correct Answer: A

Rationale: A thrill is a palpable murmur. It signifies turbulent blood flow and accompanies loud murmurs. The absence of a thrill does not rule out the presence of a murmur.

Cognitive Level: Knowledge

35. An S4 heart sound is:
    A. heard at the onset of atrial diastole.
    B. usually a normal finding in the elderly.
    C. heard at the end of ventricular diastole.
    D. heard best over the 2nd left intercostal space with the individual sitting upright.

Correct Answer: C

Rationale: An S4 heart sound is heard at the end of

diastole when the atria contract (atrial systole) and when the ventricle is resistant to filling. The S4 occurs just before the S1.

Cognitive Level: Comprehension

36. Which of the following statements is true regarding the apical impulse?
    A. It should be normally palpable in the anterior axillary line.
    B. It is palpable in all adults.
    C. The apical impulse occurs with the onset of diastole.
    D. Location of the apical impulse may be indicative of heart size.

Correct Answer: D

Rationale: The apical impulse is palpable in about 50% of adults. It is located in the 5th left intercostal space in the midclavicular line. Horizontal or downward displacement of the apical impulse may indicate an enlargement of the left ventricle.

Cognitive Level: Comprehension

37. A heart sound heard during the interval between the second heart sound (S2) and the next first sound (S1) is a(n):
    A. diastolic sound.
    B. systolic sound.
    C. ventricular contraction sound.
    D. atrial filling sound.

Correct Answer: A

Rationale: S2 signifies the onset of diastole. Any sound heard between S2 and the next first heart sound (S1) is a diastolic sound. A sound heard between S1 and S2 is a systolic sound.

Cognitive Level: Comprehension

38. While auscultating over the 2nd left intercostal space, you hear S2 louder than S1. What should be your response?
    A. Ask the patient to turn on his or her left side to assess whether the S2 sound changes.
    B. Expect that the S2 sound will muffle during inspiration.
    C. Consider this a normal finding and proceed with the examination.
    D. Continue with the examination and refer the patient for additional cardiac evaluation.

Correct Answer: C

Rationale: It is normal to hear the S2 sound louder or more emphasized at the base of the heart—the 2nd right and left intercostal spaces at the sternal border. S1 should be louder or more emphasized at the apex of the heart.

Cognitive Level: Analysis

Chapter 18

Peripheral Vascular System and Lymphatic System

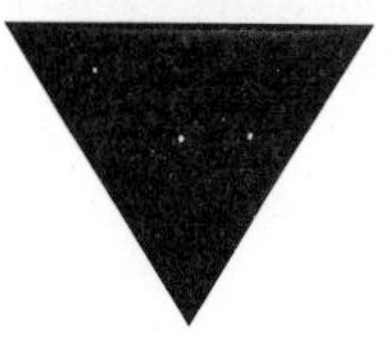

1. Which of the following statements is true regarding the arterial system?
   A. The arterial system is a high pressure system.
   B. Arteries are large diameter vessels.
   C. The walls of arteries are thinner than those of veins.
   D. Arteries can expand greatly to accommodate a large blood volume increase.

Correct Answer: A

Rationale: The pumping heart makes the arterial system a high-pressure system.

Cognitive Level: Knowledge

2. The major artery supplying the arm is the:
   A. ulnar artery.
   B. radial artery.
   C. brachial artery.
   D. deep palmar artery.

Correct Answer: C

Rationale: The major artery supplying the arm is the brachial artery.

Cognitive Level: Knowledge

3. To assess the dorsalis pedis artery, you would palpate:
   A. in the groove behind the medial malleolus.
   B. lateral to the extensor tendon of the great toe.
   C. over the lateral malleolus.
   D. behind the knee.

Correct Answer: B

Rationale: The dorsalis pedis artery is located on the dorsum of the foot. Palpate just lateral to and parallel with the extensor tendon of the big toe.

Cognitive Level: Application

4. J.L., a 65-year-old male, is experiencing pain in his left calf when he exercises, which disappears after resting for a few minutes. This description is most consistent with:
   A. ischemia due to complete blockage of an artery supplying the left leg.
   B. ischemia due to partial blockage of an artery supplying the left leg.
   C. claudication due to venous abnormalities in the left leg.
   D. venous obstruction of the left leg.

Correct Answer: B

Rationale: Ischemia is a deficient supply of oxygenated arterial blood to a tissue. A partial blockage creates an insufficient supply, and the ischemia may only be apparent at exercise when oxygen needs increase.

Cognitive Level: Analysis

5. Which of the following statements best describes the mechanism(s) by which venous blood returns to the heart?
   A. Increased thoracic pressure and decreased abdominal pressure facilitate venous return to the heart.
   B. Contracting skeletal muscles milk blood distally toward the veins.
   C. Intraluminal valves ensure unidirectional flow toward the heart.
   D. The high pressure system of the heart helps to facilitate venous return.

Correct Answer: C

Rationale: Blood moves through the veins by: (1) contracting skeletal muscles that milk the blood proximally; (2) pressure gradients caused by breathing, in which inspiration makes the thoracic pressure decrease and the abdominal pressure increase; and (3) the intraluminal valves, which ensure unidirectional flow.

Cognitive Level: Comprehension

6. The veins in the arms responsible for most of the venous return are the _____ veins.

A. deep
B. superficial
C. subclavian
D. ulnar

Correct Answer: B

Rationale: The superficial veins of the arms are in the subcutaneous tissue and are responsible for most of the venous return.

Cognitive Level: Knowledge

7. A 70-year-old male is scheduled for open heart surgery. The physicians plan to use the great saphenous vein for the coronary bypass grafts. The patient asks you, "What happens to my circulation when the veins are removed?" You reply:
   A. "You will probably experience decreased circulation after the veins are removed."
   B. "Oh we have lots of veins, you won't even notice that it has been removed."
   C. "As long as the deeper veins in your leg are in good condition, this vein can be removed without harming your circulation."
   D. "Venous insufficiency is a common problem after this type of surgery."

Correct Answer: C

Rationale: As long as the femoral and popliteal veins remain intact, the superficial veins can be excised without harming the circulation.

Cognitive Level: Analysis

8. Which of the following situations best describes a person at risk for developing venous disease?
   A. A person with a 30-year, 1 PPD smoking history
   B. An elderly person taking anticoagulant medication
   C. An individual who has been hospitalized and on bedrest for 3 days
   D. A woman in her fifth month of pregnancy

Correct Answer: C

Rationale: At risk for venous disease are people who undergo prolonged standing, sitting, or bedrest. Hypercoagulable states and vein wall trauma also place the person at risk for venous disease.

Cognitive Level: Analysis

9. Which of the following statements regarding the lymphatic system is true?
   A. The flow of lymph is slow compared with that of the blood.
   B. Lymph flow is propelled by the contraction of the heart.
   C. One of the functions of the lymph is to absorb lipids from the biliary tract.
   D. Lymph vessels have no valves, so there is a free flow of lymph fluid from the tissue spaces into blood stream and back again.

Correct Answer: A

Rationale: The flow of lymph is slow compared with that of the blood.

Cognitive Level: Comprehension

10. When performing an assessment on a patient, you note the presence of an enlarged right epitrochlear lymph node. You would carefully examine which of the following areas?
   A. Ask additional history questions regarding any recent ear infections or sore throats.
   B. Carefully assess the cervical lymph nodes, checking for any enlargement.
   C. Examine the patient's lower arm and hand, checking for the presence of infection or lesions.
   D. Assess the patient's abdomen, noting any tenderness.

Correct Answer: C

Rationale: The epitrochlear nodes are located in the antecubital fossa and drain the hand and lower arm.

Cognitive Level: Application

11. W.P., a 35-year-old male, is seen in the clinic for an "infection in my left foot." Which of the following would you expect to find during your assessment of this patient?
   A. Enlarged and tender inguinal nodes
   B. Hard and fixed cervical nodes
   C. "Pellet-like" nodes in the supraclavicular region
   D. Bilateral enlargement of the popliteal nodes

Correct Answer: A

Rationale: The inguinal nodes in the groin drain most of the lymph of the lower extremity. With local inflammation, the nodes in that area become swollen and tender.

Cognitive Level: Application

12. Which of the following would be considered a normal finding when assessing the lymphatic system of a healthy 3-year-old child?
    A. Excessive swelling and hyperplasia of the lymph nodes
    B. The presence of palpable lymph nodes
    C. Fewer numbers and a decrease in size of lymph nodes when compared to an adult
    D. No nodes palpable due to the immature immune system of a child

Correct Answer: B

Rationale: Lymph nodes are relatively large in children, and the superficial ones often are palpable even when the child is healthy.

Cognitive Level: Application

13. Which of the following is a normal physiologic change associated with the aging process?
    A. Hormonal changes causing vasodilation and a resulting drop in blood pressure
    B. Narrowing of the inferior vena cava causing low blood flow and increases in venous pressure resulting in varicosities
    C. Peripheral blood vessels growing more rigid with age producing a rise in systolic blood pressure
    D. Progressive atrophy of the intramuscular calf veins causing venous insufficiency

Correct Answer: C

Rationale: Peripheral blood vessels grow more rigid with age, resulting in a rise in systolic blood pressure.

Cognitive Level: Comprehension

14. A 67-year-old patient states that he recently began to develop pain in his left calf when climbing the 10 stairs to his apartment. This pain is relieved by sitting for about 2 minutes; then he is able to resume his activities. This patient is most likely experiencing:
    A. muscle cramps related to musculoskeletal problems.
    B. sore muscles from overexertion.
    C. venous insufficiency.
    D. claudication.

Correct Answer: D

Rationale: Intermittent claudication feels like a "cramp," usually relieved by rest within 2 minutes.

Cognitive Level: Analysis

15. A patient complains of leg pain that wakes him at night. He states that he "has been having problems" with his legs. He develops pain in his legs when they are elevated, which disappears when he dangles them. He recently noticed "a sore" on the inner aspect of the right ankle. Based on this history information, the patient is most likely experiencing:
    A. pain related to lymphatic abnormalities.
    B. pain related to musculoskeletal abnormalities.
    C. problems related to arterial insufficiency.
    D. problems related to venous insufficiency.

Correct Answer: C

Rationale: Night leg pain is common in aging adults. It may indicate the ischemic rest pain of PVD. Alterations in arterial circulation cause pain that becomes worse with leg elevation and a decrease in pain when dangling the extremity.

Cognitive Level: Analysis

16. The "profile sign" is used to detect:
    A. insufficient capillary refill.
    B. pitting edema.
    C. symmetry of the fingers.
    D. early clubbing.

Correct Answer: D

Rationale: Use the profile sign (viewing the finger from the side) to detect early clubbing.

Cognitive Level: Comprehension

17. You are performing a well-child assessment on a 3-year-old child. The child's vital signs are normal. Capillary refill time is 5 seconds. You would:
    A. suspect the child has a venous insufficiency problem.
    B. ask the parent if the child has had frostbite in the past.
    C. consider this a delayed capillary refill time for a healthy child and investigate further.
    D. refer the child for circulatory evaluation.

Correct Answer: C

Rationale: Normal capillary refill time is less than 1-2 seconds. Note that these conditions can skew your findings: a cool room, decreased body temperature, cigarette smoking, peripheral edema, and anemia.

Cognitive Level: Analysis

18. When assessing a patient you document the left femoral pulse as 0/0-4+. Which of the following findings would you expect at the dorsalis pedis pulse?
   A. 0/0-4+
   B. 1+/0-4+
   C. 2+/0-4+
   D. 3+/0-4+

Correct Answer: A

Rationale: Pulsations are graded on a four-point scale: 0=absent; 1+=weak; 2+=normal; 3+=increased; 4+=bounding. If a pulse is absent at the femoral site, one would expect the dorsalis pedis pulse to also be absent.

Cognitive Level: Analysis

19. When performing a peripheral vascular assessment on a patient, you are unable to palpate the ulnar pulses. The patient's skin is warm and capillary refill time is normal. You would:
   A. refer the individual for further evaluation.
   B. consider this a normal finding and proceed with the PV evaluation.
   C. ask the patient if he/she has experienced any unusual cramping or tingling in his/her arm.
   D. check for the presence of claudication.

Correct Answer: B

Rationale: It is not usually necessary to palpate the ulnar pulses. The ulnar pulses are often not palpable.

Cognitive Level: Analysis

20. Which of the following pulses would most likely be seen in an individual with untreated hyperthyroidism?
   A. A weak, thready pulse
   B. An absent pulse
   C. A normal pulse
   D. A bounding pulse

Correct Answer: D

Rationale: A full, bounding pulse occurs with hyperkinetic states such as exercise, anxiety, fever, anemia, and hyperthyroidism.

Cognitive Level: Comprehension

21. An Allen's test is performed to determine whether there is a problem with which of the following?
   A. Arterial function
   B. Venous function
   C. Lymphatic drainage
   D. Capillary patency

Correct Answer: A

Rationale: An Allen test is done to determine the patency of the radial and ulnar arteries.

Cognitive Level: Comprehension

22. A patient has a positive Homan's sign. You know that a positive Homan's sign:
   A. is indicative of possible thrombophlebitis.
   B. occurs with venous insufficiency.
   C. indicates problems with arterial circulation.
   D. is seen in the presence of severe edema.

Correct Answer: A

Rationale: Calf pain on dorsiflexion of the foot is a positive Homan's sign, which occurs in about 35 percent of deep vein thrombosis. It also occurs with superficial phlebitis, Achilles tendinitis, gastrocnemius, and plantar muscle injury.

Cognitive Level: Application

23. A patient has been diagnosed with venous stasis. Which of the following are you most likely to observe?
   A. A unilateral cool foot
   B. A brownish discoloration to the skin of the lower leg
   C. Pallor of the toes and cyanosis of the nailbeds
   D. Thin, shiny atrophic skin

Correct Answer: B

Rationale: A brown discoloration occurs with chronic venous stasis due to hemosiderin deposits (a byproduct of red blood cell degradation). Pallor, cyanosis, atrophic skin, and unilateral coolness are all signs associated with arterial problems.

Cognitive Level: Application

24. When attempting to assess the femoral pulse in an obese patient, which of the following actions would be most appropriate?
   A. Have the patient assume a prone position.
   B. Ask the patient to bend his or her knees to the side in a froglike position.
   C. Listen with your stethoscope for pulsations, since it is very difficult to palpate the pulse.
   D. Press firmly against the bone with the patient in a semi-Fowler's position.

Correct Answer: B

Rationale: To help expose the femoral area, particularly in obese people, ask the person to bend his or her knees to the side in a froglike position.

Cognitive Level: Application

25. When auscultating over a patient's femoral arteries you note the presence of a bruit on the left side. You know that:
    A. bruits are often associated with venous disease.
    B. bruits occur with turbulent blood flow, indicating partial occlusion.
    C. hypermetabolic states will cause bruits in the femoral arteries.
    D. bruits occur in the presence of lymphadenopathy.

Correct Answer: B

Rationale: A bruit occurs with turbulent blood flow, indicating partial occlusion of the artery.

Cognitive Level: Comprehension

26. How would you document mild, slight pitting edema present at the ankles of a pregnant patient?
    A. 1+/0-4+
    B. 3+/0-4+
    C. 4+/0-4+
    D. edema present

Correct Answer: A

Rationale: If pitting edema is present, grade it on a scale of 1+(mild) to 4+(severe).

Cognitive Level: Application

27. A patient has pitting edema of the left foot and ankle. You know that:
    A. pitting edema often occurs with venous insufficiency.
    B. alterations in arterial function will cause pitting edema.
    C. longstanding lymphatic obstruction will cause pitting edema.
    D. phlebitis of a superficial vein will cause bilateral edema.

Correct Answer: A

Rationale: Unilateral edema occurs with occlusion of a deep vein and unilaterally with lymphatic obstruction. With these factors, it is nonpitting and feels hard to the touch. Chronic venous problems produce edema.

Cognitive Level: Application

28. When assessing a patient's pulse you note that the amplitude is weaker during inspiration, and stronger during expiration. When measuring the blood pressure, the reading decreases 20 mm Hg during inspiration and increases with expiration. This patient is experiencing:
    A. pulsus bisferiens.
    B. pulsus alternans.
    C. pulsus paradoxus.
    D. pulsus bigeminus.

Correct Answer: C

Rationale: Beats have a weaker amplitude with inspiration, stronger with expiration. It is best determined during blood pressure measurement; reading decreases (>10 mm Hg) during inspiration and increases with expiration.

Cognitive Level: Analysis

29. You are performing a peripheral vascular assessment on a bedridden patient. You note the following findings in the right leg: increased warmth, swelling, redness, tenderness to palpation, and a positive Homan's sign. You would:
    A. consider this a normal finding for a bedridden patient.
    B. re-evaluate the patient in a few hours.
    C. ask the patient to raise his leg off of the bed and check for pain on elevation.
    D. seek emergent referral due to the risk of pulmonary embolism.

Correct Answer: D

Rationale: Increased warmth, swelling, redness, and tenderness requires emergency referral due to risk of pulmonary embolism.

Cognitive Level: Analysis

30. You have elevated a patient's legs 12 inches off the table and have had him wiggle his feet to drain off venous blood. Now you have helped him to sit up and dangle his legs over the side of the table. A normal finding at this point would be:
    A. marked elevational pallor.
    B. venous filling within 15 seconds.
    C. color returning to the feet within 20 seconds of assuming a sitting position.
    D. pain in the feet and lower legs when assuming a sitting position.

Correct Answer: B

Rationale: In this test it normally takes 10 seconds or less for the color to return to the feet and 15 seconds for the veins of the feet to fill.

Cognitive Level: Application

31. An individual has bilateral pitting edema of the feet. In your assessment of the peripheral vascular system, the primary focus should be:
    A. arterial function of the lower extremities.
    B. venous function of the lower extremities.
    C. oxygenation of the lower extremities.
    D. possible thrombophlebitis of the lower extremities.

Correct Answer: B

Rationale: Bilateral pitting edema of the lower extremities occurs with heart failure, venous disease, or lymphatic obstruction.

Cognitive Level: Analysis

32. Which of the following is a true statement regarding the manual compression test?
    A. The test assesses whether the valves of varicosity are competent when the person is in the supine position.
    B. Competent valves in the veins will transmit a wave to the distal fingers.
    C. A palpable wave transmission occurs when the valves are incompetent.
    D. Rapid filling of the veins indicates incompetent veins.

Correct Answer: C

Rationale: With the manual compression test, a palpable wave transmission occurs when the valves are incompetent.

Cognitive Level: Application

33. When performing the Trendelenburg test, which of the following findings is a normal finding?
    A. There is evidence of rapid filling of the veins from above.
    B. The saphenous veins fill slowly from below in about 30 seconds.
    C. Venous filling occurs in the upper thigh first, then the lower leg.
    D. A palpable wave is transmitted from one hand to the other.

Correct Answer: B

Rationale: With the Trendelenburg test, the individual assumes a supine position, the involved leg is elevated 90 degrees until the veins empty, and a tourniquet is placed on the thigh. The nurse watches for venous filling when the individual stands. Normally, the saphenous veins should fill slowly from below in about 30 seconds.

Cognitive Level: Application

34. Which of the following statements is true regarding assessment of the Ankle-Brachial Index (ABI)?
    A. The ABI is a reliable measurement of peripheral vascular disease in diabetic individuals.
    B. The normal ankle pressure is slightly lower than the brachial pressure.
    C. Normal ABI indices are from 0.50 to 1.0.
    D. An ABI of 0.90 to 0.70 indicates the presence of peripheral vascular disease and mild claudication.

Correct Answer: D

Rationale: Use of the Doppler stethoscope is a noninvasive way to determine the extent of peripheral vascular disease. The normal ankle pressure is slightly greater than or equal to the brachial pressure. An ABI of 0.90 to 0.70 indicates the presence of peripheral vascular disease and mild claudication.

Cognitive Level: Application

35. You are performing a well child check on Johnny Jones, age 5. He has no current history that would lead you to suspect illness. His past medical history is unremarkable. He did receive immunizations 1 week ago. Which of the following findings would be considered normal in this situation?
    A. Palpable firm, small, shotty, mobile, nontender lymph nodes
    B. Enlarged, warm, tender nodes
    C. Lymphadenopathy of the cervical nodes
    D. Firm, rubbery, large nodes, somewhat fixed to the underlying tissue

Correct Answer: A

Rationale: Palpable lymph nodes are often normal in children and infants. They are small, firm, shotty, mobile, and nontender. Vaccinations can produce lymphadenopathy. Enlarged, warm, tender nodes indicate current infection.

Cognitive Level: Analysis

Chapter 19

Abdomen

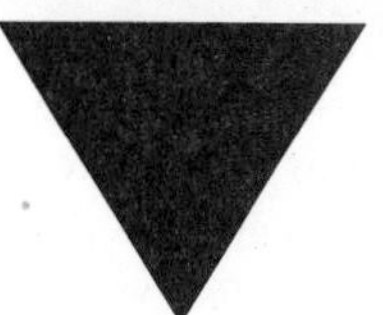

1. Tenderness on light palpation in the RLQ could indicate a disorder of the:
   A. spleen.
   B. sigmoid.
   C. gallbladder.
   D. appendix.

Correct Answer: D

Rationale: The appendix is located in the right lower quadrant, and tenderness upon light palpation may indicate an inflammation.

Cognitive Level: Comprehension

2. It would be normal to elicit a _____ percussion note in the 7th RICS at the MCL because this is the location of the __________.
   A. dull, liver
   B. dull, heart
   C. tympanic, stomach
   D. resonant, lung

Correct Answer: A

Rationale: The liver is located in the RUQ and would elicit a dull percussion note.

Cognitive Level: Application

3. Which structure would not be located in the RUQ of the abdomen?
   A. Sigmoid colon
   B. Liver
   C. Duodenum
   D. Gallbladder

Correct Answer: A

Rationale: The sigmoid colon is located in the left lower quadrant of the abdomen.

Cognitive Level: Comprehension

4. Ms. S. is having difficulty swallowing her medications and her food. In your charting, you would say that Ms. S. is experiencing:
   A. aphasia.
   B. dysphasia.
   C. dysphagia.
   D. myophagia.

Correct Answer: C

Rationale: Dysphagia is a condition that occurs with disorders of the throat or esophagus, and results in difficulty swallowing.

Cognitive Level: Application

5. You are suspicious that Mrs. B. has a distended bladder. How would you assess for this condition?
   A. Inspect and palpate in the epigastric region.
   B. Auscultate and percuss in the inguinal region.
   C. Percuss and palpate in the hypogastric region.
   D. Percuss and palpate in the lumbar region.

Correct Answer: C

Rationale: Dull percussion sounds would be elicited over a distended bladder, and the hypogastric area would seem firm to palpation.

Cognitive Level: Application

6. A change that may occur in the gastrointestinal system of an elderly patient is:
   A. increased salivation.
   B. decreased gastric acid secretion.
   C. enhanced esophageal emptying.
   D. decreased peristalsis.

Correct Answer: B

Rationale: During aging salivation decreases, esophageal emptying is delayed, and peristalsis is thought to remain fairly constant throughout life. Decreased peristalsis may be due to decreased bulk in diet, decreased fluid intake, or laxative abuse.

Cognitive Level: Comprehension

7. B.T. comes to the clinic for an examination after falling off his motorcycle and landing on his left side on the handlebars. You suspect that he may have injured his spleen. Which of the following is not true in regards to assessment of the spleen?
   A. The spleen must be enlarged three times its normal size to be felt.
   B. The spleen is located in the LUQ of the abdomen.
   C. The spleen can be enlarged with mononucleosis and trauma.
   D. Thoroughly palpating the enlarged spleen is appropriate and necessary for a complete assessment.

Correct Answer: D

Rationale: If you feel an enlarged spleen, refer the person but do not continue to palpate it. An enlarged spleen is friable and can rupture easily with overpalpation.

Cognitive Level: Application

8. An abdomen that is bulging and stretched in appearance is described as:
   A. rounded.
   B. herniated.
   C. scaphoid.
   D. protuberant.

Correct Answer: D

Rationale: Refer to illustration in chapter.

Cognitive Level: Knowledge

9. A scaphoid contour of the abdomen depicts:
   A. a convex profile to the horizontal plane.
   B. a concave profile to the horizontal plane.
   C. a flat profile to the horizontal plane.
   D. a bulging profile to the horizontal plane.

Correct Answer: B

Rationale: Contour describes the profile of the abdomen from the rib margin to the pubic bone, and scaphoid contour is one that is concave from a horizontal plane.

Cognitive Level: Application

10. While examining a patient you observe abdominal pulsations between the xiphoid and umbilicus. You would suspect that this is:
   A. increased peristalsis due to a bowel obstruction.
   B. normal abdominal aortic pulsations.
   C. pulsations of the renal arteries.
   D. pulsations of the inferior vena cava.

Correct Answer: B

Rationale: Normally, you may see the pulsations from the aorta beneath the skin in the epigastric area, particularly in thin persons with good muscle wall relaxation.

Cognitive Level: Application

11. Which of the following would be classed as a symptom?
   A. Striae
   B. Dysphagia
   C. Ascites
   D. Cyanosis

Correct Answer: B

Rationale: Dysphagia occurs with disorders of the throat or esophagus, and is related to difficulty swallowing. The patient would have to tell you that he/she was having difficulty swallowing, making this a symptom.

Cognitive Level: Application

12. The main reason auscultation precedes percussion and palpation of the abdomen is:
   A. to allow the patient more time to relax and, therefore, be more comfortable with the physical examination.
   B. to prevent distortion of vascular sounds such as bruits and hums that might occur after percussion and palpation.
   C. to prevent distortion of bowel sounds that might occur after percussion and palpation.
   D. to determine areas of tenderness before employing percussion and palpation.

Correct Answer: C

Rationale: This is done because percussion and palpation can increase peristalsis, which would give a false interpretation of bowel sounds.

Cognitive Level: Application

13. Which of the following is true of bowel sounds?
   A. They are usually loud, high-pitched, rushing, tinkling sounds.
   B. They originate from the movement of air and fluid through the large intestine.
   C. They sound like "two pieces of leather being rubbed together."
   D. They may be absent following abdominal

surgery or with inflammation of the peritoneum.

Correct Answer: D

Rationale: Hypoactive bowel sounds signal decreased motility due to inflammation as seen with peritonitis from paralytic ileus following abdominal surgery, or from bowel obstruction.

Cognitive Level: Knowledge

14. Borborygmi could best be described as:
    A. a loud continuous hum.
    B. a peritoneal friction rub.
    C. hyperactive bowel sounds.
    D. hypoactive bowel sounds.

Correct Answer: C

Rationale: Borborygmi is the term used for hyperperistalsis when the person/patient actually feels his/her stomach growling.

Cognitive Level: Comprehension

15. Which of the following is a normal finding in the abdominal assessment?
    A. The presence of a bruit in the femoral area
    B. A palpable spleen between the 9th and 11th ribs in LMAL
    C. A dull percussion note in the LUQ at the MCL
    D. A tympanic percussion note in the umbilical region

Correct Answer: D

Rationale: Tympany should predominate in all four quadrants of the abdomen because air in the intestines rises to the surface when the person is supine.

Cognitive Level: Comprehension

16. Mrs. T. is complaining of morning sickness, pyrosis, and constipation. You know that these are caused by:
    A. HBG, gastrointestinal reflux, and increased water absorption in the colon.
    B. HCR, pyrogastro subflex, and increased peristaltic movement.
    C. HCG, esophageal reflux, and increased water absorption from the colon.
    D. HCG, retrogastric influx, and increased sodium absorption from the colon.

Correct Answer: C

Rationale: Morning sickness may be due to production of human chorionic gonadotropin (hCG), heartburn (pyrosis) caused by esophageal reflux, and constipation caused by decreased motility and more water reabsorbed from the colon.

Cognitive Level: Analysis

17. Percussion notes heard during the abdominal assessment may include:
    A. resonance, hyperresonance, and flatness.
    B. tympany, hyperresonance, and dullness.
    C. resonance, dullness, and tympany.
    D. flatness, resonance, and dullness.

Correct Answer: B

Rationale: Percussion notes normally heard during the abdominal assessment may include tympany, which should predominate because air in the intestines rises to the surface when the person is supine; hyperresonance may be present with gaseous distension, and dullness may be palpated over a distended bladder, enlarged spleen or liver.

Cognitive Level: Comprehension

18. Mrs. P., a 90-year-old female, has been diagnosed with pernicious anemia. You know that this could be related to:
    A. decreased gastric acid secretion.
    B. increased gastric acid secretion.
    C. delayed gastrointestinal emptying time.
    D. increased gastrointestinal emptying time.

Correct Answer: A

Rationale: Gastric acid secretion decreases with aging, and this may cause pernicious anemia (because it interferes with vitamin B-12 absorption), iron deficiency anemia, and malabsorption of calcium.

Cognitive Level: Application

19. Mr. T. is complaining of tenderness along the costovertebral angles. This is most often indicative of:
    A. liver enlargement.
    B. spleen enlargement.
    C. kidney inflammation.
    D. ovary infection.

Correct Answer: C

Rationale: Tenderness along the CVA occurs with inflammation of the kidney or paranephric area.

Cognitive Level: Application

20. Which of the following is the cause of ascites?
    A. Flatus
    B. Feces
    C. Fluid
    D. Fibroid tumors

Correct Answer: C

Rationale: Ascites occurs with congestive heart failure, portal hypertension, cirrhosis, hepatitis, pancreatitis, and cancer.

Cognitive Level: Knowledge

21. Deep palpation is used to determine:
    A. organomegaly.
    B. overall impression of skin surface and superficial musculature.
    C. bowel motility.
    D. superficial tenderness.

Correct Answer: A

Rationale: With deep palpation, note the location, size, consistency, and mobility of any palpable organs and the presence of any abnormal enlargement, tenderness, or masses.

Cognitive Level: Comprehension

22. D.B. comes to your clinic complaining of abdominal tenderness. You know that during your examination you would not be focusing on examination of:
    A. local inflammation.
    B. inflammation of the peritoneum.
    C. an enlarged organ whose capsule is stretched.
    D. enlarged epitrochlear nodes.

Correct Answer: D

Rationale: Epitrochlear nodes are located between the triceps and biceps in the arm. Tenderness occurs with local inflammation of the peritoneum or underlying organ, and with an enlarged organ whose capsule is stretched.

Cognitive Level: Application

23. Tenderness on light palpation in the RLQ could indicate a disorder of which of the following structures?
    A. Spleen
    B. Sigmoid
    C. Gallbladder
    D. Appendix

Correct Answer: D

Rationale: The appendix is located in the RLQ and when the iliopsoas muscle is inflamed (which occurs with an inflamed or perforated appendix), pain is felt in the right lower quadrant.

Cognitive Level: Application

24. Which of the following statements is not true of the aging adult?
    A. The abdominal musculature is thinner.
    B. The abdominal tone is decreased.
    C. The abdominal rigidity with acute abdominal conditions is more pronounced.
    D. The abdominal complaints of pain are usually fewer.

Correct Answer: C

Rationale: Abdominal rigidity with acute abdominal conditions is less common in aging persons.

Cognitive Level: Application

25. In the newborn, pyloric stenosis is manifested by:
    A. hypoactive bowel activity.
    B. pronounced peristaltic waves crossing from right to left.
    C. projectile vomiting.
    D. palpable olive-sized mass in RLQ.

Correct Answer: C

Rationale: Marked peristalsis together with projectile vomiting in the newborn suggests pyloric stenosis. After feeding, pronounced peristaltic waves cross from left to right, leading to projectile vomiting. One can also palpate an olive-sized mass in the RUQ.

Cognitive Level: Application

26. To detect diastasis recti abdominous, you should have the patient perform which of the following maneuvers?
    A. Relax in the supine position.
    B. Raise arms in the left lateral position.
    C. Raise arms over the head while supine.
    D. Raise the head and shoulders while remaining supine.

Correct Answer: D

Rationale: Diastasis recti is a separation of the abdominal rectus muscles, which can occur congenitally, as a result of pregnancy, or marked obesity. This is assessed by having the patient raise the head and shoulders while remaining supine.

Cognitive Level: Application

27. Which of the following statements would not be true of aortic aneurysms?
    A. You will hear a bruit.
    B. More than 95 percent are located below the umbilicus.
    C. Femoral pulses are decreased.
    D. Aortic aneurysms may rupture.

Correct Answer: B

Rationale: Most aortic aneurysms (more than 95 percent) are located below the renal arteries and extend to the umbilicus. You will hear a bruit. Femoral pulses are present but decreased.

Cognitive Level: Comprehension

28. You suspect that Ms. W. is suffering from appendicitis. Which of the following procedures would not be helpful in assessing for appendicitis?
    A. Murphy's sign
    B. Rebound tenderness
    C. Obturator test
    D. Iliopsoas muscle test

Correct Answer: A

Rationale: Murphy's sign is used to assess for an inflamed gallbladder or cholecystitis.

Cognitive Level: Analysis

29. The test utilized to assess for inflammation of the gallbladder or cholecystitis is:
    A. Murphy's sign.
    B. rebound tenderness.
    C. iliopsoas muscle test.
    D. obturator test.

Correct Answer: A

Rationale: Normally, palpating the liver causes no pain. In a person with inflammation of the gallbladder or cholecystitis, pain occurs as the descending liver pushes the inflamed gallbladder onto the examining hand during inspiration. The person feels sharp pain and abruptly stops inspiration midway.

Cognitive Level: Knowledge

30. Mrs. O. brings her newborn in for a check-up and asks you to teach her about the umbilical cord. You would tell her:
    A. at birth, the cord is a bluish color.
    B. it contains two veins and one artery.
    C. it falls off by 10-14 days.
    D. in girls, the cord is approximately 10 inches longer at birth.

Correct Answer: C

Rationale: At birth, the umbilical cord is white and contains two umbilical arteries and one vein inside the Warton's jelly. The umbilical stump dries within a week, hardens, and falls off by 10 to 14 days.

Cognitive Level: Application

31. Which of the following percussion findings would be found in a patient with a large amount of ascites?
    A. Tympany in the right and left lower quadrants
    B. Hyperresonance in the LUQ
    C. Flatness in the RUQ
    D. Dullness across the abdomen

Correct Answer: D

Rationale: The presence of fluid causes a dull sound to percussion. A large amount of ascitic fluid would produce a dull sound to percussion.

Cognitive Level: Comprehension

32. M.J., a 40-year-old male, states that his doctor told him that he has a hernia. He asks you to briefly explain what a hernia is. Which course of action should you take?
    A. Refer him to his physician for additional consultation, since he or she made the initial diagnosis.
    B. Explain that a hernia is a loop of bowel protruding through a weak spot in the muscles of the abdomen.
    C. Explain that hernias that occur in adulthood are often the result of prenatal growth abnormalities.
    D. Tell M.J. not to worry, that most men his age develop hernias.

Correct Answer: B

Rationale: A hernia is a protrusion of the abdominal viscera through an abnormal opening in the muscle wall.

Cognitive Level: Application

33. Mr. Jones is 45 years old and has come to the clinic for an abdominal assessment. Upon percussion, you note an area of dullness above the right costal margin of about 10 cm. You would:
    A. consider this a normal finding and proceed with the examination.
    B. describe this as an enlarged liver and refer him to a physician.
    C. document the presence of hepatomegaly.
    D. ask additional history questions regarding his alcohol intake.

Correct Answer: A

Rationale: The average liver span in the midclavicular line is 6-12 cm. Men and taller individuals are at the upper end of this range. Women and shorter individuals are at the lower end of this range. A liver span of 10 cm is within normal limits for this individual.

Cognitive Level: Analysis

34. When palpating the abdomen of a 20-year-old female patient, you note the presence of tenderness in the LUQ with deep palpation. Which of the following structures is most likely to be involved?
    A. Appendix
    B. Spleen
    C. Sigmoid
    D. Gallbladder

Correct Answer: B

Rationale: The spleen is located in LUQ of the abdomen.

Cognitive Level: Application

Chapter 20

Musculoskeletal System

1. Mr. I. is being assessed for range of joint movement. You ask him to move his arm in towards the center of his body. This movement is called:
   A. flexion.
   B. extension.
   C. adduction.
   D. abduction.

Correct Answer: C

Rationale: Moving a limb toward the midline of the body is called adduction; abduction is moving a limb away from the midline of the body.

Cognitive Level: Application

2. Mrs. P. tells you that she is having a hard time bringing her hand to her mouth. You know that in order for her to move her hand to her mouth, she must perform the following movement:
   A. flexion.
   B. extension.
   C. adduction.
   D. abduction.

Correct Answer: A

Rationale: Flexion, or bending a limb at a joint, would be required to move your hand to your mouth.

Cognitive Level: Application

3. The functional units of the musculoskeletal system are the:
   A. muscles.
   B. bones.
   C. joints.
   D. tendons.

Correct Answer: C

Rationale: Joints are the functional units of the musculoskeletal system because they permit the mobility needed for activities of daily living.

Cognitive Level: Knowledge

4. Hematopoiesis takes place in the:
   A. kidneys.
   B. liver.
   C. spleen.
   D. bone marrow.

Correct Answer: D

Rationale: The musculoskeletal system functions to encase and protect inner vital organs, supports the body, produces red blood cells in the bone marrow, and stores minerals.

Cognitive Level: Application

5. Fibrous bands running directly from one bone to another that strengthen the joint and help prevent movement in undesirable directions are called:
   A. cartilage.
   B. bursa.
   C. tendons.
   D. ligaments.

Correct Answer: D

Rationale: Fibrous bands running directly from one bone to another that strengthen the joint and help prevent movement in undesirable directions are called ligaments.

Cognitive Level: Knowledge

6. You notice that Ms. Q. is unable to jump rope. You know that in order to jump rope, your shoulder has to be capable of:
   A. inversion.
   B. protraction.
   C. circumduction.
   D. supination.

Correct Answer: C

Rationale: Circumduction is defined as moving the arm in a circle around the shoulder.

Cognitive Level: Application

7. The articulation of the mandible and the temporal bone is the:
   A. condyle of the mandible.
   B. zygomatic arch of the temporal bone.
   C. temporomandibular joint.
   D. intervertebral foramen.

Correct Answer: C

Rationale: The articulation of the mandible and the temporal bone is the temporomandibular joint.

Cognitive Level: Comprehension

8. The temporomandibular joint can be palpated by placing the fingers in the depression:
   A. posterior to the tragus of the ear.
   B. anterior to the tragus of the ear.
   C. distal to the helix of the ear.
   D. proximal to the helix of the ear.

Correct Answer: B

Rationale: The temporomandibular joint can be felt in the depression anterior to the tragus of the ear.

Cognitive Level: Application

9. Of the 33 vertebrae in the spinal column, there are:
   A. 5 thoracic.
   B. 12 cervical.
   C. 7 sacral.
   D. 5 lumbar.

Correct Answer: D

Rationale: There are 7 cervical, 12 thoracic, 5 lumbar, 5 sacral, and 304 coccygeal vertebrae.

Cognitive Level: Comprehension

10. An imaginary line connecting the highest point on each iliac crest would cross:
   A. the 12th thoracic vertebra.
   B. the 7th cervical vertebra.
   C. the 4th lumbar vertebra.
   D. the 1st sacral vertebra.

Correct Answer: C

Rationale: An imaginary line connecting the highest point on each iliac crest crosses the 4th lumbar vertebra.

Cognitive Level: Comprehension

11. You are explaining to Mr. B. that there are "shock absorbers" in his back to cushion the spine and to help it move. You are referring to his:
   A. nucleus pulposus.
   B. vertebral foramen.
   C. intervertebral discs.
   D. costal facets.

Correct Answer: C

Rationale: Intervertebral discs are elastic fibrocartilaginous plates that cushion the spine like shock absorbers and help it move.

Cognitive Level: Application

12. Mr. R. has been diagnosed with a rotator cuff injury and has been sent to you for patient education. You would tell him that a rotator cuff injury involves:
   A. the medial epicondyle.
   B. the glenohumoral joint.
   C. the articular process.
   D. nucleus pulposus.

Correct Answer: B

Rationale: A rotator cuff injury involves the glenohumeral joint, which is enclosed by a group of four powerful muscles and tendons that support and stabilize it.

Cognitive Level: Application

13. Mrs. B. comes in for an evaluation and states, "I can feel this bump on the top of both of my shoulders—it doesn't hurt but I am curious about what it might be." You would tell her:
   A. "That is your subacromial bursa."
   B. "That is the greater tubercle of your humerus."
   C. "That is your acromion process."
   D. "That is your glenohumeral joint."

Correct Answer: C

Rationale: You can feel the bump of the scapula's acromion process at the very top of the shoulder.

Cognitive Level: Application

14. The wrist is capable of the following movements:
   A. flexion, extension, supination, and pronation.
   B. flexion, extension, inversion, and eversion.
   C. elevation, depression, inversion, and eversion.
   D. elevation, depression, supination, and pronation.

Correct Answer: A

Rationale: The wrist joint is capable of flexion, extension, supination, and pronation (Figure 20-10).

Cognitive Level: Comprehension

15. Mr. C. comes to you for an evaluation of a swollen knuckle—you notice that the knuckle above his ring on the left hand is swollen and he is unable to remove his wedding ring. This joint is called the:
    A. interphalangeal joint.
    B. metacarpophalangeal joint.
    C. tarsometatarsal joint.
    D. talocalcaneonavicular joint.

Correct Answer: B

Rationale: Figure 20-10.

Cognitive Level: Application

16. You are assessing Mr. O.'s ischial tuberosity. In order to palpate the ischial tuberosity, it is best to:
    A. have the person stand.
    B. have the person flex his hip.
    C. have the person flex his knee.
    D. have the person in the supine position.

Correct Answer: B

Rationale: The ischial tuberosity lies under the gluteus maximus muscle, and is palpable when the hip is flexed.

Cognitive Level: Application

17. The knee joint is the articulation of the femur, the tibia, and the:
    A. fibula.
    B. patella.
    C. radius.
    D. humerus.

Correct Answer: B

Rationale: The knee joint is the articulation of three bones, including the femur, the tibia, and the patella (kneecap) in one common articular cavity.

Cognitive Level: Knowledge

18. The ankle joint is the articulation of the tibia, fibula, and the:
    A. calcaneus.
    B. cuboid.
    C. talus.
    D. talocalcaneonavicular joint.

Correct Answer: C

Rationale: The ankle or tibiotalar joint is the articulation of the tibia, fibula, and talus.

Cognitive Level: Knowledge

19. You are explaining the mechanism of the growth of long bones to Mrs. R. You know that bones increase in width or diameter by deposition of new bony tissue around the shafts. You also know that lengthening occurs at the:
    A. bursa.
    B. epiphyses.
    C. calcaneus.
    D. tuberosities.

Correct Answer: B

Rationale: Long bones grow in two dimensions: first in width or diameter by deposition of new bony tissue around the shafts. Lengthening occurs at the epiphyses, or growth plates.

Cognitive Level: Comprehension

20. Mrs. T. is 8 months pregnant and she is complaining of a change in posture and lower back pain. You tell her that during pregnancy, women have a posture shift to compensate for the enlarging fetus. This shift in posture is called:
    A. scoliosis.
    B. ankylosis.
    C. kyphosis.
    D. lordosis.

Correct Answer: D

Rationale: Lordosis compensates for the enlarging fetus, which would shift the center of balance forward. This shift is balance in turn creates strain on the low back muscles, felt as low back pain during late pregnancy in some women.

Cognitive Level: Application

21. Mr. P., a 90-year-old gentleman, comes to you for information on why he seems to be getting shorter as he ages. You would explain that decreased height occurs with aging because:
    A. long bones tend to shorten with age.
    B. there is a thickening of the intervertebral discs.
    C. there is a significant loss of subcutaneous fat.
    D. of the shortening of the vertebral column.

Correct Answer: D

Rationale: Postural changes are evident with aging, and decreased height is most noticeable, and is due to shortening of the vertebral column.

Cognitive Level: Application

22. Osteoporosis can be defined as:
    A. loss of bone matrix.
    B. new, weaker bone growth.
    C. loss of bone density.
    D. increased phagocytic activity.

Correct Answer: C

Rationale: Osteoporosis is the loss of bone density.

Cognitive Level: Knowledge

23. M.O. is a 28-year-old jogger who is complaining of increased foot problems while running. You know that in this cultural group, M.O. has a high chance of having:
    A. convex anterior curvature of the femur.
    B. 25 vertebrae.
    C. a second toe that is longer than the great toe.
    D. a missing peroneus teritus.

Correct Answer: C

Rationale: Table 20-1.

Cognitive Level: Application

24. The muscle responsible for wrist flexion, and absent in 12 to 20 percent of all whites, is the:
    A. palmaris longus.
    B. peroneus tertius.
    C. lateral meniscus.
    D. talocalcaneal interosseous.

Correct Answer: A

Rationale: Table 20-1.

Cognitive Level: Application

25. K.P. has arrived complaining of pain in her left wrist. She has been playing basketball and fell, landing on her left hand. You examine her hand, and expect a fracture if:
    A. she complains of a dull ache.
    B. she complains that the pain in her wrist is deep.
    C. she complains of sharp pain that increases with movement.
    D. she complains of dull throbbing pain that increases with rest.

Correct Answer: C

Rationale: A fracture causes sharp pain that increases with movement.

Cognitive Level: Analysis

26. M.Y. is complaining of pain in his joints that is worse in the morning, is better after he has moved around for awhile, and then gets worse again if he sits for long periods of time. You suspect that M.Y. may have:
    A. tendinitis.
    B. osteoarthritis.
    C. intermittent claudication.
    D. rheumatoid arthritis.

Correct Answer: D

Rationale: Rheumatoid arthritis (RA) is worse in the morning when the person gets up. Movement increases most joint pain except in RA, in which movement decreases pain.

Cognitive Level: Analysis

27. V.P. states that "she can hear a crunching or grating sound when she kneels." She also states that "it is very difficult to get out of bed in the morning because of stiffness and pain in her joints." You suspect that the sound she hears is:
    A. crepitation.
    B. a tendon or ligament slipping over bone when she kneels.
    C. a small amount of fluid in the knee joint.
    D. a bone spur on the patella.

Correct Answer: A

Rationale: Crepitation is an audible and palpable crunching or grating that accompanies movement and occurs when articular surfaces in the joints are roughened as with rheumatoid arthritis.

Cognitive Level: Analysis

28. Mr. P. is able to flex his right arm forward without difficulty or pain, but is unable to abduct his arm because of pain and muscle spasms, and you suspect:
    A. rotator cuff lesions.
    B. rheumatoid arthritis.
    C. crepitation.
    D. dislocated shoulder.

Correct Answer: A

Rationale: Rotator cuff lesions may cause limited range of motion and pain and muscle spasm during abduction, whereas forward flexion stays fairly normal.

Cognitive Level: Analysis

29. C.G., a professional tennis player, comes in complaining of a sore elbow. You suspect that he has tenderness at:
    A. the medial and lateral epicondyle.
    B. the base of the radius.
    C. the olecranon bursa.
    D. annular ligament.

Correct Answer: A

Rationale: Epicondyle, head of radius, and tendons are common sites of inflammation and local tenderness, or "tennis elbow."

Cognitive Level: Analysis

30. You suspect that M.B. has carpal tunnel syndrome, and so you ask her to perform the phalen's test. To perform this test, M.B. would:
    A. dorsiflex her foot.
    B. hyperextend her wrists, with the palmar surface of both hands touching and wait for 60 seconds.
    C. hold both hands back to back while flexing the wrists 90 degrees for 60 seconds.
    D. plantarflex her foot.

Correct Answer: C

Rationale: Ask the person to hold both hands back to back while flexing the wrists 90 degrees.

Cognitive Level: Application

31. Mrs. P., an 80-year-old female, comes to your clinic for a check-up. You are looking for motor dysfunction in her hip and so you would have her:
    A. abduct her hip while she is lying on her back.
    B. adduct her hip while she is lying on her back.
    C. internally rotate her hip while she is sitting.
    D. externally rotate her hip while she is standing.

Correct Answer: A

Rationale: Limitation of abduction of the hip while supine is the most common motion dysfunction found in hip disease.

Cognitive Level: Analysis

32. You have completed your musculoskeletal examination, and have found a positive bulge sign. You suspect:
    A. soft tissue swelling in the joint.
    B. swelling from fluid in the suprapatellar pouch.
    C. irregular bony margins.
    D. swelling from fluid in the epicondyle.

Correct Answer: B

Rationale: For swelling in the suprapatellar pouch, the bulge sign confirms the presence of fluid.

Cognitive Level: Analysis

33. You are examining Mr. O., and when you ask him to bend forward from the waist, you notice lateral tilting and when you raise his leg straight up, he complains of a pain going down his buttock into his leg. You suspect:
    A. meniscus tear.
    B. herniated nucleus pulposus.
    C. scoliosis.
    D. spasm of paravertebral muscles.

Correct Answer: B

Rationale: Lateral tilting and forward bending occur with a herniated nucleus pulposus.

Cognitive Level: Analysis

34. You are examining 3-month-old baby J., and you flex her knees holding your thumbs on the inner mid-thighs, and your fingers outside on the hips touching the greater trochanter, you adduct the legs until your thumbs touch and abduct the legs until the knees touch the table. You do not notice any "clunking," and so you are confident in recording a:
    A. negative Ortolani.
    B. positive Allis.
    C. positive Ortolani.
    D. negative Allis.

Correct Answer: A

Rationale: With a positive Ortolani, you will feel and hear a clunk as the head of the femur pops back into place.

Cognitive Level: Analysis

35. Baby T. has six toes on her left foot. You would record this as:
    A. syndactyly.
    B. polydactyly.

C. unidactyly.
D. multidactyly.

Correct Answer: B

Rationale: Polydactyly is the presence of extra fingers or toes.

Cognitive Level: Comprehension

36. Mrs. J. brings newborn baby P. in for her check-up, and tells you that she doesn't seem to be moving her right arm as much as her left, and that she seems to have pain when Mrs. J. lifts her up under the arms. You suspect a fractured clavicle and you would:
    A. observe for limited ROM during the Moro reflex.
    B. observe for a positive Ortolani sign.
    C. observe for a negative Allis sign.
    D. observe for limited ROM during the LaSegue's reflex.

Correct Answer: A

Rationale: Observe limited arm ROM and unilateral response to the Moro reflex.

Cognitive Level: Analysis

37. Mr. G., a 40-year-old male, has come into the clinic with complaints of "severe crushing pain in his toes, that seem to be a little swollen." His complaints would suggest:
    A. ankylosing spondylitis.
    B. degenerative joint disease.
    C. gouty arthritis.
    D. osteoporosis.

Correct Answer: C

Rationale: Gout occurs primarily in men over 40 years of age and the deposits of urate crystals in joints lead to inflammation, cartilage damage, and severe crushing pain.

Cognitive Level: Analysis

38. J.J., a young swimmer, comes to you complaining of a very sore shoulder. He was running at the pool, slipped on some wet concrete, and tried to catch himself with his outstretched hand. He landed on his outstretched hand and has not been able to move his shoulder since. You suspect:
    A. joint effusion.
    B. adhesive capsulitis.
    C. tear of rotator cuff.
    D. dislocated shoulder.

Correct Answer: D

Rationale: Dislocated shoulder occurs with trauma involving abduction, extension, and external rotation, e.g., falling on an outstretched arm or diving into a pool.

Cognitive Level: Analysis

39. B.P. has come in for an assessment of her rheumatoid arthritis, and you note raised, firm nontender nodules at the olecranon bursa and along the ulna. These nodules are most commonly diagnosed as:
    A. olecranon bursitis.
    B. gouty arthritis.
    C. subcutaneous nodules.
    D. epicondylitis.

Correct Answer: C

Rationale: Raised, firm nontender nodules occur with rheumatoid arthritis, and are in the olecranon bursa and along the extensor surface of ulna.

Cognitive Level: Analysis

40. Mrs. A. has had arthritis for years, and is starting to notice that her fingers are drifting to the side. This is commonly referred to as:
    A. ulnar deviation.
    B. radial drift.
    C. dupuytren's contracture.
    D. swan neck deformity.

Correct Answer: A

Rationale: Fingers drift to the ulnar side because of stretching of the articular capsule and muscle imbalance caused by chronic rheumatoid arthritis.

Cognitive Level: Analysis

41. P.R. complains of stiffness in the morning when rising out of bed, which improves over the course of the day with movement. She has also noticed changes in her hands. Possible changes she might report could include:
    A. heberden's nodes.
    B. swan-neck deformities.
    C. dupuytren's contractures.
    D. bouchard's nodules.

Correct Answer: B

Rationale: Conditions caused by chronic rheumatoid arthritis include swan neck and boutonniere deformities.

Cognitive Level: Analysis

42. J.S.'s annual physical examination reveals a lateral curvature of the thoracic and lumbar segments of his spine; however, this curvature disappears with forward bending. This abnormality of the spine would be called:
    A. dislocated nucleus pulposus.
    B. herniated nucleus pulposus.
    C. structural scoliosis.
    D. functional scoliosis.

Correct Answer: D

Rationale: Functional scoliosis is flexible; it is apparent with standing and disappears with forward bending.

Cognitive Level: Analysis

43. S.S., a 14-year-old male diagnosed with Osgood-Schlatter disease, reports painful swelling just below the knee x 5 months. You reply:
    A. "Your disease is due to repeated stress on the patellar tendon. It is usually self limited, and your symptoms should resolve with rest."
    B. "Increasing your activity and performing knee strengthening exercises will help to decrease the inflammation and maintain mobility in the knee."
    C. "If these symptoms persist, you may need arthroscopic surgery."
    D. "You are experiencing degeneration of your knee which may not resolve."

Correct Answer: A

Rationale: Osgood-Schlatter disease is painful swelling of the tibial tubercle just below the knee. It is most likely due to repeated stress on the patellar tendon. It is usually self limited, occurring during rapid growth and most often in males. The symptoms resolve with rest.

Cognitive Level: Application

44. When assessing muscle strength, you observed that your patient had complete range of motion against gravity with full resistance. What would you record using a 0–5+ scale?
    A. 2+
    B. 3+
    C. 4+
    D. 5+

Correct Answer: D

Rationale: Complete range of motion against gravity is normal muscle strength and is recorded as 5+ muscle strength.

Cognitive Level: Application

45. You are examining a 6-month-old baby. You place the baby's feet flat on the table and flex his knees up. You note that the right knee is significantly lower than the left. Which of the following is true of this finding?
    A. This is a normal finding for the Allis test for an infant of this age.
    B. This is a positive Allis sign and suggests hip dislocation.
    C. The infant probably has a dislocated patella on the right.
    D. The infant should return to the clinic in 2 weeks to see if this has changed.

Correct Answer: B

Rationale: Finding one knee significantly lower than the other is a positive Allis sign and suggests hip dislocation.

Cognitive Level: Analysis

46. You are assessing a 1-week-old infant and testing his muscle strength. When you lift the infant with your hands under the axillae, you note that the infant starts to "slip" between your hands. You:
    A. consider this a normal finding because the musculature of an infant this age is undeveloped.
    B. suspect that the infant may have weakness of the shoulder muscles.
    C. consider that the infant may have a deformity of the spine.
    D. suspect a fractured clavicle.

Correct Answer: B

Rationale: A baby who starts to "slip" between your hands shows weakness of the shoulder muscles.

Cognitive Level: Analysis

Chapter 21

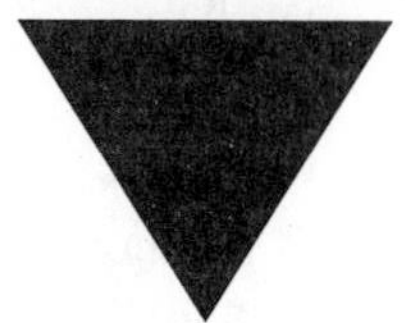

Neurologic System

1. The two parts of the nervous system are the:
   A. peripheral and autonomic.
   B. central and peripheral.
   C. hypothalamus and cerebral.
   D. motor and sensory.

Correct Answer: B

Rationale: The nervous system can be divided into two parts—central and peripheral. The central nervous system (CNS) includes the brain and spinal cord. The peripheral nervous system includes the 12 pairs of cranial nerves, the 31 pairs of spinal nerves, and all their branches.

Cognitive Level: Knowledge

2. The wife of a 65-year-old male tells you she is concerned because she has noted a change in his personality and ability to understand. He also cries and becomes angry very easily. The cerebral lobe responsible for these changes is the _____ lobe.
   A. parietal
   B. occipital
   C. temporal
   D. frontal

Correct Answer: D

Rationale: The frontal lobe has areas concerned with personality, behavior, emotions, and intellectual function.

Cognitive Level: Analysis

3. Which of the following statements is accurate concerning areas of the brain?
   A. The hypothalamus controls temperature and regulates sleep.
   B. Motor pathways of the spinal cord and brain stem synapse in the thalamus.
   C. The basal ganglia are responsible for controlling voluntary movements.
   D. The cerebellum is the center for speech and emotions.

Correct Answer: A

Rationale: The hypothalamus is a vital area with many important functions: Temperature control, sleep center, anterior and posterior pituitary gland regulator, and coordinator of autonomic nervous system activity and emotional status.

Cognitive Level: Comprehension

4. The area of the nervous system that is responsible for mediating reflexes is the:
   A. cerebellum.
   B. medulla.
   C. spinal cord.
   D. cerebral cortex.

Correct Answer: C

Rationale: It is the main highway for ascending and descending fiber tracts that connect the brain to the spinal nerves, and it mediates reflexes.

Cognitive Level: Knowledge

5. You have just pricked yourself with a sharp needle. In order for you to be able to interpret this sensation, which of the following areas must be intact?
   A. anterior spinothalamic tract, basal ganglia, and sensory cortex
   B. lateral spinothalamic tract, thalamus, and sensory cortex
   C. corticospinal tract, medulla, and basal ganglia
   D. pyramidal tract, hypothalamus, and sensory cortex

Correct Answer: B

Rationale: The spinothalamic tract contains sensory fibers that transmit the sensations of pain, temperature, and crude or light touch. Fibers carrying pain and temperature sensations ascend the lateral spinothalamic tract, whereas those of crude touch form the anterior spinothalamic tract.

At the thalamus, the fibers synapse with another sensory neuron, which carries the message to the sensory cortex for full interpretation.

Cognitive Level: Application

6. A patient with lack of oxygen to his heart will present with pain in his chest as well as shoulder, arms, or jaw. Which of the following best explains why this occurs?
   A. The lack of oxygen in his heart has resulted in decreased amount of oxygen to these areas.
   B. There is a problem with the sensory cortex and its ability to discriminate the location.
   C. The sensory cortex does not have the ability to localize pain in the heart so the pain is referred.
   D. There is a lesion in the dorsal root that is preventing the sensation from being transmitted normally.

Correct Answer: C

Rationale: The sensory cortex is arranged in a specific pattern, forming a corresponding "map" of the body. Pain in the right hand is perceived at a specific spot on the map. Some organs are absent from the brain map, such as the heart, liver, or spleen. Pain originating in these organs is referred, because no felt image exists in which to have pain. Pain is felt "by proxy" by another body part that does have a felt image.

Cognitive Level: Application

7. The ability that humans have to perform very skilled movements such as writing is controlled by the:
   A. corticospinal tract.
   B. extrapyramidal tract.
   C. basal ganglia.
   D. spinothalamic tract.

Correct Answer: A

Rationale: Corticospinal fibers mediate voluntary movement, particularly very skilled, discrete, purposeful movements, such as writing. The corticospinal tract is a newer, "higher," motor system that humans have that permits very skilled and purposeful movements.

Cognitive Level: Comprehension

8. A 30-year-old female tells you she has been very unsteady and has had difficulty maintaining her balance. Which area of the brain would you be concerned about with these findings?
   A. Extrapyramidal tract
   B. Thalamus
   C. Brain stem
   D. Cerebellum

Correct Answer: D

Rationale: This motor system coordinates movement, maintains equilibrium, and helps maintain posture.

Cognitive Level: Comprehension

9. Which of the following statements about the peripheral nervous system is correct?
   A. The peripheral nerves are inside the CNS and carry impulses via their motor fibers.
   B. The cranial nerves enter the brain via the spinal cord.
   C. The peripheral nerves carry input to the CNS by afferent fibers and away by efferent fibers.
   D. Efferent fibers carry sensory input to the CNS through the spinal cord.

Correct Answer: C

Rationale: A nerve is a bundle of fibers outside the CNS. The peripheral nerves carry input to the CNS via their sensory afferent fibers, and deliver output from the CNS via the efferent fibers.

Cognitive Level: Knowledge

10. Your patient has a severed spinal nerve due to trauma. Which of the following do you know is true?
    A. The dermatome served by this nerve will no longer experience any sensation.
    B. This will only affect motor function of the patient as spinal nerves have no sensory component.
    C. Since there are 31 pairs of spinal nerves there is no effect if only one is severed.
    D. The adjacent spinal nerves will continue to carry sensations for the dermatome served by the severed nerve.

Correct Answer: D

Rationale: A dermatome is a circumscribed skin area that is supplied mainly from one spinal cord segment through a particular spinal nerve. The dermatomes overlap, which is a form of biologic insurance. That is, if one nerve is severed most of the sensations can be transmitted by the one above and the one below.

Cognitive Level: Application

11. A 21-year-old female has a head injury secondary to trauma and is unconscious. There are no other injuries. In your assessment what would you expect to find when you test her deep tendon reflexes?
    A. You will be unable to elicit any reflexes.
    B. Reflexes will be normal.
    C. All reflexes would be diminished but present.
    D. Some would be present depending on area of injury.

Correct Answer: B

Rationale: A reflex is a defense mechanism of the nervous system. It operates below the level of conscious control and permits a quick reaction to potentially painful or damaging situations. The deep tendon or stretch reflex has five components: intact sensory nerve (afferent); functional synapse in the cord, intact motor nerve fiber (efferent); neuromuscular junction, competent muscle.

Cognitive Level: Application

12. A mother of a 1-month old asks you why it takes so long for babies to learn to roll over. What is the reason for this?
    A. Myelin is needed to conduct the impulses and the neurons of a newborn are not myelinated.
    B. The cerebral cortex is not fully developed so control over motor function occurs gradually.
    C. The spinal cord is controlling the movement because the cerebellum is not yet fully developed.
    D. There must be a demyelinating process occurring with her baby.

Correct Answer: A

Rationale: The infant's sensory and motor development proceeds along with the gradual acquisition of myelin, because myelin is needed to conduct most impulses. The process of myelinization follows a cephalocaudal and proximodistal order (head, neck, trunk, and extremities). This is just the order we observe the infant gaining motor control (lifts head, lifts head and shoulders, rolls over, moves whole arm, uses hands, walks).

Cognitive Level: Application

13. In your assessment of an 80-year-old male you note the following: inability to identify vibrations at the ankle and to identify position of big toe; decreased muscle tone in face and neck; irregular shaped pupils. All other neurologic findings are normal. What would be your assessment of these findings?
    A. Lesion in the cerebral cortex
    B. Normal changes due to aging
    C. Demyelinization of nerves due to lesion
    D. Cranial nerve dysfunction

Correct Answer: B

Rationale: The aging process causes a steady loss of neurons. Neuron loss occurs in the brain and spinal cord. It leads many people over 65 to show signs that, in the younger adult, would be considered abnormal, such as general loss of muscle bulk, loss of muscle tone in the face, neck, and around the spine, loss of vibratory sense at the ankle, loss of position sense at the big toe, loss of ankle jerk, and irregular pupil shape (Carter, 1986). As long as no other symptoms or evidence of neurologic disease is present, these signs are attributed to the expected aging process.

Cognitive Level: Analysis

14. A 70-year-old female tells you that every time she gets up in the morning or after she's been sitting she gets "really dizzy." She feels like she is going to fall over. What would be your response?
    A. "I'll refer you for a complete neurological examination."
    B. "You probably just need to drink more liquids."
    C. "Have you been extremely tired lately?"
    D. "You need to get up slowly when you've been lying or sitting."

Correct Answer: D

Rationale: Aging is accompanied by a progressive decrease in cerebral blood flow. In some people this causes dizziness and a loss of balance with position change. These people need to be taught to get up slowly.

Cognitive Level: Analysis

15. During the history, a patient tells you that "it feels like the room is spinning around me." You

would document this as:
A. dizziness.
B. vertigo.
C. syncope.
D. seizure activity.

Correct Answer: B

Rationale: True vertigo is rotational spinning caused by neurologic dysfunction or a problem in the vestibular apparatus or the vestibular nuclei in brain stem.

Cognitive Level: Application

16. When doing the history on a patient with a seizure disorder you are assessing whether they have an aura. Which of the following would be the best question for obtaining this information?
A. "Does your muscle tone seem tense or limp?"
B. "After the seizure, do you spend a lot of time sleeping?"
C. "Do you have any warning sign before your seizure starts?"
D. "Do you experience any color change or incontinence during the seizure?"

Correct Answer: C

Rationale: Aura is a subjective sensation that precedes a seizure; it could be auditory, visual or motor.

Cognitive Level: Application

17. While obtaining a history of a 3-month old from the mother, you ask about the baby's ability to suck and grasp the mother's finger. What are you assessing?
A. Reflexes
B. Cerebral cortex function
C. Cranial nerves
D. Intelligence

Correct Answer: A

Rationale: Reflexes—What have you noticed about the baby's behavior? Do the baby's sucking and swallowing seem coordinated? Does the baby grasp your finger?

Cognitive Level: Application

18. In obtaining a history on a 74-year-old patient you note the following: he drinks alcohol daily; he has noticed a tremor in his hands that affects his ability to hold things. With this information, what should your response be?
A. "You really shouldn't drink so much alcohol; it may be causing your tremor."
B. "Does the tremor change when you drink the alcohol?"
C. "Does your family know you are drinking every day?"
D. "We'll do some tests to see what is causing the tremor."

Correct Answer: B

Rationale: Senile tremor is relieved by alcohol, although this is not a recommended treatment. Assess whether the person is abusing alcohol in an effort to relieve tremor.

Cognitive Level: Analysis

19. A 50-year-old female is here for "weakness in her left arm and leg for past week." What type of neurologic examination would be appropriate?
A. Screening neurologic examination
B. Glasgow coma scale
C. Complete neurologic examination
D. Neurologic recheck examination

Correct Answer: C

Rationale: Perform a complete neurologic examination on persons who have neurologic concerns (e.g., headache, weakness, loss of coordination) or who have shown signs of neurologic dysfunction.

Cognitive Level: Application

20. During your assessment of the cranial nerves, you find the following: lack of blink in right eye with corneal reflex; intact ability to sense light touch on face; loss of movement with facial features on right side. This would indicate dysfunction of which of the following cranial nerves?
A. Motor component of V
B. Motor and sensory of XI
C. Motor of X and sensory of VII
D. Motor of VII

Correct Answer: D

Rationale: Motor function. Note mobility and facial symmetry. Loss of movement and asymmetry of movement occur with both central nervous system lesions and peripheral nervous system lesions. The corneal reflex tests the sensory afferent in cranial nerve V and the motor efferent in cranial nerve VII.

Cognitive Level: Analysis

21. You are testing the function of cranial nerve XI. Which of the following best describes the response you would expect if the nerve is intact?
    A. Sticks tongue out midline without tremors or deviation
    B. Moves head and shoulders against resistance with equal strength
    C. Follows an object with eyes without nystagmus or strabismus
    D. Demonstrates full range of motion of the neck

Correct Answer: B

Rationale: Examine the sternomastoid and trapezius muscles for equal size. Check equal strength by asking the person to rotate the head forcibly against resistance applied to the side of the chin. Then ask the person to shrug the shoulders against resistance. These movements should feel equally strong on both sides.

Cognitive Level: Application

22. During the neurologic assessment of a "healthy" 35-year-old patient you ask him to relax his muscles completely. You then move each extremity through full range of motion. Which of the following would you expect to find?
    A. Slight pain with some directions of movement
    B. Firm, rigid resistance to movement
    C. Mild, even resistance to movement
    D. Hypotonic muscles due to total relaxation

Correct Answer: C

Rationale: Tone is the normal degree of tension (contraction) in voluntarily relaxed muscles. It shows a mild resistance to passive stretch. Normally, you will note a mild, even resistance to movement.

Cognitive Level: Application

23. When you ask your 68-year-old patient to stand with feet together and arms at his side with his eyes closed, he starts to sway and moves his feet further apart. You would document this as a:
    A. negative Homan's sign.
    B. positive Romberg's sign.
    C. ataxia.
    D. lack of coordination.

Correct Answer: B

Rationale: Abnormal findings for Romberg's test: patient sways; falls; widens base of feet to avoid falling. Positive Romberg's sign is loss of balance that is increased by closing of the eyes.

Cognitive Level: Analysis

24. You are doing an assessment on a 29-year-old female here for "always dropping things and falling down." While testing rapid alternating movements you notice she is unable to pat both her knees. Her response is very slow and she misses frequently. What might you suspect?
    A. Dysfunction of the cerebellum
    B. Vestibular disease
    C. Lesion of cranial nerve IX
    D. Inability to understand directions

Correct Answer: A

Rationale: In rapid, alternating movements, slow, clumsy, and sloppy response occurs with cerebellar disease.

Cognitive Level: Analysis

25. During the history of a 78-year-old male, his wife states that he is having problems with periodic short-term memory loss and confusion: "He can't even remember how to button his shirt." In doing the assessment of his sensory system, which of the following would be most accurate?
    A. You would proceed with the explanations of each test making sure the wife understands.
    B. You would not do this part of the exam as results would not be valid.
    C. You would perform the tests knowing that mental status does not affect sensory ability.
    D. Before testing you would assess patient's mental status and ability to follow directions at this time.

Correct Answer: D

Rationale: Ensure validity of sensory system testing by making sure the person is alert, cooperative, and comfortable and has an adequate attention span. Otherwise, you may get misleading and invalid results.

Cognitive Level: Analysis

26. Your assessment of a 60-year-old patient has taken longer than you anticipated. In testing his pain perception you decide to complete test as quickly as possible. When you applied the sharp point of the pin on his arm several times, he was only able to identify these as one "very sharp

prick." What would be the most accurate explanation for this?

A. You were probably not poking hard enough with the pin in the other areas.
B. The patient most likely has analgesia in some areas of arm and hyperalgesia in others.
C. This is most likely the result of the summation effect.
D. Patient has hyperesthesia due to the aging process.

Correct Answer: C

Rationale: Let at least 2 seconds elapse between each stimulus to avoid summation. With summation, frequent consecutive stimuli are perceived as one strong stimulus.

Cognitive Level: Analysis

27. You are performing a neurologic assessment on a 41-year-old female with a history of diabetes. When testing her ability to feel the vibrations of a tuning fork you note the following: unable to feel vibrations on the great toe or ankle bilaterally; is able to feel vibrations of both patellae. Given this information, what would you suspect?

A. Hyperesthesia
B. Peripheral neuropathy
C. Inconsistent function of tuning fork
D. Lesion of sensory cortex

Correct Answer: B

Rationale: Loss of vibration sense occurs with peripheral neuropathy, e.g., diabetes and alcoholism. Peripheral neuropathy is worse at the feet and gradually improves as you move up leg, as opposed to a specific nerve lesion, which has a clear zone of deficit for its dermatome.

Cognitive Level: Analysis

28. You place a key in the hand of a patient and he identifies it as a penny. What term would you use to describe this?

A. Astereognosis
B. Graphesthesia
C. Tactile discrimination
D. Extinction

Correct Answer: A

Rationale: Stereognosis. Test the person's ability to recognize objects by feeling their forms, sizes and weights. Astereognosis—unable to identify objects correctly. Occurs in sensory cortex lesions.

Cognitive Level: Application

29. You are testing the deep tendon reflexes of a 30-year-old female here for her "annual physical." When striking the achilles and quadriceps, you are unable to elicit a reflex. What would be an appropriate response?

A. Document these reflexes as "0" on a scale of 0 to 4+.
B. Complete exam, then test these reflexes again.
C. Ask patient to lock her fingers and "pull."
D. Refer the patient to a specialist for further testing.

Correct Answer: C

Rationale: Sometimes the reflex response fails to appear. Try further encouragement of relaxation, varying the person's position or increasing the strength of the blow. Reinforcement is another technique to relax the muscles and enhance the response. Ask the person to perform an isometric exercise in a muscle group somewhat away from the one being tested. For example, to enhance a patellar reflex, ask the person to lock the fingers together and "pull."

Cognitive Level: Application

30. In assessing a 70-year-old patient with a recent cerebrovascular accident, you note right-sided weakness. What might you expect to find when you test his reflexes on the right side?

A. Lack of reflexes
B. Normal reflexes
C. Diminished reflexes
D. Hyperactive reflexes

Correct Answer: D

Rationale: Hyperreflexia is the exaggerated reflex seen when the monosynaptic reflex arc is released from the influence of higher cortical levels. This occurs with upper motor neuron lesions, e.g., a cerebrovascular accident.

Cognitive Level: Application

31. When testing the triceps reflex, what is the expected response?

A. Flexion of the hand
B. Extension of the forearm
C. Flexion and supination of the forearm
D. Pronation of the hand

Correct Answer: B

Rationale: The normal response is extension of the forearm.

Cognitive Level: Knowledge

32. You are testing superficial reflexes on an adult patient. When you stroke up the lateral side of the sole and across the ball of the foot, you notice plantar flexion of the toes. How would you document this finding?
    A. Plantar reflex "2+" on a scale from "0 to 4+"
    B. Positive Babinski sign
    C. Plantar reflex present bilaterally
    D. Plantar reflex abnormal

Correct Answer: C

Rationale: With the same instrument, draw a light stroke up the lateral side of the sole of the foot and across the ball of the foot, like an upside-down "J." The normal response is plantar flexion of the toes and sometimes of the whole foot.

Cognitive Level: Analysis

33. In the assessment of a 1-month-old infant you note a lack of response to noise or stimulation. The mother reports that in the last week he has been sleeping all the time and when awake all he does is cry. When the baby cries it is very high pitched and shrill. What would be an appropriate response to these findings?
    A. Nothing; these are expected findings for an infant this age.
    B. Refer the infant for further testing.
    C. Talk with the mother about eating habits.
    D. Tell the mother to bring baby back in a week for a recheck.

Correct Answer: B

Rationale: A high-pitched shrill cry or cat-sounding screech occurs with CNS damage. Lethargy, hyporeactivity, hyperirritability, and parent's report of significant change in behavior all warrant referral.

Cognitive Level: Analysis

34. Which of the following would you use to test the motor coordination of an 11-month old?
    A. Denver II
    B. Deep tendon reflexes
    C. Rapid alternating movements
    D. Stereognosis

Correct Answer: A

Rationale: To screen gross and fine motor coordination, use the Denver II with its age-specific developmental milestones.

Cognitive Level: Application

35. To assess the head control of a 4-month-old, you lift him up in a prone position while supporting his chest. What should the infant's response be?
    A. Holds head at 45 degrees and keeps back straight.
    B. Flexes knees and elbows with back straight.
    C. Raises head and arches back.
    D. Extends arms and drops head down.

Correct Answer: C

Rationale: Second, lift up the baby in a prone position, with one hand supporting the chest. At 3 months of age, the baby raises the head and arches the back as in a swan dive. This is the Landau reflex, which persists until 1½ years of age.

Cognitive Level: Application

36. While assessing a 7-month-old infant you make a loud noise and note the following response: Abduction and flexion of arms and legs; fanning of fingers and curling of index and thumb in C position; followed by infant bringing in arms and legs to body. What do you know about this response?
    A. This is an expected startle response at this age.
    B. This could indicate brachial nerve palsy.
    C. It is normal as long as movements are symmetrical bilaterally.
    D. This reflex should disappear between 1 and 4 months of age.

Correct Answer: D

Rationale: The Moro reflex is present at birth and disappears at 1 to 4 months. Absence of the Moro reflex in the newborn or persistence after 5 months of age indicates severe CNS injury.

Cognitive Level: Application

37. To test for gross motor skill and coordination of a 6-year-old, which of the following techniques would be appropriate?
    A. Ask child to hop on one foot.
    B. Have child touch finger to his nose.
    C. Have the child make "funny" faces at you.

D. Have the child stand on his head.

Correct Answer: A

Rationale: Normally, the child can balance on one foot for about 5 seconds by 4 years of age, for 8 to 10 seconds at 5 years of age, and can hop at 4 years. Children enjoy performing these tests. Failure to hop after 5 years of age indicates incoordination of gross motor skill.

Cognitive Level: Application

38. During the assessment of an 80-year-old male, you note that his hands tremor when he reaches for something and his head is always nodding. There is no associated rigidity with movement. Which of the following statements is most accurate?
    A. These are the result of degenerative arthropathy.
    B. These are normal findings due to aging.
    C. This patient should be evaluated for a cerebellar lesion.
    D. These could be related to hyperthyroidism.

Correct Answer: B

Rationale: Senile tremors occasionally occur. These benign tremors include an intention tremor of the hands, head nodding (as if saying yes or no), and tongue protrusion.

Cognitive Level: Analysis

39. While you take the history of a 68-year-old patient who sustained a head injury 3 days earlier, he tells you he is on a cruise ship and is 30 years old. What would this be indicative of?
    A. Inability to understand question
    B. A great sense of humor
    C. Decreased level of consciousness
    D. Uncooperative behavior

Correct Answer: C

Rationale: A change in consciousness may be subtle. Note any decreasing level of consciousness, disorientation, memory loss, uncooperative behavior, or even complacency in a previously combative person.

Cognitive Level: Application

40. You are caring for a patient who has just had neurosurgery. To assess for increased intracranial pressure, what would you include in your assessment?
    A. Level of consciousness, motor function, pupillary response, and vital signs
    B. Deep tendon reflexes, vital signs, and coordinated movements
    C. Cranial nerves, motor function, and sensory function
    D. Mental status, deep tendon reflexes, sensory function, and pupillary response

Correct Answer: A

Rationale: Some hospitalized persons have head trauma or a neurologic deficit due to a systemic disease process. These people must be monitored closely for any improvement or deterioration in neurologic status and for any indication of increasing intracranial pressure. Use an abbreviation of the neurologic examination in the following sequence: level of consciousness, motor function, pupillary response, and vital signs.

Cognitive Level: Application

41. In your assessment of a 22-year-old female who has a head injury from a car accident 4 hours ago, you note the following change: pupils were equal, now right is fully dilated and nonreactive, left is 4 mm and reacts to light. What would this suggest?
    A. Test was not performed accurately
    B. Increased intracranial pressure
    C. Normal response following a head injury
    D. Injury to the right eye

Correct Answer: B

Rationale: In a brain-injured person, a sudden, unilateral, dilated and nonreactive pupil is ominous. Cranial nerve III runs parallel to the brain stem. When increasing intracranial pressure pushes the brain stem down (uncal herniation), it puts pressure on cranial nerve III, causing pupil dilation.

Cognitive Level: Analysis

42. Throughout your assessment of a 52-year-old male with blindness in his right eye, you notice he never looks to the right and seems to ignore environmental stimuli that come from his right side. The appropriate diagnosis for this would be:
    A. impaired motor coordination.
    B. sensory perceptual alteration.
    C. unilateral neglect.
    D. body image disturbance.

Correct Answer: C

Rationale: Unilateral neglect. Does not look toward

affected side; consistent inattention to stimuli on affected side; leaves food on plate on the affected side; inadequate self-care, positioning, and/or safety precautions in regard to affected side.

Cognitive Level: Application

43. A 32-year-old female tells you that she has noticed "very sudden, jerky movements" mainly in her hands and arms. "They seem to come and go, primarily when I am trying to do something. I haven't noticed them when I'm sleeping." This description suggests:
    A. chorea.
    B. athetosis.
    C. Parkinson's.
    D. myoclonus.

Correct Answer: A

Rationale: Chorea. Sudden, rapid, jerky, purposeless movement, involving limbs, trunk, or face. Occurs at irregular intervals, not rhythmic or repetitive, more convulsive than a tic. Some are spontaneous, and some are initiated; all are accentuated by voluntary acts. Disappears with sleep.

Cognitive Level: Analysis

44. In your assessment of a 62-year-old male you note the following: stooped posture; walks with shuffling, short steps; very rigid; flat facial expression; fingers move as if rolling a pill with them. These findings would be consistent with:
    A. cerebellar ataxia.
    B. cerebral palsy.
    C. muscular dystrophy.
    D. Parkinsonism.

Correct Answer: D

Rationale: Parkinsonism. Body tends to stay immobile; facial expression is flat, staring, expressionless; excessive salivation occurs; reduced eye blinking. Posture is stooped; equilibrium is impaired; loses balance easily. Parkinsonian tremor; cogwheel rigidity on passive range of motion.

Cognitive Level: Analysis

45. When assessing a 32-year-old patient with a recent head injury, he responds to pain by extending, adducting and internally rotating his arms. His palms pronate. His lower extremities extend as well with plantar flexion. Which of the following statements is accurate?
    A. This is a normal response and will go away in 24 to 48 hours.
    B. This is a very ominous sign and may indicate brain stem injury.
    C. This indicates a lesion of the cerebral cortex.
    D. This indicates a completely nonfunctional brain stem.

Correct Answer: B

Rationale: Decerebrate rigidity. Upper extremities are stiffly extended, adducted, internal rotation, palms pronated. Lower extremities stiffly extended, plantar flexion; teeth clenched. More ominous that decorticate rigidity; indicates lesion in brain stem at midbrain or upper pons.

Cognitive Level: Analysis

46. A 78-year-old male has a past history of a CVA. You note that when he walks, his left arm is immobile against the body, with flexion of the shoulder, elbow, wrist and fingers, and adduction of the shoulder. His left leg is stiff and extended and circumducts with each step. What type of gait disturbance is this individual experiencing?
    A. Cerebellar ataxia
    B. Parkinsonian gait
    C. Spastic hemiparesis
    D. Scissors gait

Correct Answer: C

Rationale: With spastic hemiparesis, the arm is immobile against the body. There is flexion of the shoulder, elbow, wrist, fingers, and adduction of the shoulder. The leg is stiff and extended and circumducts with each step. Causes of this type of gait include CVA.

Cognitive Level: Analysis

47. In an individual with an upper motor neuron lesion such as a CVA, which of the following physical assessment findings would you expect to see?
    A. Loss of muscle tone and flaccidity
    B. Atrophy and wasting of the muscles
    C. Hyperreflexia
    D. Fasciculations

Correct Answer: C

Rationale: Hyperreflexia, diminished or absent superficial reflexes, increased muscle tone or spasticity can be expected with upper motor neuron lesions.

Cognitive Level: Application

48. Mr. J., a 59-year-old male, has herniated his intervertebral disk. Which of the following findings would you expect to see on physical assessment of this individual?
    A. Increased muscle tone
    B. Hyporeflexia
    C. The presence of pathologic reflexes
    D. A positive Babinski sign

Correct Answer: B

Rationale: With a herniated intervertebral disk or lower motor neuron lesion, there is loss of tone, flaccidity, atrophy, fasciculations, and hyporeflexia or areflexia.

Cognitive Level: Application

49. A patient is not able to perform rapid alternating movements such as patting her knees rapidly. You would document this as:
    A. a probable abnormality in the cerebellum.
    B. the presence of dysdiadochokinesia.
    C. ataxia.
    D. asterognosis.

Correct Answer: B

Rationale: Slow clumsy movements and the inability to perform rapid alternating movements occurs with cerebellar disease. It is termed dysdiadochokinesia.

Cognitive Level: Application

50. Determining whether an individual is oriented to his or her surroundings will test the functioning of which of the following structures?
    A. Cerebellum
    B. Medulla oblongata
    C. Cerebrum
    D. Cranial nerves

Correct Answer: C

Rationale: The cerebral cortex is responsible for thought, memory, reasoning, sensation and voluntary movement.

Cognitive Level: Comprehension

Chapter 22

Male Genitalia

1. The external male genital structures include the:
   A. testis.
   B. epididymis.
   C. vas deferens.
   D. scrotum.

Correct Answer: D

Rationale: The external male genital structures include the penis and scrotum.

Cognitive Level: Knowledge

2. An accessory glandular structure for the genitals is:
   A. the prostate.
   B. the penis.
   C. the testis.
   D. the vas deferens.

Correct Answer: A

Rationale: Glandular structures accessory to the genital organs are the prostate, seminal vesicles and bulbourethral glands.

Cognitive Level: Knowledge

3. Which of the following statements is true regarding the male penis?
   A. The penis is composed of two cylindrical columns of erectile tissue.
   B. The corpus spongiosum expands into a cone of erectile tissue called the glans.
   C. The prepuce is the fold of foreskin covering the shaft of the penis.
   D. The urethral meatus is located on the ventral side of the penis.

Correct Answer: B

Rationale: The penis is composed of three cylindrical columns of erectile tissue. At the distal end of the shaft, the corpus spongiosum expands into a cone of erectile tissue, the glans.

Cognitive Level: Knowledge

4. When performing a genital examination on a 20-year-old male, you note deeply pigmented, wrinkled scrotal skin with large sebaceous follicles. Based on this information you would:
   A. consider this a normal finding and proceed with the examination.
   B. obtain a more detailed history focusing on any scrotal abnormalities the patient has noticed.
   C. squeeze the glans checking for the presence of discharge.
   D. assess the testicles for the presence of masses or painless lumps.

Correct Answer: A

Rationale: After adolescence, the scrotal skin is deeply pigmented and has large sebaceous follicles . . . the scrotal skin looks corrugated.

Cognitive Level: Application

5. Which of the following statements about the testes is true?
   A. The vas deferens is located along the inferior portion of each testis.
   B. The lymphatics of the testes drain into the abdominal lymph nodes.
   C. The cremaster muscle contracts in response to cold and draws the testicles closer to the body.
   D. The right testis is lower than the left because the right spermatic cord is longer.

Correct Answer: C

Rationale: When it is cold, the cremaster muscle contracts, raising the sac and bringing the testes closer to the body to absorb heat necessary for sperm viability.

Cognitive Level: Knowledge

6. Sperm production occurs in the:
   A. testes.

B. prostate.
C. epididymis.
D. vas deferens.

Correct Answer: A

Rationale: Sperm production occurs in the testes.

Cognitive Level: Knowledge

7. M.J., a 62-year-old male, states that his doctor told him that he has an "inguinal hernia." He asks you to explain what a hernia is. You:
   A. refer him to his physician for additional consultation, since he or she made the initial diagnosis.
   B. explain that a hernia is a loop of bowel protruding through a weak spot in the muscles of the abdomen.
   C. explain that a hernia is often the result of prenatal growth abnormalities.
   D. tell M.J. not to worry and that most men his age develop hernias.

Correct Answer: B

Rationale: A hernia is a loop of bowel protruding through a weak spot in the musculature.

Cognitive Level: Application

8. The mother of a 10-year-old boy asks you to discuss the recognition of puberty. You reply:
   A. "Puberty usually begins about age 15."
   B. "The development of pubic hair precedes testicular or penis enlargement."
   C. "Penis size does not increase until about the age of 16."
   D. "The first sign of puberty is enlargement of the testes."

Correct Answer: D

Rationale: Puberty begins sometime between ages 9½ and 13½. The first sign is enlargement of the testes. Next, pubic hair appears, then penis size increases.

Cognitive Level: Application

9. Normal changes in the aging adult include:
   A. declining testosterone production.
   B. difficulty in maintaining an erection.
   C. premature ejaculation.
   D. a decreased refractory state after ejaculation.

Correct Answer: A

Rationale: After age 55-60 years, testosterone production declines.

Cognitive Level: Comprehension

10. In the absence of disease, a withdrawal from sexual activity later in life may be due to:
   A. decreased pleasure from sexual intercourse.
   B. decreased libido with aging.
   C. side effects of medications.
   D. decreased sperm production.

Correct Answer: C

Rationale: In the absence of disease, a withdrawal from sexual activity may be due to side effects of medications such as antihypertensives, antidepressants, sedatives.

Cognitive Level: Comprehension

11. Indications for circumcision include the following:
   A. the prevention of paraphimosis.
   B. cultural beliefs.
   C. prevention of testicular cancer.
   D. decreasing the transmission of the AIDS virus during sexual intercourse.

Correct Answer: B

Rationale: Indications for circumcision include cultural reasons, the prevention of phimosis, decreasing the incidence of cancer of the penis, and decreasing the incidence of urinary tract infections in infancy.

Cognitive Level: Comprehension

12. Mr. R.O., a 59-year-old patient, has been diagnosed with prostatitis and is being seen at the clinic for complaints of burning and pain during urination. Mr. R.O. is experiencing:
   A. nocturia.
   B. dysuria.
   C. polyuria.
   D. hematuria.

Correct Answer: B

Rationale: Dysuria or burning is common with acute cystitis, prostatitis, and urethritis.

Cognitive Level: Analysis

13. L.W., a 45-year-old carpenter, is seen at the clinic for complaints of "losing my urine when I lift heavy objects." L.W. is most likely experiencing:
   A. urgency incontinence.

B. urinary hesitancy.
C. stress incontinence.
D. frequency.

Correct Answer: C

Rationale: Stress incontinence is loss of urine with physical strain due to weakness of sphincters. The individual accidentally urinates when sneezing, laughing, coughing, or bearing down.

Cognitive Level: Analysis

14. When eliciting an initial sexual history from an adolescent, which of the following statements is most appropriate?
    A. "Often boys your age have questions about sexual activity."
    B. "You don't masturbate, do you?"
    C. "Do you use condoms?"
    D. "Have you had sex in the last 6 months?"

Correct Answer: A

Rationale: Start the interview with a permission statement. This conveys that it is normal and all right to think or feel a certain way. Avoid sounding judgmental.

Cognitive Level: Analysis

15. Which of the following statements is most appropriate when obtaining a genitourinary history from an elderly male?
    A. "Do you know how to perform Testicular Self Examination?"
    B. "Do you experience nocturnal emissions, or 'wet dreams'?"
    C. "Do you need to get up at night to urinate?"
    D. "Has anyone ever touched your genitals and you did not want them to?"

Correct Answer: C

Rationale: The elderly patient is asked about the presence of nocturia. This may be due to diuretic medication, fluid retention from mild heart failure or varicose veins, or fluid ingestion.

Cognitive Level: Analysis

16. When performing a genital examination on a patient, he experiences an erection. The most appropriate action or response is to:
    A. ask the patient if he would like a male nurse to examine him.
    B. continue with the examination as though nothing has happened.
    C. stop the examination and tell the patient that you will return at a later time.
    D. reassure the patient that this is a normal response and continue with the examination.

Correct Answer: D

Rationale: When the male patient develops an erection, reassure the patient that this is a normal physiologic response to touch and proceed with the rest of the examination.

Cognitive Level: Application

17. Which of the following is a normal finding when examining the glans?
    A. The skin is wrinkled and without lesions.
    B. Smegma may be present under the foreskin of an uncircumcised male.
    C. The dorsal vein may be visible.
    D. Hair is without pest inhabitants.

Correct Answer: B

Rationale: The glans looks smooth and without lesions. Some cheesy smegma may have collected under the foreskin of an uncircumcised male.

Cognitive Level: Comprehension

18. When performing a genitourinary assessment, you note that the urethral meatus is positioned ventrally. This is:
    A. probably due to a stricture.
    B. often associated with aging.
    C. the result of phimosis.
    D. called hypospadius.

Correct Answer: D

Rationale: Hypospadius is the ventral location of the urethral meatus.

Cognitive Level: Analysis

19. You are performing a genital examination on Mr. D. and note urethral drainage. When collecting urethral discharge for microscopic examination and culture, you should:
    A. insert a cotton-tipped applicator into the urethra.
    B. compress the glans between your thumb and forefinger, collecting any discharge.
    C. ask the patient to urinate into a sterile cup.
    D. ask the patient to obtain a specimen of semen.

Correct Answer: B

Rationale: If urethral discharge is noted, collect a smear for microscopic examination and culture by compressing the glans anteroposteriorly between your thumb and forefinger.

Cognitive Level: Application

20. When assessing the scrotum of a male patient, you note the presence of multiple firm, nontender, yellow 1-cm nodules. These are most likely:
    A. subcutaneous plaques.
    B. due to urethritis.
    C. due to inflammation of the epididymis.
    D. sebaceous cysts.

Correct Answer: D

Rationale: Sebaceous cysts are commonly found on the scrotum. These are yellowish, 1-cm nodules and are firm, nontender, and often multiple.

Cognitive Level: Analysis

21. When performing a scrotal assessment, you note that the scrotal contents transilluminate and show a red glow. Based on this finding you would:
    A. consider this normal and proceed with the examination.
    B. suspect the presence of serous fluid in the scrotum.
    C. refer the patient for evaluation of a mass in the scrotum.
    D. assess the patient for the presence of a hernia.

Correct Answer: B

Rationale: Normal scrotal contents do not transilluminate. Serous fluid does transilluminate and shows as a red glow.

Cognitive Level: Analysis

22. Which of the following statements is true when performing a genital examination?
    A. Palpate for the vertical chain of lymph nodes along the groin inferior to the inguinal ligament.
    B. Palpate the inguinal canal only if there is a bulge present in the inguinal region during inspection.
    C. When palpating for a hernia on the right side, have the patient shift his weight onto the left (unexamined) leg.
    D. Auscultate for the presence of bowel sounds over the scrotum in all-male patients.

Correct Answer: C

Rationale: When palpating for the presence of a hernia on the right side, ask the male to shift his weight onto the left (unexamined) leg.

Cognitive Level: Application

23. Which of the following statements is true regarding the incidence of testicular cancer?
    A. Testicular cancer is the most common cancer in men ages 30-50.
    B. Males with a history of cryptorchidism are at greatest risk of developing testicular cancer.
    C. The early symptoms of testicular cancer are pain and induration.
    D. Nonwhite males are four times more likely to develop testicular cancer than white males.

Correct Answer: B

Rationale: Males with undescended testicles (cryptorchidism) are at greatest risk of developing testicular cancer.

Cognitive Level: Comprehension

24. You are describing how to perform a testicular self-examination to a patient. Which of the following statements is most appropriate?
    A. "A good time to examine your testicles is just before you take a shower."
    B. "The testicle is egg shaped and moveable. It feels firm and has a lumpy consistency."
    C. "If you notice an enlarged testicle or a painless lump, call your health care provider."
    D. "Perform testicular exam at least once a week, to detect the early stages of testicular cancer."

Correct Answer: C

Rationale: If the patient notices a firm painless lump, a hard area, or an overall enlarged testicle, call your health care provider for further evaluation.

Cognitive Level: Application

25. T.O., a 2-month-old, uncircumcised male, is here for a "well-baby check-up." How would you proceed with the genital examination?
    A. Assess the glans for redness or lesions.
    B. Note any dirt or smegma that has collected under the foreskin.

C. Elicit the cremasteric reflex.
D. Avoid retracting the foreskin until the infant is 3 months old.

Correct Answer: D

Rationale: If uncircumcised, the foreskin is normally tight during the first 3 months, and should not be retracted because of the risk of tearing the membrane attaching the foreskin to the shaft.

Cognitive Level: Application

26. R.J., a 2-year-old male, has been diagnosed with "physiologic cryptorchidism." Given this diagnosis, during assessment, you will most likely observe:
   A. an atrophic scrotum and absence of the testis bilaterally.
   B. an absence of the testis in the scrotum, but the testis can be milked down.
   C. testis that migrate into the abdomen when the child squats or sits cross-legged.
   D. testes that are hard and painful to palpation.

Correct Answer: B

Rationale: Migratory testes (physiologic cryptorchidism) are common because of the strength of the cremasteric reflex and the small mass of the prepubertal testes. The affected side has a normally developed scrotum and the testis can be milked down.

Cognitive Level: Application

27. A common assessment finding in a boy under 2 years old is:
   A. the presence of a hernia in the scrotum.
   B. the presence of a hydrocele, or fluid in the scrotum.
   C. a penis that looks large in relation to the scrotum.
   D. an inflamed and tender spermatic cord.

Correct Answer: B

Rationale: A common scrotal finding in the boy under 2 years of age is a hydrocele, or fluid in the scrotum.

Cognitive Level: Application

28. Which of the following is considered a normal finding when assessing an aging adult male?
   A. Enlargement of the testes and scrotum
   B. An increase in the number of rugae over the scrotal sac
   C. A decrease in the size of the penis
   D. A decrease in scrotal color

Correct Answer: C

Rationale: In the older male, you may note thinner, graying pubic hair and a decrease in the size of the penis.

Cognitive Level: Application

29. When performing a genital assessment on a 34-year-old male you note the following: multiple soft, moist, painless papules in the shape of cauliflower-like patches scattered across the shaft of the penis. These lesions are characteristic of:
   A. condylomata acuminata.
   B. syphilitic chancres.
   C. carcinoma.
   D. herpes progenitalis.

Correct Answer: A

Rationale: The lesions of condylomata acuminata are soft, pointed, moist, fleshy, painless papules that may be single or multiple in a cauliflower-like patch. They occur on the shaft of the penis, behind the corona, or around the anus where they may grow into large grape-like clusters.

Cognitive Level: Analysis

30. A 15-year-old male is seen in the clinic for complaints of "dull pain and pulling" in the scrotal area. On examination you palpate a soft, irregular mass posterior to and above the testis on the left. This mass collapses when the patient is supine and refills when he is upright. This description is consistent with:
   A. testicular torsion.
   B. spermatic cord varicocele.
   C. epididymitis.
   D. spermatocele.

Correct Answer: B

Rationale: A varicocele is dilated, tortuous varicose veins in the spermatic cord due to incompetent valves within the vein. Symptoms include dull pain, constant pulling or dragging feeling; or the individual may be asymptomatic. When palpating the mass, the examiner will feel a soft, irregular mass posterior to and above the testis that collapses when the individual is supine and refills when the individual is upright.

Cognitive Level: Analysis

31. When performing a genitourinary assessment on a 16-year-old male you notice a swelling in the scrotum that increases with increased intra-abdominal pressure and decreases when lying down. The patient complains of pain when straining. This description is most consistent with:
   A. an indirect inguinal hernia.
   B. a direct inguinal hernia.
   C. a femoral hernia.
   D. an incisional hernia.

Correct Answer: A

Rationale: With indirect inguinal hernias there is pain with straining; a soft swelling that increases with increased intra-abdominal pressure, which may decrease when lying down. This is the most common type of hernia. It is more common in infants <1 year and in males 16 to 20 years of age.

Cognitive Level: Analysis

32. When performing a testicular examination on a 25-year-old male, which of the following findings is considered within normal limits?
   A. Non-tender subcutaneous plaques are normal and are an expected finding.
   B. The scrotal area should be dry, scaly and nodular.
   C. The testes should feel ovoid, movable, and be slightly sensitive to compression.
   D. A single, hard, circumscribed, movable mass, less than 1 cm under the surface of the testes is a normal finding.

Correct Answer: C

Rationale: The testes should feel ovoid, movable, and may be slightly sensitive to compression.

Cognitive Level: Application

33. You are inspecting the scrotum and testes of a 43-year-old male. Which finding would require additional follow-up and evaluation?
   A. The left testicle hangs lower than the right testicle.
   B. The scrotum is a darker color than the general skin color.
   C. The skin on the scrotum is shiny and smooth.
   D. The testes move closer to the body in response to cold temperatures.

Correct Answer: C

Rationale: Scrotal swelling may cause the skin to become shiny and smooth. Normal scrotal skin is rugated.

Cognitive Level: Analysis

34. A 55-year-old male is experiencing severe pain of sudden onset in the scrotal area. It is somewhat relieved by elevation. On examination you note an enlarged, red scrotum that is very tender to palpation. It is difficult to distinguish the epididymis from the testis and the scrotal skin is thick and edematous. This description is consistent with which of the following?
   A. Testicular torsion
   B. Varicocele
   C. Spermatocele
   D. Epididymitis

Correct Answer: D

Rationale: Epididymitis presents as severe pain of sudden onset in scrotum, that is somewhat relieved by elevation. On examination, the scrotum is enlarged, reddened, exquisitely tender. The epididymis is enlarged, indurated and may be hard to distinguish from the testis. The overlying scrotal skin may be thick and edematous.

Cognitive Level: Analysis

35. You are performing a genitourinary assessment on a 50-year-old obese male laborer. On examination you note a painless round swelling close to the pubis in the area of the internal inguinal ring that is easily reduced when the individual is supine. These findings are most consistent with which of the following conditions?
   A. A femoral hernia
   B. A direct inguinal hernia
   C. A scrotal hernia
   D. An indirect inguinal hernia

Correct Answer: B

Rationale: Direct inguinal hernias occur most often in men over the age of 40. It is an acquired weakness brought on by heavy lifting, obesity, chronic cough, or ascites. The direct inguinal hernia is usually a painless, round swelling close to the pubis in the area of the internal inguinal ring that is easily reduced when the individual is supine.

Cognitive Level: Analysis

Chapter 23

Anus, Rectum, and Prostate

1. Which of the following statements is true? The anal canal:
   A. contains hair and sebaceous glands.
   B. is the outlet for the gastrointestinal tract.
   C. slants backward toward the sacrum.
   D. is about 2 cm long in the adult.

Correct Answer: B

Rationale: The anal canal is the outlet of the gastrointestinal tract, and it is about 3.8 cm long in the adult.

Cognitive Level: Knowledge

2. Which of the following statements about the sphincters is correct?
   A. The internal sphincter is under voluntary control.
   B. Both sphincters remain slightly relaxed at all times.
   C. The external sphincter is under voluntary control.
   D. The internal sphincter surrounds the external sphincter.

Correct Answer: C

Rationale: The external sphincter surrounds the internal sphincter but also has a small section overriding the tip of the internal sphincter at the opening. It is under voluntary control.

Cognitive Level: Knowledge

3. When performing an examination of the anus and rectum, which of the following is important to remember?
   A. The anorectal junction cannot be palpated.
   B. There are no sensory nerves in the anal canal or rectum.
   C. The rectum is about 8 cm long.
   D. Above the anal canal, the rectum turns anteriorly.

Correct Answer: A

Rationale: These extend vertically down from the rectum and end in the anorectal junction. This junction is not palpable, but it is visible on proctoscopy.

Cognitive Level: Knowledge

4. The structure that secretes a thin, milky alkaline fluid to enhance the viability of sperm is the:
   A. Cowper gland.
   B. prostate gland.
   C. median sulcus.
   D. seminal vesicle.

Correct Answer: B

Rationale: In the male, the prostate gland lies in front of the anterior wall of the rectum. It surrounds the bladder neck and the urethra, and it secretes a thin milky alkaline fluid that helps sperm viability.

Cognitive Level: Knowledge

5. A 46-year-old male requires assessment of his sigmoid colon. The technique utilized should be:
   A. a rectal exam utilizing an examining finger.
   B. a proctoscope.
   C. an ultrasound.
   D. a sigmoidoscope.

Correct Answer: D

Rationale: It is 40 cm long and is accessible to examination only through the sigmoidoscope.

Cognitive Level: Comprehension

6. Thirty hours after birth, the newborn you are caring for passes a dark green meconium stool. Why is this important?
   A. The dark green color could indicate occult blood in the stool.
   B. The newborn should have passed the first stool within 12 hours after birth.

C. This stool would indicate anal patency.
D. Meconium stool can be reflective of distress in the newborn.

Correct Answer: C

Rationale: The first stool passed by the newborn is dark green meconium and occurs within 24 to 48 hours of birth, indicating anal patency.

Cognitive Level: Comprehension

7. During the assessment of an 18-month-old, the mother expresses concern about the infant's inability to toilet train. What would be your best response?
   A. "Some children are just more difficult to train, so I wouldn't worry about it yet."
   B. "The nerves that will allow your baby to have control over the passing of stools are not developed until at least 18 to 24 months of age."
   C. "Have you considered reading any of the books on toilet training? They can be very helpful."
   D. "This could mean there is a problem in your baby's development. We'll watch her closely for the next few months."

Correct Answer: B

Rationale: The infant passes stools by reflex. Voluntary control of the external anal sphincter cannot occur until the nerves supplying the area have become fully myelinated, usually around 1½ to 2 years of age. Toilet training usually starts after age 2 years.

Cognitive Level: Application

8. A 60-year-old male has just been told he has benign prostatic hypertrophy. He has a friend who just died from cancer of the prostate and is concerned this will happen to him. How would you respond?
   A. "The enlargement of your prostate is caused by hormone changes and not cancer."
   B. "We will treat you with chemotherapy so we can control the cancer."
   C. "It would be very unusual for a man your age to have cancer of the prostate."
   D. "The swelling in your prostate is only temporary and will go away."

Correct Answer: A

Rationale: The prostate gland commonly starts to enlarge during the middle adult years. This benign prostatic hypertrophy (BPH) is present in 1 out of 10 males at the age of 40 years and increases with age. It is thought that the hypertrophy is caused by hormonal imbalance that leads to the proliferation of benign adenomas.

Cognitive Level: Application

9. A 30-year-old female is here for "pain in her bottom when she has a bowel movement." Which of the following would you want to assess for?
   A. Food poisoning
   B. Hemorrhoids
   C. Fecal incontinence
   D. Pinworms

Correct Answer: B

Rationale: Dyschezia. Pain may be due to a local condition (hemorrhoid, fissure) or constipation.

Cognitive Level: Application

10. A patient here for "stomach pains for 2 weeks" describes his stools as being "soft and black" for about the last 10 days. He denies taking any medications. This is most indicative of:
    A. increase in bile pigment secondary to liver problems.
    B. excessive fat caused by malabsorption.
    C. increased iron intake secondary to change in diet.
    D. occult blood resulting from gastrointestinal bleeding.

Correct Answer: D

Rationale: Black stools may be tarry due to occult blood (melena) from gastrointestinal bleeding, or nontarry from ingestion of iron medications.

Cognitive Level: Analysis

11. After doing the assessment of a 60-year-old male with a family history of colon cancer you discuss with him early detection measures for colon cancer. You are sure to include:
    A. stool test for blood every 6 months.
    B. annual proctoscopy.
    C. sigmoidoscopy every 3 to 5 years.
    D. digital rectal examinations every 2 years.

Correct Answer: C

Rationale: Early detection for cancer: Digital rectal examination performed annually after age 40; stool blood test annually after age 50; sigmoidoscopy every 3 to 5 years after age 50; prostate specific antigen blood test annually for men over 50.

Cognitive Level: Application

12. The mother of a 5-year-old girl tells you she has noticed her daughter "scratching at her bottom a lot the last few days." During her assessment, you find redness and raised skin in the anal area. This most likely indicates:
    A. pinworms.
    B. bacterial infection.
    C. chickenpox.
    D. child abuse.

Correct Answer: A

Rationale: In children, pinworms are a common cause of intense itching and irritated anal skin.

Cognitive Level: Analysis

13. When examining only the rectal area of a female what position should she be in?
    A. The lithotomy position
    B. Bending over the table while standing
    C. Lying in the prone position
    D. Left lateral decubitus position

Correct Answer: D

Rationale: Place the female in lithotomy position if examining genitalia as well; use the left lateral decubitus position for the rectal area alone.

Cognitive Level: Comprehension

14. While doing an assessment of the perianal area of a patient, you note the following: pigmentation of anus is darker than surrounding skin; anal opening closed; a skin sac which is shiny and blue. Patient stated he had pain with bowel movements and noted some spots of blood occasionally. What would this assessment and history be most likely to indicate?
    A. Anal fistula
    B. Rectal prolapse
    C. Thrombosed hemorrhoid
    D. Pilonidal cyst

Correct Answer: C

Rationale: The anus normally looks moist and hairless, with coarse folded skin that is more pigmented than the perianal skin. The anal opening is tightly closėd. Shiny blue skin sac—thrombosed hemorrhoid.

Cognitive Level: Analysis

15. Which of the following techniques is correct for palpation of the rectum?
    A. Insert your extended index finger at a right angle to the anus.
    B. Instruct the patient first that this will be a painful procedure.
    C. Flex your finger and insert slowly toward the umbilicus.
    D. Place your finger directly into the anus to overcome the tight sphincter.

Correct Answer: C

Rationale: Place the pad of your index finger gently against the anal verge. You will feel the sphincter tighten, then relax. As is relaxes, flex the tip of your finger and slowly insert it into the anal canal in a direction toward the umbilicus. Never approach the anus at right angles with your index finger extended.

Cognitive Level: Comprehension

16. While performing a rectal examination, you note a firm, irregularly-shaped mass. What would be an appropriate response?
    A. Report finding and refer the patient to a specialist for further examination.
    B. Continue with exam and note finding in chart.
    C. Instruct patient to return for repeat assessment in 1 month.
    D. Tell patient you felt a mass but it is nothing to worry about.

Correct Answer: A

Rationale: A firm or hard mass with irregular shape or rolled edges may signify carcinoma. Promptly report any mass you discover for further examination.

Cognitive Level: Application

17. When testing stool for occult blood, which of the following might give you a false-positive?
    A. Increased ingestion of iron medication
    B. Absent bile pigment
    C. Increased fat content
    D. Large amount of red meat within last 3 days

Correct Answer: D

Rationale: If the stool is hematest positive, it indicates occult blood. Note that a false-positive finding may occur if the person has ingested significant amounts of red meat within 3 days of the test.

Cognitive Level: Comprehension

18. In assessment of the newborn what do you expect to see when you lightly stroke the anal area?
    A. A quick contraction of the sphincter
    B. A jerking of the legs
    C. Relaxation of the external sphincter
    D. Flexion of the knees

Correct Answer: A

Rationale: To assess sphincter tone, check the anal reflex. Gently stroke the anal area and note a quick contraction of the sphincter.

Cognitive Level: Comprehension

19. A 13-year-old female is here for a "sports physical." Which of the following would be important to include in her exam?
    A. Internal palpation of the anus
    B. Inspection of the perianal area
    C. Test for occult blood
    D. The Valsalva maneuver

Correct Answer: B

Rationale: Inspect the perianal region of the school-aged child and adolescent during examination of the genitalia. Internal palpation is not performed routinely.

Cognitive Level: Application

20. In your assessment of a 20-year-old male you note a small, palpable lesion with a tuft of hair located directly over the coccyx. You know that this would most likely be a:
    A. pruritus ani.
    B. benign tumor.
    C. pilonidal cyst.
    D. polyp.

Correct Answer: C

Rationale: Pilonidal cyst or sinus. A hair containing cyst or sinus located in the midline over the coccyx or lower sacrum. Often opens as a dimple with visible tuft of hair and, possibly, an erythematous halo.

Cognitive Level: Application

21. While performing the Valsalva maneuver, you notice your patient has a moist, red doughnut shape protruding from the anus. This would be consistent with:
    A. hemorrhoids.
    B. rectal fissure.
    C. rectal polyp.
    D. rectal prolapse.

Correct Answer: D

Rationale: Rectal prolapse. The rectal mucous membrane protrudes through the anus, appearing as a moist red doughnut with radiating lines. Occurs following a Valsalva maneuver, such as straining at stool, or with exercise.

Cognitive Level: Comprehension

22. A 70-year-old male is here for "difficulty passing urine." In the history he indicates he has to urinate frequently, especially at night. He has burning when he urinates and has noticed pain in his back. Given this history, what might you expect to find during the physical assessment?
    A. Occult blood and perianal pain to palpation
    B. Asymmetrical, hard, fixed prostate gland
    C. A soft nodule protruding from rectal mucosa
    D. Symmetrically enlarged, soft prostate gland

Correct Answer: B

Rationale: Carcinoma of the prostate. S: Frequency, nocturia, hematuria, weak stream, hesitancy, pain or burning on urination, continuous pain in lower back, pelvis and thighs. O: A malignant neoplasm often starts as a single hard nodule on the posterior surface, producing asymmetry and a change in consistency. As it invades normal tissue, multiple hard nodules appear, or the entire gland feels stone hard and fixed.

Cognitive Level: Analysis

23. Mr. Jones, a white, 51-year-old male, is at the clinic for a routine physical examination. The results of his examination are within normal limits. What would you recommend for Mr. Jones regarding early detection for prostate cancer, according to the American Cancer guidelines?
    A. Digital rectal examination performed every 6 months after age 50
    B. Prostate specific antigen test annually for men over age 50
    C. Sigmoidoscopy or colonoscopy every 3 years
    D. Fecal occult blood test beginning at age 45

Correct Answer: B

Rationale: The ACS recommends the following: a digital rectal examination annually after age 50; fecal occult blood test annually after age 50; sigmoidoscopy every 5 years or colonoscopy every 10 years after age 50; prostate specific antigen test annually for men over 50, except black men beginning at age 45.

Cognitive Level: Application

24. A mother brings her 4-year-old child to the clinic because of frequent itching and irritation in the anal area. On examination you note excoriation and evidence of itching and erythema. Which of the following is the most likely cause of the symptoms in a child of this age?
    A. Urinary incontinence
    B. Constipation
    C. Pinworms
    D. Hemorrhoids

Correct Answer: C

Rationale: In children, pinworms are a common cause of intense itching and irritated anal skin.

Cognitive Level: Analysis

25. While performing an assessment of the perianal area of a patient, you note the following: inflammation, swelling, tenderness and a tuft of hair at the tip of the coccyx. What does this assessment data most likely indicate?
    A. Anal fistula
    B. Inflamed hemorrhoid
    C. Pilonidal cyst
    D. Fissure

Correct Answer: C

Rationale: Inflammation or tenderness, swelling, a tuft of hair, or dimple at the tip of the coccyx may indicate a pilonidal cyst.

Cognitive Level: Analysis

26. A 62-year-old male is experiencing fever, chills, malaise, urinary frequency and urgency. He also reports urethral discharge and a dull aching pain in the perineal and rectal area. These symptoms are most consistent with which of the following?
    A. Benign prostatic hypertrophy (BPH)
    B. Carcinoma of the prostate
    C. Prostatitis
    D. Urinary tract infection

Correct Answer: C

Rationale: The common presenting symptoms of prostatitis are fever, chills, malaise, urinary frequency and urgency. The individual may also experience dysuria, urethral discharge and a dull aching pain in the perineal and rectal area.

Cognitive Level: Analysis

Chapter 24

Female Genitalia

1. The female structure that is homologous with the male penis is called the:
   A. clitoris.
   B. prepuce.
   C. frenulum.
   D. labia.

Correct Answer: A

Rationale: The clitoris is a small, pea-shaped erectile body, homologous with the male penis and highly sensitive to tactile stimulation.

Cognitive Level: Knowledge

2. When observing the vestibule, you should be able to see the:
   A. urethral meatus and paraurethral (Skene's) glands.
   B. vaginal orifice and vestibular (Bartholin's) glands.
   C. urethral meatus and vaginal orifice.
   D. paraurethral (Skene's) and vestibular (Bartholin's) glands.

Correct Answer: C

Rationale: The labial structures encircle a boat-shaped space, or cleft, termed the vestibule. Within it are numerous openings. The urethral meatus appears as a dimple 2.5-cm posterior to the clitoris. Surrounding the urethral meatus are the tiny, multiple paraurethral (Skene's) glands. Their ducts are not visible but open posterior to the urethra at the 5 and 7 o'clock positions. The vaginal orifice is posterior to the urethral meatus. On either side and posterior to the vaginal orifice are two vestibular (Bartholin's) glands, which secrete a clear lubricating mucus during intercourse. Their ducts are not visible but open in the groove between the labia minora and the hymen.

Cognitive Level: Comprehension

3. At the end of the vagina, you would expect to see the:
   A. uterus.
   B. cervix.
   C. fallopian tubes.
   D. ovaries.

Correct Answer: B

Rationale: At the end of the canal, the uterine cervix projects into the vagina.

Cognitive Level: Knowledge

4. The uterus is usually positioned tilting forward and superior to the bladder. This position is known as:
   A. retroverted and anteflexed.
   B. retroverted and retroflexed.
   C. superior-verted and anteflexed.
   D. anteverted and anteflexed.

Correct Answer: D

Rationale: The uterus is a pear-shaped, thick-walled, muscular organ. It is freely movable, not fixed, and usually tilts forward and superior to the bladder (a position labeled as anteverted and anteflexed).

Cognitive Level: Knowledge

5. M.R., 11 years old, is in your clinic for a sports physical. You notice that she has begun to develop breasts and during your conversation she reveals that she is unsure about the progression of development. Which of the following would best assist her in understanding the expected sequence for development?
   A. You could use Tanner's table on the five stages of sexual development.
   B. You could describe her development and compare it with other girls her age.
   C. You could reassure her that her development is within normal limits and tell her not to worry about the next step.
   D. You could use Jacobsen's table on expected development based on height and weight data.

Correct Answer: A

Rationale: Tanner's table on the five stages of pubic hair development is helpful in teaching girls the expected sequence of sexual development.

Cognitive Level: Application

6. Mrs. W. is 8 weeks pregnant. You read on her chart that her cervix is softened and looks cyanotic. You know that she is exhibiting which of the following signs?
   A. Chadwick's sign and Hegar's sign
   B. Goodell's sign and Chadwick's sign
   C. Hegar's sign and Goodell's sign
   D. Tanner's sign and Hegar's sign

Correct Answer: B

Rationale: Shortly after the first missed menstrual period, the female genitalia show signs of the growing fetus. The cervix softens (Goodell's sign) at 4 to 6 weeks, and the vaginal mucosa and cervix look cyanotic (Chadwick's sign) at 8 to 12 weeks. These changes occur because of increased vascularity and edema of the cervix, and hypertrophy and hyperplasia of the cervical glands. The isthmus of the uterus softens (Hegar's sign) at 6 to 8 weeks.

Cognitive Level: Comprehension

7. Mrs. F. is 22 weeks pregnant. She is fearful that she will develop a vaginal infection that may harm her growing fetus. You explain that:
   A. a thick mucus plug forms that protects the fetus from infection.
   B. the acidic pH of vaginal secretions promote the growth of pathogenic bacteria.
   C. the mucus plug that forms in the cervical canal is a good medium for bacterial growth.
   D. if intercourse is avoided, the risk for infection is minimal.

Correct Answer: A

Rationale: A clot of thick, tenacious mucus forms in the spaces of the cervical canal (the mucus plug), which protects the fetus from infection. Cervical and vaginal secretions increase during pregnancy and are thick, white, and more acidic. The increased acidity occurs because of the action of Lactobacillus acidophilus, which changes glycogen into lactic acid. The acidic pH keeps pathogenic bacteria from multiplying in the vagina, but the increase in glycogen increases the risk of candidiasis (commonly called a yeast infection) during pregnancy.

Cognitive Level: Comprehension

8. The changes normally associated with menopause occur generally because:
   A. the cells in the reproductive tract are aging.
   B. the cells in the reproductive tract are becoming fibrous.
   C. the cells in the reproductive tract are estrogen dependent.
   D. the cells in the reproductive tract are less able to respond to estrogen.

Correct Answer: C

Rationale: Since cells in the reproductive tract are estrogen-dependent, decreased estrogen levels during menopause bring dramatic physical changes.

Cognitive Level: Comprehension

9. Which of the following are changes associated with menopause?
   A. Cervical hypertrophy, ovarian atrophy, and increased acidity of vaginal secretions
   B. Uterine and ovarian atrophy along with thinning vaginal epithelium
   C. Vaginal mucosa fragility, increased acidity of vaginal secretions, and uterine hypertrophy
   D. Ovarian atrophy, increased vaginal secretions, and increasing clitoral size

Correct Answer: B

Rationale: The uterus shrinks in size because of its decreased myometrium. The ovaries atrophy to 1 to 2 cm and are not palpable after menopause. The sacral ligaments relax, and the pelvic musculature weakens, so the uterus droops. The cervix shrinks and looks paler with a thick glistening epithelium. The vaginal epithelium atrophies, becoming thinner, drier, and itchy. This results in a fragile mucosal surface that is at risk for bleeding and vaginitis.

Cognitive Level: Comprehension

10. Mrs. G. is in your office for a yearly physical examination. She is 54 years old and has just completed menopause. You should plan to explain that:
   A. a postmenopausal woman has only stopped menstruating; there really are no other signif-

icant changes that she should be concerned with.
B. A postmenopausal woman is likely to have difficulty with sexual pleasure due to drastic changes in the female sexual response cycle.
C. A postmenopausal woman should be aware that she is at increased risk for dyspareunia due to decreased vaginal secretions.
D. A postmenopausal woman is not at any greater risk for heart disease than a younger woman.

Correct Answer: C

Rationale: Decreased vaginal secretions leave the vagina dry and at risk for irritation and pain with intercourse (dyspareunia).

Cognitive Level: Comprehension

11. Ms. J. is in your clinic for gynecologic examination. You should plan to begin your interview with:
   A. menstrual history because it is generally nonthreatening.
   B. obstetric history because it is the most important information.
   C. urinary system history since it is generally not a routine part of a gynecologic check-up.
   D. sexual history since it is fairly threatening and you can get it over with before rapport building.

Correct Answer: A

Rationale: Menstrual history is usually nonthreatening, thus it is a good place to start history.

Cognitive Level: Application

12. Mrs. F. has had three pregnancies and two live births. How would you record this information?
   A. Gravida 2, Para 2, AB 1
   B. Gravida 3, Para 3, 1 AB
   C. Gravida 3, Para 2, AB 1
   D. Gravida 3, Para 2, AB 0

Correct Answer: C

Rationale: Gravida is number of pregnancies. Para is number of births. Abortions are interrupted pregnancies, including elective abortions and spontaneous miscarriages.

Cognitive Level: Application

13. During your interview with Mrs. K. you gather data that leads you to believe that she is perimenopausal. Which of the following statements made by Mrs. K. led to this conclusion?
   A. "I have noticed that my muscles ache at night when I go to bed."
   B. "I have only been pregnant twice but both times I had breast tenderness as my first symptom."
   C. "I have been noticing that I sweat a lot more than I used to, especially at night."
   D. "I will be very happy when I can stop worrying about having a period."

Correct Answer: C

Rationale: Any associated symptoms of menopause, e.g., hot flash, numbness and tingling, headache, palpitations, drenching sweats, mood swings, vaginal dryness, itching? Menopause—cessation of menstruation. Perimenopausal period, from 40-55 years of age, has hormone shifts, resulting in vasomotor instability.

Cognitive Level: Analysis

14. Ms. S., 50 years old, calls your clinic because she has noticed some changes in her body and breasts and wonders if they could be due to the estrogen replacement therapy she started 3 months ago. You tell her:
   A. "Estrogen replacement therapy is at such a low dose that side effects are very unusual."
   B. "Estrogen replacement therapy has several side effects including fluid retention, breast tenderness or enlargement, and vaginal bleeding."
   C. "It would be very unusual to have vaginal bleeding with estrogen replacement therapy and I suggest you contact your doctor immediately to have this evaluated."
   D. "It sounds as if your dose of estrogen is too high, I think you should decrease the amount you take and then call me back in a month to let me know how you're feeling."

Correct Answer: B

Rationale: Side effects of estrogen replacement therapy include fluid retention, breast pain or enlargement, vaginal bleeding.

Cognitive Level: Application

15. Mrs. G., a 52-year-old patient, states that when she sneezes or coughs she "wets herself a little." She is very concerned that something may be wrong with her. You know that:
   A. this is called true urinary incontinence and

may mean that she has a kidney infection.
B. this is called stress incontinence and is usually due to muscle weakness.
C. this is called urgency incontinence and she should empty her bladder before she sneezes or coughs.
D. this is called hematuria and usually needs to be evaluated by a urologist.

Correct Answer: B

Rationale: True incontinence—loss of urine without warning. Urgency incontinence—sudden loss, as with acute cystitis. Urination with a sneeze, laugh, cough, or bearing down. Stress incontinence—loss of urine with physical strain due to muscle weakness.

Cognitive Level: Comprehension

16. During the interview your patient reveals that she has some vaginal discharge. She is worried that it may be a sexually transmitted disease. Your most appropriate response to this would be:
A. "Have you been engaging in unprotected sexual intercourse?"
B. "Oh, don't worry. Some cyclic vaginal discharge is normal."
C. "I'd like some information about the discharge. What color is it?"
D. "Have you had any urinary incontinence associated with the discharge?"

Correct Answer: C

Rationale: Any unusual vaginal discharge? Increased amount? Character or color: white, yellow-green, gray, curd-like, foul smelling? Normal discharge is small, clear or cloudy, and always nonirritating. Suggests vaginal infection; character of discharge often suggests causative organism.

Cognitive Level: Analysis

17. Ms. T. states that 2 weeks ago she had a urinary tract infection that was treated with an antibiotic. As a part of your interview, you would definitely want to ask:
A. "Have you noticed a change in your vaginal pH?"
B. "Have you noticed any unusual vaginal discharge or itching?"
C. "Have you noticed any excessive vaginal bleeding?"
D. "Have you noticed any changes in your desire for intercourse?"

Correct Answer: B

Rationale: Taking any medications? Factors that increase the risk of vaginitis: Oral contraceptives increase glycogen content of vaginal epithelium, providing fertile medium for some organisms. Broad-spectrum antibiotics alter balance of normal flora.

Cognitive Level: Application

18. Which statement would be most appropriate when introducing the topic of sexual relationships during an interview?
A. "Most women your age have had more than one sexual partner. How many would you say you have had?"
B. "Women often feel dissatisfied with their sexual relationships. It would be okay to discuss this now."
C. "Now it is time to talk about your sexual history. When did you first have intercourse?"
D. "Often women have a question about their sexual relationship and how it affects their health. Do you?"

Correct Answer: D

Rationale: Begin with an open-ended question to assess individual needs. Include appropriate questions as a routine part of the history: Communicates that you accept individual's sexual activity and believe it is important. Your comfort with discussion prompts person's interest and possibly relief that the topic has been introduced. Establishes a database for comparison with any future sexual activities. Provides opportunity to screen sexual problems.

Cognitive Level: Application

19. Ms. D. has been considering using oral contraceptives. As a part of her history, you should ask:
A. "If you use tobacco, or smoke, how many cigarettes would you say you smoke per day?"
B. "Will you be in a monogamous relationship?"
C. "Do you have a history of heart murmurs?"
D. "I wonder if you have thought this choice through carefully."

Correct Answer: A

Rationale: If oral contraceptives are used, assess smoking history. Cigarettes increase cardiovascular side effects of oral contraceptives.

Cognitive Level: Application

20. Mr. and Mrs. Y. have come to your clinic seeking advice on pregnancy. They have been trying to conceive for 6 months and have not been successful. What might you do first?
    A. Explain that couples are considered infertile after 6 months of engaging in unprotected intercourse and that you will refer them to a fertility expert.
    B. Explain that couples are considered infertile after 1 year of unprotected intercourse.
    C. Ascertain if either of them have been using broad-spectrum antibiotics.
    D. Immediately refer Mrs. Y. to an expert in pelvic inflammatory disease—the most common cause of infertility.

Correct Answer: B

Rationale: Have you ever had any problems becoming pregnant? Infertility is considered after 1 year of engaging in unprotected sexual intercourse without conceiving.

Cognitive Level: Application

21. In assessing risk of contracting an STD, an appropriate question would be:
    A. "Do you use a condom with each episode of sexual intercourse?"
    B. "You use condoms don't you?"
    C. "Since you are in a monogamous relationship, are you worried about contracting an STD?"
    D. "I am worried that you may have an STD. I'd like to ask you a few questions about your sexual behavior and patterns."

Correct Answer: A

Rationale: STD risk reduction. Any precautions to reduce risk of STDs? Use condoms at each episode of sexual intercourse.

Cognitive Level: Comprehension

22. When asking questions of a preadolescent girl, which opening statement would be least threatening?
    A. "Do you have any questions about growing up?"
    B. "When did you notice that your body was changing?"
    C. "What has your mother told you about growing up?"
    D. "I remember being very scared when I got my period. How do you think you'll feel?"

Correct Answer: B

Rationale: Try the open-ended, "When did you . . ." rather than "Do you . . ." This is less threatening because it implies that the topic is normal and unexceptional.

Cognitive Level: Comprehension

23. When discussing sexuality and sexual issues with adolescents, a permission statement helps to convey that it is normal to think or feel a certain way. Which of the following is the best example of a permission statement?
    A. "It is okay that you have become sexually active."
    B. "If it is okay with you. I'd like to ask you some questions about your sexual history."
    C. "Often girls your age have questions about sexual activity. Have you?"
    D. "Often girls your age engage in sexual activity. It is okay to tell me if you have had intercourse."

Correct Answer: C

Rationale: Start with a permission statement, "Often girls your age experience . . ." This conveys that it is normal to think or feel a certain way.

Cognitive Level: Comprehension

24. Which of the following statements is true with regard to the history of a postmenopausal woman?
    A. Once a woman reaches menopause, you don't have to ask any further history questions.
    B. You should ask a postmenopausal woman if she ever experiences vaginal bleeding.
    C. Postmenopausal women very often experience uterine prolapse and should be screened for this.
    D. Postmenopausal women are not at risk for contracting STDs and thus these questions can be omitted.

Correct Answer: B

Rationale: Postmenopausal bleeding warrants further work-up and referral.

Cognitive Level: Comprehension

25. During the examination portion of Mrs. F.'s visit, she will be in lithotomy position. Which statement below reflects some things that you can do

to make this more comfortable for her?
  A. Ask her to place her hands and arms behind her head.
  B. Allow her to keep her buttocks about 6 inches from the edge of the table to prevent her from feeling as if she will fall off.
  C. Elevate her head and shoulders to maintain eye contact.
  D. Allow her to choose to have her feet in the stirrups or have them resting side by side on the edge of the table.

Correct Answer: C

Rationale: The arms should be at the woman's sides or across the chest, not over the head, because this position only tightens the abdominal muscles. You can help the woman relax, decrease her anxiety, and retain a sense of control by employing these measures. Have her empty the bladder before the examination. Elevate her head and shoulders to maintain eye contact. Pull out the stirrups so the legs are not abducted too far. Explain each step in the examination before you do it. Assure the woman she can stop the examination at any point should she feel any discomfort. Touch the inner thigh before you touch the vulva. Communicate throughout the examination. Maintain a dialogue to share information. Use the techniques of the educational or mirror pelvic examination.

Cognitive Level: Application

26. K.C., an 18-year-old, is having her first pelvic examination. It would be appropriate to:
  A. avoid the lithotomy position this first time since it can be uncomfortable and embarrassing.
  B. raise the head of the examination table and give K.D. a mirror so that she can see and learn about her anatomy.
  C. drape K.C. fully, leaving the drape between her legs elevated to avoid embarrassing her with eye contact.
  D. invite K.C.'s mother to be present during the examination.

Correct Answer: B

Rationale: Use the techniques of the educational or mirror pelvic examination. This is a routine examination with some modifications in attitude, position, and communication. First, the woman is considered an active participant, one who is interested in learning and in sharing decisions about her own health care. The woman props herself up on one elbow, or the head of the table is raised. Her other hand holds a mirror between her legs, above the examiner's hands. The woman can see all that the examiner is doing and has a full view of her genitalia. The mirror works well for teaching normal anatomy and its relation to sexual behavior.

Cognitive Level: Application

27. Which of the following would be a description of a finding within normal limits during the inspection of the external genitalia?
  A. Multiple sebaceous cysts that are yellow, nontender, firm, 1-cm nodules
  B. Swelling of the perineum prior to onset of menses
  C. Redness of the labia majora
  D. Discharge that is sticky and yellow-green

Correct Answer: A

Rationale: There should be no lesions, except for occasional sebaceous cysts. These are yellowish, 1-cm nodules that are firm, nontender, and often multiple.

Cognitive Level: Comprehension

28. The order of examination of the internal genitalia is important. Which statement best describes the proper order of examination?
  A. Bimanual examination, speculum examination, rectovaginal examination
  B. Speculum examination, rectovaginal examination, bimanual examination
  C. Speculum examination, bimanual examination, rectovaginal examination
  D. Rectovaginal examination, bimanual examination, speculum examination

Correct Answer: C

Rationale: Speculum Examination: Select the proper-sized speculum. Warm and lubricate the speculum under warm running water. Avoid gel lubricant at this point because it is bacteriostatic and would distort cells in the cytology specimen you will collect. Bimanual Examination: Use both hands to palpate the internal genitalia to assess their location, size, and mobility, and to screen for any tenderness or mass. Lubricate the first two fingers of your gloved intravaginal hand. Rectovaginal Examination: Use this technique to assess the rectovaginal septum, posterior uterine wall, cul-de-sac, and rectum. Change gloves to avoid spreading any possible infection. Lubricate the first two fingers. Instruct the woman that this may feel uncomfortable and will mimic the feeling of moving her bowels.

Cognitive Level: Analysis

29. Which of the following is an example of correct technique for insertion of the speculum?
    A. Instruct the woman to bear down, open the speculum blades, and apply in a swift, upward movement.
    B. Push the introitus down and open, instruct the woman to bear down, and insert the speculum with the width of the blades at an oblique angle, applying any pressure downward.
    C. Insert the blades of the speculum on a horizontal plane, turning them to a 45-degree angle as you continue to insert them. Ask the woman to bear down to ease insertion.
    D. Lock the blades open by turning the thumbscrew. Once you have them open, apply pressure to the introitus and insert the blades at a 45-degree angle downward to bring the cervix into view.

Correct Answer: B

Rationale: Hold the speculum in your right hand with the index and the middle fingers surrounding the blades and your thumb under the thumbscrew. This prevents the blades from opening painfully during insertion. With your left index and middle fingers, push the introitus down and open to relax the pubococcygeal muscle. Tilt the width of the blades obliquely and insert the speculum past your left fingers, applying any pressure downward. This avoids pressure on the sensitive urethra above it. Ease insertion by asking the woman to bear down. This method relaxes the perineal muscles and opens the introitus. (With experience, you can combine speculum insertion with assessing the support of the vaginal muscles.) As the blades pass your left fingers, withdraw your fingers. Now turn the width of the blades horizontally, and continue to insert in a 45-degree angle downward toward the small of the woman's back. This matches the natural slope of the vagina.

Cognitive Level: Application

30. You are examining Mrs. E. You note that she has had two full-term pregnancies, both babies delivered vaginally. You observe the following upon internal examination: Cervical os is a horizontal slit with some healed lacerations. The cervix has some Nabothian cysts that are small, smooth, and yellow. In addition, you notice that the cervical surface is granular and red, especially around the os. Finally, you note the presence of stringy, opaque, odorless secretions. Which of these findings are abnormal?
    A. The cervical os is a horizontal slit.
    B. The presence of Nabothian cysts.
    C. The cervical surface is granular and red.
    D. The presence of stringy and opaque secretions.

Correct Answer: C

Rationale: Color. Normally the cervical mucosa is pink and even. During the second month of pregnancy it looks blue (Chadwick's sign) and after menopause it is pale. Surface. This is normally smooth but cervical eversion, or ectropion, may occur normally after vaginal deliveries. Abnormal findings: Surface reddened, granular, and asymmetric, particularly around os.

Cognitive Level: Analysis

31. Mrs. K. calls you for instructions prior to having a Papanicolaou (Pap) smear. The most appropriate instructions are:
    A. "If you are menstruating, please use pads to avoid placing anything into the vagina."
    B. "Avoid intercourse, inserting anything into the vagina, or douching within 24 hours of your scheduled examination."
    C. "If you suspect that you have a vaginal infection, please gather a sample of the discharge to bring with you."
    D. "We would like you to use a mild saline douche prior to your examination. You may pick this up in our office."

Correct Answer: B

Rationale: The Papanicolaou, or Pap, smear screens for cervical cancer. Do not obtain during the woman's menses or if a heavy infectious discharge is present. Instruct the woman not to douche, have intercourse, or put anything into the vagina within 24 hours before collecting the specimens.

Cognitive Level: Application

32. Which of the following cervical smears and cultures are routinely collected if you do not suspect an STD?

A. Pap smear, endocervical specimen, KOH prep, and five-percent acetic acid wash
B. Endocervical specimen, cervical scrape, and vaginal pool
C. Papanicolaou smear, KOH prep, Gonorrhea culture, five-percent acetic acid wash
D. Endocervical specimen, vaginal pool, and five-percent acetic acid wash

Correct Answer: B

Rationale: Obtain cervical smears and cultures. Obtain the Pap smear before other specimens so you will not disrupt or remove cells. Laboratories may vary in method, but usually the test consists of three specimens: Endocervical specimen, Cervical Scrape, Vaginal Pool. To screen for STDs or if you note any abnormal vaginal discharge, obtain the following samples: Saline Mount, or "Wet Prep." KOH Prep. Gonorrhea ("GC") Culture. Anal Culture. Five-percent Acetic Acid Wash.

Cognitive Level: Comprehension

33. In performing the bimanual examination, you note that the cervix feels smooth and firm, is round, and is fixed in place (doesn't move). Your cervical palpation produces some pain. Which of the following statements is true regarding these results?
A. These findings are all within normal limits.
B. It is unusual to have pain when palpating the cervix, but the rest of the findings are within normal limits.
C. The cervix should move when palpated, an immobile cervix may indicate malignancy.
D. The cervical consistency should be soft and velvety—not firm.

Correct Answer: C

Rationale: Note these characteristics of a normal cervix: Consistency: Feels smooth and firm, as the consistency of the tip of the nose. It softens and feels velvety at 5 to 6 weeks of pregnancy (Goodell's sign). Contour: Evenly rounded. Mobility: With a finger on either side, move the cervix gently from side to side. Normally, this produces no pain. Abnormal Findings: Hard with malignancy. Nodular. Irregular. Immobile with malignancy. Painful with inflammation or ectopic pregnancy.

Cognitive Level: Analysis

34. You are palpating Mrs. W.'s adnexa. Your findings include: a firm, smooth uterine wall, the ovaries are palpable and feel smooth and firm. The fallopian tube is firm and pulsating. Your most appropriate course of action would be to:
A. give her an immediate referral to a gynecologist.
B. tell Mrs. W. that her examination was normal.
C. tell Mrs. W. that her examination was a bit unusual and you would like her to return in 1 month for a recheck..
D. tell Mrs. W. that you suspect that she has an ovarian cyst and that she should have this evaluated.

Correct Answer: A

Rationale: Palpate the uterine wall with your fingers in the fornices. Normally, it feels firm and smooth, with the contour of the fundus rounded. It softens during pregnancy. Often, you cannot feel the ovary. When you can, it normally feels smooth, firm, almond shaped, and is highly moveable, sliding through the fingers. It is slightly sensitive but not painful. The fallopian tube is not palpable normally. No other mass or pulsation should be felt. Pulsation or palpable fallopian tube suggests ectopic pregnancy; This warrants immediate referral.

Cognitive Level: Application

35. Mrs. C., a 65-year-old, is in your office for routine gynecologic care. She had a complete hysterectomy 3 months ago. Which of the following statements is true with regard to this visit?
A. Mrs. C. will not have a cervix and thus does not need to have a Pap smear done.
B. You should plan to lubricate your instruments and examining hand well to avoid a painful examination.
C. You can expect that Mrs. C. will have a somewhat enlarged uterus and small, hard ovaries.
D. Mrs. C.'s cervical mucosa will be red and dry-looking.

Correct Answer: B

Rationale: Natural lubrication is decreased; to avoid a painful examination, take care to lubricate instruments and the examining hand adequately. Menopause and the resulting decrease in estrogen production shows numerous physical changes. The cervix shrinks and looks pale and glistening. With the bimanual examination, the uterus feels smaller and firmer and the ovaries are not palpable normally.

Cognitive Level: Comprehension

36. You are preparing to examine the external genitalia of a school-age female. Which of the following positions would be most appropriate in this situation?
   A. Lying flat on the examining table with legs extended
   B. In the lithotomy position with the feet in stirrups
   C. In a frog-leg position on the examining table
   D. In the parent's lap

Correct Answer: C

Rationale: For a school-age child it is best to place them on the examining table in a frog leg position. With toddlers and preschoolers, it is best to have the child on the parent's lap in a frog leg position.

Cognitive Level: Application

37. When assessing a newborn female's genitalia, you note that the genitalia are somewhat engorged. The labia majora are swollen, the clitoris looks large and the hymen is thick. The vaginal opening is difficult to visualize. The infant's mother states that she is worried about the labia being swollen. You reply:
   A. "We will need to keep close watch over the next few days to see if the genitalia decrease in size."
   B. "This could possibly indicate an abnormality and may need to be evaluated by a physician."
   C. "This is a normal finding in newborns and should resolve within a few weeks."
   D. "We will need to have estrogen levels evaluated to make sure that they are within normal limits."

Correct Answer: C

Rationale: It is normal for a newborn's genitalia to be somewhat engorged. A sanguineous vaginal discharge and or leukorrhea are normal during the first few weeks because of the maternal estrogen effect. During the early weeks, the genital engorgement resolves, and the labia minora atrophy and remain small until puberty.

Cognitive Level: Application

38. On vaginal examination of a 38-year-old female, you note the following: the vulva and vagina are erythematous and edematous with thick, white, curdlike discharge adhering to the vaginal walls. The woman reports intense pruritus and thick white discharge from her vagina. These history and physical examination findings are most consistent with which of the following?
   A. Atrophic vaginitis
   B. Trichomoniasis
   C. Bacterial vaginosis
   D. Candidiasis

Correct Answer: D

Rationale: Intense pruritus and thick white discharge are often reported by the woman with candidiasis. The vulva and vagina are erythematous and edematous. The discharge is usually thick, white and curdlike.

Cognitive Level: Analysis

39. M.J., a 22-year-old female, is being seen at the clinic for problems with vulvar pain, dysuria, and fever. On physical examination, you note the following: clusters of small, shallow vesicles with surrounding erythema on the labia. There is also inguinal lymphadenopathy present. The most likely cause of these lesions is:
   A. pediculosis pubis.
   B. contact dermatitis.
   C. human papillomavirus.
   D. herpes simplex virus-type 2.

Correct Answer: D

Rationale: Herpes simplex virus-type 2 presents with clusters of small, shallow vesicles with surrounding erythema which erupt on the genital areas. There is also the presence of inguinal lymphadenopathy. The individual reports local pain, dysuria, and fever.

Cognitive Level: Analysis

40. When performing an external genitalia examination of a 10-year-old female, you note the following: no pubic hair, the mons and the labia are covered with fine vellus hair. These findings are consistent with which stage of sexual maturity, according to the Sexual Maturity Rating (SMR) scale?
   A. Stage 1
   B. Stage 2
   C. Stage 3
   D. Stage 4

Correct Answer: A

Rationale: SMR stage 1 is the preadolescent. There is no pubic hair. The mons and labia are covered with fine vellus hair as on the abdomen.

Cognitive Level: Application

Chapter 25

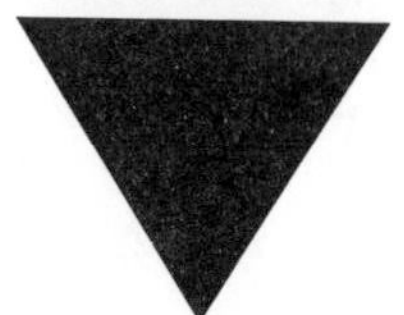

The Pregnant Woman

1. Which of the following best describes the action of the hormone progesterone during pregnancy?
   A. It stimulates the duct formation in the breast.
   B. It produces the hormone hCG, which is responsible for maintenance of the pregnancy.
   C. It maintains the endometrium around the fetus.
   D. It promotes sloughing of the endometrial wall.

Correct Answer: C.

Rationale: Progesterone prevents the sloughing of the endometrial wall and maintains the endometrium around the fetus. Progesterone increases the alveoli in the breast and keeps the uterus in a quiescent state.

Cognitive Level: Knowledge

2. Ms. J. is experiencing nausea and amenorrhea. Her last menstrual period was 6 weeks ago. What is Ms. J. experiencing?
   A. Probable signs of pregnancy
   B. Presumptive signs of pregnancy
   C. Positive signs of pregnancy
   D. Possible signs of pregnancy

Correct Answer: B

Rationale: Presumptive signs of pregnancy include amenorrhea and nausea. Probable signs are those which are detected by the examiner, such as an enlarged uterus or changes in the cervix. Positive signs of pregnancy are those which document direct evidence of the fetus such as fetal heart tones.

Cognitive Level: Application

3. When performing the examination of a woman who is 8 weeks pregnant, you note that the cervix is a bluish or cyanotic color. You would document this finding as:
   A. Hegar's sign.
   B. Chadwick's sign.
   C. Goodell's sign.
   D. Homan's sign.

Correct Answer: B

Rationale: During pregnancy, the uterus becomes globular in shape, softens and flexes over the cervix (Hegar's sign). The cervix softens (Goodell's sign) and becomes bluish or cyanotic in color (Chadwick's sign).

Cognitive Level: Application

4. Ms. K. is 8 weeks pregnant. Her systolic blood pressure is 30 mm Hg higher than her pre-pregnancy blood pressure. You would:
   A. consider this a normal finding.
   B. recommend that Ms. K. decrease her salt intake in an attempt to decrease her peripheral vascular resistance.
   C. consider this an abnormal finding since blood pressure is typically lower at this point in the pregnancy.
   D. expect the blood pressure to decrease as the estrogen levels increase throughout the pregnancy.

Correct Answer: C

Rationale: During the seventh gestational week, blood pressure begins to drop as a result of falling peripheral vascular resistance. Early in the first trimester blood pressure values are similar to those of pre-pregnancy measurements.

Cognitive Level: Analysis

5. Ms. G. is being seen at the clinic for her 10-week prenatal visit. She asks when you can hear the baby's heart beat. You reply:
   A. "Heart tones may be audible anywhere from the 9th to the 12th week."
   B. "Heart tones are not usually heard until the

second trimester."
C. "It is normal to hear the heart beat at 6 weeks. We may be able to hear it today."
D. "It is often difficult to hear the heart beat at this point in time, but we will try."

Correct Answer: A

Rationale: Fetal heart tones can heard by doppler between 9 and 12 weeks.

Cognitive Level: Application

6. Ms. X. is in her first trimester of pregnancy. She is experiencing significant nausea and vomiting and asks when it will improve. You reply:
   A. "At about the time you begin to feel the baby move, the nausea and vomiting subside."
   B. "Many women experience nausea and vomiting until the third trimester."
   C. "Did your mother have significant nausea and vomiting?"
   D. "Usually, by the beginning of the second trimester, the nausea and vomiting improve."

Correct Answer: D

Rationale: The nausea, vomiting and fatigue of pregnancy improve by weeks 12 to 16. Fetal movement occurs at approximately 20 weeks gestation.

Cognitive Level: Analysis

7. During your examination of a woman in her second trimester of pregnancy, you note the presence of a small amount of yellow drainage from the nipples. You know that this is:
   A. most likely colostrum and considered a normal finding at this stage of the pregnancy.
   B. a sign of possible breast cancer in a pregnant woman.
   C. early in the pregnancy to begin lactation. The woman should be referred to a specialist.
   D. an indication that the woman's milk is coming in.

Correct Answer: A

Rationale: During the second trimester, colostrum, the precursor of milk, may be expressed from the nipples. Colostrum is yellow in color and contains more minerals and protein, but less sugar and fat than mature milk.

Cognitive Level: Analysis

8. A woman in her second trimester of pregnancy complains of heartburn and indigestion. Which of the following offers the best explanation for this?
   A. Lower blood pressure at this time decreases blood flow to the stomach and gastrointestinal tract.
   B. Tone and motility of the gastrointestinal tract increase during the second trimester.
   C. The enlarging uterus and altered esophageal sphincter tone predispose the woman to heartburn.
   D. Sluggish emptying of the gallbladder, due to effects of progesterone, often causes heartburn.

Correct Answer: C

Rationale: Stomach displacement due to the enlarging uterus, plus altered esophageal sphincter and gastric tone as a result of progesterone predispose the woman to heartburn.

Cognitive Level: Comprehension

9. Ms. A. is 20 weeks pregnant. She reports that she feels more shortness of breath as her pregnancy progresses. Which of the following is true?
   A. Feelings of shortness of breath are abnormal during pregnancy.
   B. Ms. A. should get more exercise in an attempt to increase her respiratory reserve.
   C. The hormones of pregnancy cause an increased respiratory effort by the woman.
   D. High levels of estrogen cause shortness of breath.

Correct Answer: C

Rationale: Progesterone and estrogen cause an increased respiratory effort during pregnancy by increasing tidal volume.

Cognitive Level: Comprehension

10. You auscultate a functional systolic murmur, grade ii/iv, on a woman in week 30 of her pregnancy. The remainder of her physical assessment is within normal limits. You would:
    A. consider this an abnormal finding and refer her for additional consultation.
    B. ask the woman to run in place and auscultate the murmur again, assessing for an increase in intensity of the murmur.
    C. know that this is a normal finding due to the increase in blood volume during pregnancy.
    D. ask the woman to restrict her activities and

return to the clinic in 1 week for re-evaluation.

Correct Answer: C

Rationale: Due to the increase in blood volume, a functional systolic murmur, grade ii/iv or less, can be heard in 95% of pregnant women.

Cognitive Level: Analysis

11. Ms. Z. is a 28-week pregnant woman who is experiencing edema in her lower legs bilaterally after working 8 hours a day as a cashier at a local grocery store. What would you recommend to this patient?
   A. "Edema is usually the result of too much salt and fluids in your diet. You may need to try to cut down on salty foods."
   B. "I would like to listen to your heart sounds. Edema can indicate a problem with your heart."
   C. "Edema during pregnancy often occurs with prolonged standing. As your baby grows, it slows blood return from your legs."
   D. "You will be at risk for developing varicose veins when your legs are edematous."

Correct Answer: C

Rationale: Edema of the lower extremities occurs due to the enlarging fetus, which impairs venous return. Prolonged standing worsens the edema. Typically, the bilateral, dependent edema experienced with pregnancy is not the result of cardiac pathology.

Cognitive Level: Application

12. Which of the following are the classic symptoms associated with preeclampsia?
   A. Elevated blood pressure, proteinuria, and edema
   B. Proteinuria and headaches
   C. Neurologic signs, elevated blood pressure, and edema
   D. Elevated liver enzymes and low platelets

Correct Answer: A

Rationale: The classic triad of symptoms of preeclampsia include elevated blood pressure, proteinuria, and edema. HELLP syndrome is a variant of preeclampsia and involves hemolysis, elevated liver enzymes, and low platelets.

Cognitive Level: Knowledge

13. When would be the best time to assess a woman's blood pressure during an initial prenatal visit?
   A. At the beginning of the interview as a nonthreatening method of gaining rapport
   B. During the middle of the physical examination when she is the most comfortable
   C. Before beginning the pelvic examination since her blood pressure will be higher after the pelvic examination
   D. At the end of the examination when she will be the most relaxed

Correct Answer: D

Rationale: Assess the woman's blood pressure at the end of the examination, when it is hoped that she will be most relaxed.

Cognitive Level: Application

14. When examining the face of a 28-week pregnant woman, you note the presence of a butterfly-shaped increase in pigmentation on the face. You would document this as the presence of:
   A. linea nigra.
   B. chloasma.
   C. striae.
   D. the mask of pregnancy.

Correct Answer: B

Rationale: Chloasma is a butterfly-shaped increase in pigmentation on the face. It is known as the mask of pregnancy, but when documenting, the nurse should use the correct medical term, "chloasma."

Cognitive Level: Application

15. Which of the following is considered a normal and expected finding when performing a physical examination on a pregnant woman?
   A. Pale, hypertrophied mucous membranes of the mouth
   B. Spontaneously bleeding gingiva
   C. A palpable, full thyroid
   D. Significant diffuse enlargement of the thyroid

Correct Answer: C

Rationale: The thyroid may be palpable during pregnancy. It should feel full, but smooth. Significant diffuse enlargement occurs with hyperthyroidism, thyroiditis, and hypothyroidism.

Cognitive Level: Application

16. When auscultating the anterior thorax of a pregnant woman, you note the presence of a murmur over the 2nd, 3rd, and 4th intercostal spaces. It is continuous, but can be obliterated by pressure with the stethoscope or finger on the thorax just lateral to the murmur. You know that this is:
    A. the murmur of aortic stenosis.
    B. associated with aortic insufficiency.
    C. indication of a patent ductus arteriosis.
    D. most likely a mammary souffle.

Correct Answer: D

Rationale: Often blood flow through the blood vessels, specifically the internal mammary artery, can be heard over the 2nd, 3rd, and 4th intercostal spaces. This is called a mammary souffle, but may be mistaken for a cardiac murmur.

Cognitive Level: Analysis

17. When assessing the deep tendon reflexes (DTRs) on a 32-week pregnant woman, which of the following would be considered a normal finding, using a 0–4+ scale?
    A. Absent DTRs
    B. 2+
    C. 4+
    D. Brisk reflexes and the presence of clonus

Correct Answer: B

Rationale: Normally, during pregnancy, the DTRs are 1+ to 2+. Brisk or greater than 2+ DTRs and the presence of clonus are abnormal and may be associated with an elevated blood pressure and cerebral edema in the pre-eclamptic woman.

Cognitive Level: Application

18. When performing an examination of a 34-week pregnant woman, you note that as the woman raises her head and shoulders off of the bed there is a midline linear protrusion in the abdomen over the area of the rectus abdominis muscles. You would:
    A. document the presence of diastasis rectus abdominis.
    B. suspect that the woman has a hernia due to the increased pressure within the abdomen from pregnancy.
    C. discuss this condition with the physician since it will most likely need to be surgically repaired.
    D. tell the woman that she may have a difficult time with delivery due to the weakness in her abdominal muscles.

Correct Answer: A

Rationale: The separation of the abdominal muscles is called diastasis rectus abdominis. It frequently occurs during pregnancy. The rectus abdominis muscles will return together after pregnancy with abdominal exercise. This condition is not a true hernia.

Cognitive Level: Application

19. When palpating the fundus, you know that:
    A. fundal height is usually less than the number of weeks gestation, unless there is an abnormal condition such as too much amniotic fluid present.
    B. it should be hard and slightly tender to palpation during the first trimester.
    C. after 20 weeks gestation, the number of centimeters should approximate the number of weeks gestation.
    D. fetal movement should be felt by the examiner at the beginning of the second trimester.

Correct Answer: C

Rationale: After 20 weeks, the number of centimeters should approximate the number of weeks gestation. Also, at 20 weeks the examiner may feel fetal movement and the head can be balloted.

Cognitive Level: Knowledge

20. You are palpating the abdomen of a woman who is 35 weeks pregnant and note that the fetal head is facing downward toward the pelvis. You would document this as:
    A. fetal lie.
    B. fetal presentation.
    C. fetal attitude.
    D. fetal variety.

Correct Answer: B

Rationale: Fetal presentation describes the part of the fetus that is entering the pelvis first. Fetal lie is orientation of the fetal spine to the maternal spine. Attitude is the position of fetal parts in relation to each other and fetal variety is the location of the fetal back to the maternal pelvis.

Cognitive Level: Application

21. A 38-week pregnant woman reports a "watery" discharge. A sterile speculum examination is performed to visualize the cervix. Which of the fol-

lowing findings most likely indicates the possibility of ruptured membranes?

A. When touching the vaginal fluid to nitrazine paper, the paper turns a green color.
B. When examining the vaginal fluid under a microscope, budding yeast and hyphae are present.
C. When the woman coughs, fluid is visualized coming from the cervical os.
D. The cervix is irregular with a small laceration.

Correct Answer: C

Rationale: Four signs of ruptured membranes include the following: (1) When the woman coughs, the examiner can see fluid coming from the cervical os. (2) Nitrazine paper turns from yellow to a royal blue color in the presence of mucus, blood, lubricant, and semen. (3) Pooling of fluid in the posterior blade is evident. (4) Ferning is observed when the fluid is examined under the microscope.

Cognitive Level: Comprehension

22. Which of the following findings would be most consistent with an 8-week pregnant uterus?

A. The uterus seems slightly enlarged and softened.
B. It is about the size of an avocado, approximately 8 cm across the fundus.
C. It reaches to the pelvic brim and is about the size of a grapefruit.
D. It rises above the pelvic brim and is about the size of a cantaloupe.

Correct Answer: B

Rationale: The 8-week uterus is approximately the size of an avocado, approximately 7 to 8 cm across the fundus. The 6-week uterus is slightly enlarged and softened. The 10-week uterus is about the size of a grapefruit, and may reach to the pelvic brim. The 12-week uterus will fill the pelvis. At 12 weeks, the uterus is sized from the abdomen.

Cognitive Level: Knowledge

23. Ms. K. is a 28-year-old primagravida who is 20 weeks pregnant. Her pregnancy is progressing normally and she has had no problems. When should she return for her next prenatal visit?

A. In 2 weeks
B. In 4 weeks
C. In 1 week
D. In 3 weeks

Correct Answer: B

Rationale: Follow-up prenatal visits are at the following intervals: every 4 weeks until the 28th week; ever 2 weeks from weeks 28–36; and every week thereafter until delivery.

Cognitive Level: Application

Chapter 26

The Complete Health Assessment: Putting It All Together

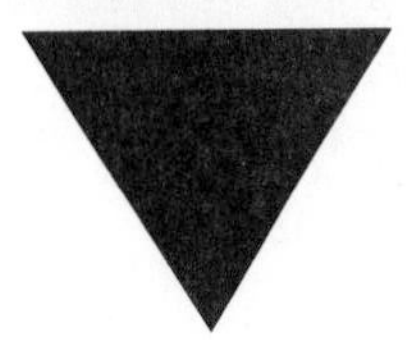

1. P.O. has come in for a physical examination, and you note that he uses a cane. As you document general appearance, this information would be written under the section that covers:
   A. posture and position.
   B. mood and affect.
   C. obvious physical deformities.
   D. mobility.

Correct Answer: D

Rationale: Use of assistive devices would be documented under the heading *Mobility.*

Cognitive Level: Knowledge

2. You are performing a vision examination on O.M. Which of the following charts is most widely used for vision examinations?
   A. Schwellon
   B. Snellen
   C. Smoollen
   D. Shetllen

Correct Answer: B

Rationale: The Snellen eye chart is most widely used for vision examinations.

Cognitive Level: Knowledge

3. After you have obtained a health history and before you begin the physical examination, you would have your patient:
   A. completely disrobe.
   B. lie on the examination table.
   C. empty his bladder.
   D. drink two full glasses of water.

Correct Answer: C

Rationale: Before you begin your examination, ask the person to empty the bladder (save the specimen if needed), disrobe except for underpants, and put on a gown sitting with legs dangling off side of the bed or table with you standing in front of the person.

Cognitive Level: Knowledge

4. While palpating the maxillary sinuses, P.Y. tells you that he is experiencing some tenderness in that area. You would proceed by:
   A. tapping on the sinus area.
   B. transilluminating the sinuses.
   C. asking P.Y. to blow his nose.
   D. auscultating the sinus area.

Correct Answer: B

Rationale: If maxillary sinuses are tender to palpation, proceed with transillumination of the sinuses.

Cognitive Level: Application

5. M.G. states "whenever I open my mouth real wide, I feel this popping sensation in front of my ears." You would:
   A. place your finger on M.G.'s temporomandibular joint (TMJ) and ask him to move his jaw from side to side.
   B. place your stethoscope over M.G.'s TMJ and listen for bruits.
   C. place one hand on M.G.'s forehead and the other on his jaw, and ask him to try to open his mouth.
   D. place your hands over M.G.'s ears and ask him to open his mouth "really wide."

Correct Answer: A

Rationale: Palpate the TMJ by placing your fingers over it, as the person opens and closes the mouth.

Cognitive Level: Application

6. You have just completed your examination of T.M.'s extraocular muscles. In your charting, you would note that you have assessed cranial nerves:
   A. 3, 4, 6
   B. 3, 4, 5
   C. 2, 4, 5
   D. 2, 3, 6

Correct Answer: A

Rationale: Extraocular muscles are innervated by cranial nerves 3, 4, and 6.

Cognitive Level: Application

7. M.M.'s uvula rises midline when she says "ahh" and she has a positive gag reflex. Which cranial nerves have you just tested?
   A. 9, 10
   B. 10, 12
   C. 11, 12
   D. 9, 12

Correct Answer: A

Rationale: Cranial nerves 9 and 10 are being tested when you have the patient say "ahh" noting the mobility of the uvula and when the patient has a positive gag reflex.

Cognitive Level: Application

8. You notice that N.P. is unable to stick out the tongue. Which cranial nerve is involved with successful performance of this task?
   A. 11
   B. 1
   C. 12
   D. 5

Correct Answer: C

Rationale: Cranial nerve number 12 enables your patient to stick out his/her tongue.

Cognitive Level: Comprehension

9. B.P. is unable to shrug her shoulders against your resistant hands. What cranial nerve is involved with successful shoulder shrugging?
   A. 11
   B. 12
   C. 9
   D. 7

Correct Answer: A

Rationale: Cranial nerve 11 enables your patient to shrug her shoulders against resistance.

Cognitive Level: Comprehension

10. C.B. has just successfully completed the finger-to-nose and the rapid-alternating-movements tests and is able to run each heel down the opposite shin for you. You believe:
   A. her cerebellar function is intact.
   B. her occipital function is intact.
   C. her cerebral function is intact.
   D. her temporal function is intact.

Correct Answer: A

Rationale: Test cerebellar function of the upper extremities using finger-to-nose test or rapid-alternating-movements test. Test cerebellar function of the lower extremities by asking the person to run each heel down the opposite shin.

Cognitive Level: Application

11. U.P. is 5 years old. You would expect him to:
   A. be able to sit on the examination table.
   B. have to be held on his mother's lap.
   C. be able to remain alone in the examination room.
   D. be able to stand on the floor for the examination.

Correct Answer: A

Rationale: At 4 or 5 years old, a child usually feels comfortable on the examination table.

Cognitive Level: Comprehension

12. Mrs. Q. tells you that she has four children and has had three pregnancies. How would you chart this?
   A. gravida 3/para 4
   B. gravida 4/para 3
   C. This is not possible to chart using gravida and para.
   D. "Mrs. Q. seems to be confused about how many times she has been pregnant."

Correct Answer: A

Rationale: Gravida refers to the number of pregnancies, and para refers to the number of children.

Cognitive Level: Application

13. During your examination, P.U. tells you that sometimes it feels as if objects are spinning around her. You would note that P.U. occasionally experiences:
   A. tinnitus.
   B. syncope.
   C. vertigo.
   D. dizziness.

Correct Answer: C

Rationale: Vertigo is the sensation of moving around

in space (subjective) or of having objects move about the person (objective) and is a result of a disturbance of equilibrator apparatus.

Cognitive Level: Application

14. M.V. tells you that "sometimes I wake up at night and I have real trouble breathing. I have to sit up in bed to get a good breath." In your charting, you would note:
   A. orthopnea.
   B. acute emphysema.
   C. paroxysmal nocturnal dyspnea.
   D. acute SOB episode.

Correct Answer: C

Rationale: Paroxysmal nocturnal dyspnea—awakened from sleep with shortness of breath and needs to be upright to achieve comfort.

Cognitive Level: Analysis

15. During your examination of D.C., you note that she has several (1-cm) small, flat macules on her posterior thorax. These macules may also be called:
   A. warts.
   B. freckles.
   C. bullas.
   D. papules.

Correct Answer: B

Rationale: A macule is solely a color change, flat and circumscribed, less than 1 cm. Examples include freckles, flat nevi, hypopigmentation, petechiae, measles, and scarlet fever.

Cognitive Level: Application

16. You notice that Mrs. A.'s legs turn white when you raise them above her head. You would suspect:
   A. chronic venous insufficiency.
   B. lymphedema.
   C. chronic arterial insufficiency.
   D. Raynaud's disease.

Correct Answer: C

Rationale: Elevational pallor (marked) indicates arterial insufficiency.

Cognitive Level: Analysis

17. You report that you have observed coarse thickened skin and brown discoloration on M.C.'s legs. This is probably the result of:
   A. chronic arterial insufficiency.
   B. chronic venous insufficiency.
   C. Raynaud's disease.
   D. lymphedema.

Correct Answer: B

Rationale: Chronic venous insufficiency would present as firm brawny edema, coarse thickened skin, normal pulses, brown discoloration, petechiae and dermatitis.

Cognitive Level: Analysis

18. You note that P.V. has ulcerations on the tips of her toes and on her lateral malleoli. This would indicate:
   A. arterial insufficiency.
   B. venous insufficiency.
   C. Raynaud's disease.
   D. lymphedema.

Correct Answer: A

Rationale: Ulcerations on the tips of the toes and lateral malleoli are indicative of arterial insufficiency.

Cognitive Level: Analysis

19. When you flexed R.B.'s knee and gently compressed her gastrocnemius muscle anteriorly against her tibia, she noticed calf pain. You would chart:
   A. positive Allen's sign.
   B. negative Allen's sign.
   C. positive Homan's sign.
   D. negative Homan's sign.

Correct Answer: C

Rationale: Calf pain with these maneuvers is a positive Homan's sign, which occurs in about 35% of cases of deep vein thrombosis.

Cognitive Level: Analysis

20. You have just recorded a positive obturator test. This test is used to confirm:
   A. enlarged gallbladder.
   B. perforated spleen.
   C. perforated appendix.
   D. inflamed liver.

Correct Answer: C

Rationale: A perforated appendix irritates the obturator muscle, producing pain.

Cognitive Level: Application

21. You are writing notes on your assessment of baby J. During the abdominal assessment, you noted a very loud splash auscultated over the upper abdomen when you rocked her from side to side. You would suspect:
   A. pyloric obstruction.
   B. hyperactive bowel sounds.
   C. hypoactive bowel sounds.
   D. epigastric hernia.

Correct Answer: A

Rationale: Unrelated to peristalsis, this very loud splash auscultated over the upper abdomen when the infant is rocked side to side indicates increased air and fluid in the stomach as seen with pyloric obstruction or large hiatus hernia.

Cognitive Level: Analysis

22. You have recorded that C.C.'s visual acuity was 20/20 O.S. This provides information about C.C.'s:
   A. vision with her glasses on.
   B. vision in her right eye.
   C. vision in her left eye.
   D. vision in both eyes.

Correct Answer: D

Rationale: A recording of "O.S." concerns both eyes.

Cognitive Level: Comprehension

23. When you record that M.B.'s visual fields are full by confrontation, you have assessed M.B.'s:
   A. EOMs.
   B. PERRLA.
   C. peripheral vision.
   D. near vision.

Correct Answer: C

Rationale: The confrontation test is a gross measure of peripheral vision.

Cognitive Level: Application

24. If you record that you performed the Hirschberg test, you have:
   A. tested the corneal light reflex.
   B. assessed for thrombophlebitis.
   C. assessed for appendicitis.
   D. tested the patellar reflex.

Correct Answer: A

Rationale: The Hirschberg test assesses the corneal light reflex.

Cognitive Level: Application

25. During your examination of R.G.'s mouth, you observe a nodular bony ridge down the middle of the hard palate. You would chart this as:
   A. leukoplakia.
   B. ankyloglossia.
   C. torus palatinus.
   D. cheilosis.

Correct Answer: C

Rationale: A normal variation of the hard palate is a nodular bony ridge down the middle of the hard palate, a torus palatinus.

Cognitive Level: Application

26. During examination, you find that R.F. is unable to distinguish objects placed in his hand, and you would chart:
   A. stereognosis.
   B. astereognosis.
   C. graphesthesia.
   D. agraphesthesia.

Correct Answer: B

Rationale: Astereognosis—unable to identify object place in hand correctly.

Cognitive Level: Application

27. After your examination of baby R., you note that you have observed opisthotonos. This often occurs in conjunction with:
   A. meningeal irritation.
   B. lower motor neuron lesion.
   C. upper motor neuron lesion.
   D. cerebral palsy.

Correct Answer: A

Rationale: Opisthotonos is a form of spasm in which the head is arched back, there is stiffness of the neck, and extension of arms and legs. It occurs with meningeal or brainstem irritation.

Cognitive Level: Analysis

28. After assessing Ms. W., you note that you observed flesh-colored, soft, pointed, moist, papules in a cauliflower-like patch around her introitus. This is most likely:
   A. syphilitic chancre.

B. urethral caruncle.
C. condylomata acuminata.
D. herpes progenitalis.

Correct Answer: C

Rationale: Condylomata acuminata appears in a flesh-colored, soft, moist, cauliflower-like patch of papules.

Cognitive Level: Analysis

29. While recording in Mr. G.'s chart, you write that his guaiac tests have been positive. This means that:
    A. there is occult blood in Mr. G.'s stool.
    B. there are parasites in Mr. G.'s stool.
    C. there are bacteria in Mr. G.'s sputum.
    D. there are crystals in Mr. G.'s urine.

Correct Answer: A

Rationale: If a stool is guaiac positive, it indicates occult blood.

Cognitive Level: Analysis

30. While examining your 48-year-old patient's eyes, you note that he had to move the handheld vision screener farther away from his face. You would suspect:
    A. presbyopia.
    B. hyperopia.
    C. omniopia.
    D. myopia.

Correct Answer: A

Rationale: Presbyopia, the decrease in power of accommodation with aging, is suggested when the handheld vision screener card is moved farther away.

Cognitive Level: Analysis

31. Which of the following is most appropriate to perform on a 9-month-old well child?
    A. Ortolani's sign
    B. Assessment for stereognosis
    C. Blood pressure measurement
    D. Assessment for the presence of the startle reflex

Correct Answer: A

Rationale: Until the age of 12 months, the infant should be assessed for Ortolani's sign. To perform this maneuver, flex the infant's knees, holding your thumbs on the inner mid-thighs, and your fingers outside on the hips touching the greater trochanter. Adduct the legs until your thumbs touch and abduct the legs until the knees touch the table. If this sign is present, it could indicate the presence of a dislocated hip.

Cognitive Level: Application

32. Which of the following statements is true regarding the complete physical assessment?
    A. The vital signs, height and weight should be obtained at the end of the exam for convenience.
    B. The patient should be in the sitting position for examination of the head and neck.
    C. The examiner should not vary the order of the assessment in order to promote consistency between patients.
    D. The male genitalia should be examined in the supine position.

Correct Answer: B

Rationale: The head and neck should be examined in the sitting position to best palpate the thyroid and lymph nodes.

Cognitive Level: Comprehension

33. Which of the following statements is true regarding the recording of data from the history and physical examination?
    A. Record the data as soon as possible after the interview and physical examination.
    B. If the information is not documented, it can be assumed that it was done as a standard of care.
    C. The examiner should avoid taking any notes during the history and examination because of possibility of decreasing rapport with the patient.
    D. Try to use long, descriptive sentences to describe your findings.

Correct Answer: A

Rationale: The data from the history and physical examination should be recorded as soon after the event as possible. From a legal perspective, if it is not documented, it was not done. Brief notes should be taken during the examination. When documenting, use short clear phrases, avoiding redundant phrases and descriptions.

Cognitive Level: Application

Chapter 27

Critical Thinking in Health Assessment

1. You have just completed your initial assessment on Mr. T. You have charted that his respirations are eupnic, and his pulse is 58. This type of data would be:
   A. subjective.
   B. reflective.
   C. objective.
   D. introspective.

Correct Answer: C

Rationale: Objective data is what you, the health professional, observe by inspecting, percussing, palpating and auscultating during the physical exam.

Cognitive Level: Comprehension

2. Mr. T. tells you that he is very nervous and that he is sweating and has a very fast pulse. This type of data would be:
   A. subjective.
   B. reflective.
   C. objective.
   D. introspective.

Correct Answer: A

Rationale: Subjective data are what the person says about himself or herself during history taking.

Cognitive Level: Comprehension

3. The patient's record, laboratory studies, objective data, and subjective data combined form the:
   A. admitting record.
   B. data base.
   C. financial statement.
   D. discharge summary.

Correct Answer: B

Rationale: Together with the patient's record and laboratory studies, the objective and subjective databases form the database.

Cognitive Level: Knowledge

4. In an ambulatory, nonemergent care setting, the first problems listed on a patient's plan of care are those concerned with:
   A. acuity of illness.
   B. payment from an insurance company.
   C. availability of care providers.
   D. the reasons the person has sought care.

Correct Answer: D

Rationale: In an ambulatory, nonemergent care setting, the first problems listed usually are those concerned with the reasons the person has sought care.

Cognitive Level: Knowledge

5. In the hospitalized, acute care settings, the order or priority of the patient's problems is usually determined by:
   A. acuity of illness.
   B. payment from an insurance company.
   C. availability of care providers.
   D. the reasons the person has sought care.

Correct Answer: A

Rationale: In the hospitalized, acute care setting, the acuity of illness often determines the order of priorities of the person's problems.

Cognitive Level: Knowledge

6. You have just admitted Mrs. Y. and she is in acute pain, has not been sleeping well lately, and is having difficulty breathing. As a nurse, you would prioritize these problems in the following order:
   A. breathing, pain, sleep.
   B. sleep, breathing, pain.
   C. sleep, pain, breathing.
   D. breathing, sleep, pain.

Correct Answer: A

Rationale: First-level priority problems are immediate priorities (remember the ABC), followed by second-level problems and then third-level problems.

Cognitive Level: Analysis

7. With ________________, nurses have the primary responsibility to diagnose the onset and monitor the changes in a person's status.
   A. collective problems
   B. collaborative problems
   C. consequential problems
   D. concentrated problems

Correct Answer: B

Rationale: With collaborative problems, nurses have the primary responsibility to diagnose the onset and monitor the changes in status.

Cognitive Level: Knowledge

8. You have developed a plan of care for Mr. Y. that includes collaborative problems that could result from Mr. Y.'s fractured leg. Collaborative problems you might include in the plan of care are:
   A. urinary retention.
   B. thrombus/embolus formation.
   C. pericarditis.
   D. paralytic ileus.

Correct Answer: B

Rationale: Potential complications for the medical diagnosis of fractures include bleeding, fracture displacement, thrombus/embolus formation, and compromised circulation.

Cognitive Level: Analysis

9. The step of the nursing process that begins with the first greeting of the patient and ends with the actual or potential nursing diagnosis is:
   A. assessment.
   B. diagnosis.
   C. implementation.
   D. planning.

Correct Answer: A

Rationale: Assessment starts with the first greeting of the patient and ends with the actual or potential nursing diagnosis.

Cognitive Level: Knowledge

10. The nursing process is a sequential method of problem-solving that includes five steps:
   A. admission, assessment, diagnosis, treatment, discharge planning.
   B. assessment, diagnosis, planning, implementation, evaluation.
   C. admission, diagnosis, treatment, evaluation, discharge planning.
   D. assessment, treatment, evaluation, discharge, follow-up.

Correct Answer: B

Rationale: The nursing process is a method of problem solving that includes assessment, diagnosis, planning, implementation, and evaluation.

Cognitive Level: Comprehension

11. As a nurse working to develop appropriate nursing interventions for your patients, you rely on the appropriateness of the:
   A. nursing diagnosis.
   B. medical diagnosis.
   C. admission diagnosis.
   D. collaborative diagnosis.

Correct Answer: A

Rationale: Nursing diagnosis provides the basis for selection of nursing interventions to achieve outcomes for which the nurse is accountable.

Cognitive Level: Comprehension

12. Novice nurses, without a background of skills and experience to draw from, are more likely to make their decisions using:
   A. intuition.
   B. a set of rules.
   C. advice from supervisors.
   D. articles in journals.

Correct Answer: B

Rationale: Novice nurses operate from a set of rules (such as the nursing process).

Cognitive Level: Comprehension

13. A nurse using diagnostic reasoning might formulate a diagnostic hypothesis, while a nurse using the nursing process would:
   A. develop interventions.
   B. develop a nursing diagnosis.
   C. do a complete assessment.
   D. evaluate the goals.

Correct Answer: B

Rationale: Diagnostic reasoning calls for the nurse to formulate a diagnostic hypothesis, while the nursing process calls for nursing diagnosis.

Cognitive Level: Comprehension

14. A tentative explanation for a cue or a set of cues that can be used as a basis for further investigation is:
    A. a diagnosis.
    B. a goal.
    C. a definition.
    D. a hypothesis.

Correct Answer: D

Rationale: A hypothesis is a tentative explanation for a cue or a set of cues that can be used as a basis for further investigation.

Cognitive Level: Knowledge

15. Expert nurses, when matched with a novice nurse, are:
    A. irritated by the questions that the novice must ask.
    B. often required to stay late in order to assist the novice with the assigned tasks.
    C. challenged by the novices' questions and are able to clarify their own thinking.
    D. often highly unorganized.

Correct Answer: C

Rationale: Expert nurses are challenged by novices' questions, clarifying their own thinking when teaching novices.

Cognitive Level: Knowledge

16. Expert nurses learn to attend to a pattern of assessment data and to act without consciously labeling it. This is referred to as:
    A. nursing process.
    B. clinical knowledge.
    C. intuition.
    D. diagnostic reasoning.

Correct Answer: C

Rationale: Intuition is characterized by pattern recognition—expert nurses learn to attend to a pattern of assessment data and act without consciously labeling it.

Cognitive Level: Comprehension

17. Critical thinking in the expert nurse is greatly enhanced from opportunities to:
    A. work with physicians to provide patient care.
    B. apply theory in real situations.
    C. follow physician orders providing patient care.
    D. develop nursing diagnoses for commonly occurring illnesses.

Correct Answer: B

Rationale: The depth and breadth of expert knowledge, largely gained from opportunities to apply theory in real situations, greatly enhances critical thinking ability.

Cognitive Level: Comprehension

18. A nursing diagnosis made by a critical thinker using a dynamic nursing process would diagnose the actual problem, and would also:
    A. reassess.
    B. predict potential problems.
    C. modify the diagnosis if necessary.
    D. check appropriateness of goals.

Correct Answer: B

Rationale: A dynamic nursing process as used by a critical thinker would include, under diagnosis, diagnoses of actual problems, prediction of potential problems, and identification of strengths.

Cognitive Level: Analysis

19. Without thinking critically, the novice nurse, when evaluating the patient's plan of care, would fail to:
    A. assess current health status.
    B. diagnose actual problems.
    C. assess readiness to act.
    D. determine goal achievement.

Correct Answer: A

Rationale: Linear nursing process followed by rote by a novice without critical thinking would fail to assess current health status and to evaluate accuracy of diagnosis when evaluating a patient's plan of care.

Cognitive Level: Comprehension

20. Which of the following is a good example of a first-level priority problem?
    A. An individual experiencing shortness of breath and respiratory distress
    B. An individual with a small laceration on the sole of his foot
    C. A patient experiencing post-operative pain

D. A newly diagnosed diabetic who need diabetic teaching

Correct Answer: A

Rationale: First-level priority problems are those that are emergent, life-threatening, and immediate; e.g., establishing an airway, supporting breathing, maintaining circulation and monitoring abnormal vital signs.

Cognitive Level: Comprehension

21. Second-level priority problems include which of the following?
    A. Severely abnormal vital signs
    B. Abnormal laboratory values
    C. Knowledge deficit
    D. Low self esteem

Correct Answer: B

Rationale: Second-level priority problems are those that require prompt intervention to forestall further deterioration. Examples include: mental status change, acute pain, abnormal laboratory values, or risks to safety or security.

Cognitive Level: Comprehension